Liver in Systemic Diseases

Editor

JORGE L. HERRERA

CLINICS IN LIVER DISEASE

www.liver.theclinics.com

Consulting Editor
NORMAN GITLIN

May 2019 • Volume 23 • Number 2

ELSEVIER

1600 John F. Kennedy Boulevard • Suite 1800 • Philadelphia, Pennsylvania, 19103-2899

http://www.theclinics.com

CLINICS IN LIVER DISEASE Volume 23, Number 2
May 2019 ISSN 1089-3261, ISBN-13: 978-0-323-67815-5

Editor: Kerry Holland
Developmental Editor: Meredith Madeira

Clinics in Liver Disease (ISSN 1089-3261) is published quarterly by Elsevier Inc., 360 Park Avenue South, New York, NY 10010-1710. Months of issue are February, May, August, and November. Business and Editorial Offices: 1600 John F. Kennedy Blvd., Ste. 1800, Philadelphia, PA 19103-2899. Customer Service Office: 3251 Riverport Lane, Maryland Heights, MO 63043. Periodicals postage paid at New York, NY and additional mailing offices. Subscription prices are $304.00 per year (U.S. individuals), $100.00 per year (U.S. student/resident), $542.00 per year (U.S. institutions), $409.00 per year (international individuals), $200.00 per year (international student/resident), $672.00 per year (international instituitions), $343.00 per year (Canadian individuals), $200.00 per year (Canadian student/resident), and $672.00 per year (Canadian institutions). Foreign air speed delivery is included in all *Clinics* subscription prices. All prices are subject to change without notice. **POSTMASTER:** Send address changes to *Clinics in Liver Disease*, Elsevier Health Sciences Division, Subscription Customer Service, 3251 Riverport Lane, Maryland Heights, MO 63043. **Customer Service: Telephone: 1-800-654-2452 (U.S. and Canada); 314-447-8871 (outside U.S. and Canada). Fax: 314-447-8029. E-mail: journalscustomer service-usa@elsevier.com (for print support); journalsonlinesupport-usa@elsevier.com (for online support).**

Reprints. For copies of 100 or more of articles in this publication, please contact the Commercial Reprints Department, Elsevier Inc., 360 Park Avenue South, New York, NY 10010-1710. Tel.: 212-633-3874; Fax: 212-633-3820; E-mail: reprints@elsevier.com.

Clinics in Liver Disease is covered in *MEDLINE/PubMed (Index Medicus)*, Science Citation Index Expanded, Journal Citation Reports/Science Edition, and Current Contents/Clinical Medicine.

Contributors

CONSULTING EDITOR

NORMAN GITLIN, MD, FRCP (LONDON), FRCPE (EDINBURGH), FAASLD, FACP, FACG
Head of Hepatology, Southern California Liver Centers, San Clemente, California, USA

EDITOR

JORGE L. HERRERA, MD
Professor of Medicine, Division of Gastroenterology, University of South Alabama College of Medicine, Mobile, Alabama, USA

AUTHORS

FARSHAD ADULI, MD
Division of Gastroenterology and Hepatology, Department of Internal Medicine, Howard University Hospital and College of Medicine, Washington, DC, USA

DANIEL BERGER, MD
Section of Gastroenterology, Division of Digestive Diseases, Department of Internal Medicine, Rush University Medical Center, Chicago, Illinois, USA

CHALERMRAT BUNCHORNTAVAKUL, MD
Division of Gastroenterology and Hepatology, Assistant Professor, Department of Medicine, Rajavithi Hospital, College of Medicine, Rangsit University, Bangkok, Thailand, Division of Gastroenterology and Hepatology, Department of Medicine, University of Pennsylvania, Philadelphia, Pennsylvania, USA

ANDRES F. CARRION, MD
Assistant Professor of Clinical Medicine, Division of Gastroenterology and Hepatology, University of Miami Miller School of Medicine, Miami, Florida, USA

AMANDA CHEUNG, MD
Clinical Assistant Professor of Medicine, Division of Gastroenterology and Hepatology, Stanford University School of Medicine, Palo Alto, California, USA

DOUGLAS T. DIETERICH, MD
Professor, Icahn School of Medicine at Mount Sinai, New York, New York, USA

STEVEN FLAMM, MD
Professor of Medicine and Surgery, Division of Gastroenterology and Hepatology, Northwestern Feinberg School of Medicine, Chicago, Illinois, USA

AGAZI GEBRESELASSIE, MD, MSc
Division of Gastroenterology and Hepatology, Department of Internal Medicine, Howard University Hospital, Washington, DC, USA

NIYATI M. GUPTA, MD
Department of Gastroenterology and Hepatology, Digestive Disease and Surgery
Institute, Cleveland Clinic Foundation, Cleveland, Ohio, USA

THEO HELLER, MD
Liver Diseases Branch, National Institute of Diabetes and Digestive and Kidney Diseases,
National Institutes of Health, Bethesda, Maryland, USA

JORGE L. HERRERA, MD
Professor of Medicine, Division of Gastroenterology, University of South Alabama College
of Medicine, Mobile, Alabama, USA

MOIRA B. HILSCHER, MD
Division of Gastroenterology and Hepatology, Mayo Clinic, Rochester, Minnesota, USA

CHARLES D. HOWELL, MD
Division of Gastroenterology and Hepatology, Department of Internal Medicine, Howard
University Hospital and College of Medicine, Washington, DC, USA

PATRICK S. KAMATH, MD
Division of Gastroenterology and Hepatology, Mayo Clinic, Rochester, Minnesota, USA

DAVID E. KLEINER, MD, PhD
Laboratory of Pathology, National Cancer Institute, National Institutes of Health,
Bethesda, Maryland, USA

CHRISTOPHER KOH, MD, MHSc
Liver Diseases Branch, National Institute of Diabetes and Digestive and Kidney Diseases,
National Institutes of Health, Bethesda, Maryland, USA

MANOJ KUMAR, MD, MPH
Assistant Professor of Medicine, Division of Gastroenterology, University of South
Alabama College of Medicine, Mobile, Alabama, USA

KAREN MA, MD
Section of Gastroenterology, Division of Digestive Diseases, Department of Internal
Medicine, Rush University Medical Center, Chicago, Illinois, USA

MAHMOUD MAHFOUZ, MD
Department of Internal Medicine, Mount Sinai Medical Center, Miami Beach, Florida, USA

MIGUEL MALESPIN, MD
Department of Medicine, University of Florida Health, Jacksonville, Florida, USA

PAUL MARTIN, MD, FRCP, FRCPI
Chief, Division of Gastroenterology and Hepatology, Professor of Medicine, University of
Miami Miller School of Medicine, Miami, Florida, USA

ARTHUR J. McCULLOUGH, MD
Department of Gastroenterology and Hepatology, Digestive Disease and Surgery Institute,
Cleveland Clinic Foundation, Department of Inflammation and Immunity, Cleveland
Clinic Lerner College of Medicine, Case Western University, Cleveland, Ohio, USA

JOSEPH A. MURRAY, MD
Division of Gastroenterology and Hepatology, Department of Medicine, Mayo Clinic
College of Medicine, Rochester, Minnesota, USA

AMMAR NASSRI, MD
Department of Medicine, University of Florida Health, Jacksonville, Florida, USA

KATERINA G. OIKONOMOU, MD, PhD
Clinical Fellow, Infectious Diseases, Icahn School of Medicine at Mount Sinai, New York, New York, USA

MALAV P. PARIKH, MD, FACP
Department of Gastroenterology and Hepatology, Digestive Disease and Surgery Institute, Cleveland Clinic Foundation, Cleveland, Ohio, USA

LORIS PIRONI, MD
Professor, Department of Medical and Surgical Science, Centre for Chronic Intestinal Failure, University of Bologna, St. Orsola-Malpighi Hospital, Bologna, Italy

NANCY REAU, MD
Section of Hepatology, Division of Digestive Diseases, Department of Internal Medicine, Rush University Medical Center, Chicago, Illinois, USA

K. RAJENDER REDDY, MD
Division of Gastroenterology and Hepatology, Ruimy Family President's Distinguished Professor, Department of Medicine, University of Pennsylvania, Philadelphia, Pennsylvania, USA

ALBERTO RUBIO-TAPIA, MD
Division of Gastroenterology and Hepatology, Department of Medicine, Mayo Clinic College of Medicine, Rochester, Minnesota, USA

SASAN SAKIANI, MD
Assistant Professor of Medicine, Division of Gastroenterology and Hepatology, University of Maryland School of Medicine, University of Maryland Medical Center, Baltimore, Maryland, USA

DOST SARPEL, MD
Assistant Professor, Icahn School of Medicine at Mount Sinai, New York, New York, USA

ANNA SIMONA SASDELLI, MD
Department of Medical and Surgical Science, Centre for Chronic Intestinal Failure, University of Bologna, St. Orsola-Malpighi Hospital, Bologna, Italy

ABID R. SUDDLE, MD, FRCP
Consultant Hepatologist, Institute of Liver Studies, King's College Hospital NHS Foundation Trust, London, United Kingdom

ELENI THEOCHARIDOU, PhD
Institute of Liver Studies, King's College Hospital NHS Foundation Trust, London, United Kingdom

EUGENIA TSAI, MD
Clinical Fellow, Liver Transplant, Icahn School of Medicine at Mount Sinai, New York, New York, USA

Contents

Preface: The Liver in Systemic Disease   xiii

Jorge L. Herrera

The Liver and Celiac Disease   167

Alberto Rubio-Tapia and Joseph A. Murray

> Celiac disease is a multisystem disorder. Celiac hepatitis characterized by gluten-responsive mild elevation of transaminases is the more common liver manifestation of celiac disease. Celiac disease may also be associated or coexist with other chronic liver disorders. Shared genetic risk and increased intestinal permeability have been suggested to be the most relevant events in the pathogenesis of liver injury in celiac disease. The aim of this article is to review the full spectrum of liver disorders in patients with celiac disease.

The Liver in Sickle Cell Disease   177

Eleni Theocharidou and Abid R. Suddle

> Patients with sickle cell disease can develop liver disease as a result of intrahepatic sickling of erythrocytes, viral hepatitis and iron overload secondary to multiple blood transfusions, and gallstone disease as a result of chronic hemolysis. The spectrum of clinical liver disease is wide and often multifactorial. Some patients develop cirrhosis that may progress to end-stage liver failure. Limited evidence exists for medical treatments. Exchange blood transfusions may improve outcomes in the acute liver syndromes. Liver transplantation may be an option for chronic liver disease. The role for prophylactic cholecystectomy in preventing complications of gallstone disease is controversial.

Hepatic Complications of Inflammatory Bowel Disease   191

Mahmoud Mahfouz, Paul Martin, and Andres F. Carrion

> Hepatobiliary disorders are commonly encountered in patients with inflammatory bowel disease (IBD). Although primary sclerosing cholangitis is the stereotypical hepatobiliary disorder associated with IBD, other diseases, including autoimmune hepatitis and nonalcoholic fatty liver disease, also are encountered in this population. Several agents used for treatment of IBD may cause drug-induced liver injury, although severe hepatotoxicity occurs infrequently. Furthermore, reactivation of hepatitis B virus infection may occur in patients with IBD treated with systemic corticosteroids and biologic agents.

The Liver in Circulatory Disturbances   209

Moira B. Hilscher and Patrick S. Kamath

> Liver diseases frequently coexist with heart disease. The causes of coexistent heart and liver disease are categorized into four groups: (1) heart

disease affecting the liver, (2) liver disease affecting the heart, (3) cardiac and hepatic manifestations of a common cause, and (4) coexistent heart and liver disease with distinct causes. Discerning the cause of cardiac and liver dysfunction is important in the management of these conditions, particularly when considering surgical intervention or heart or liver transplantation.

Hepatobiliary Complications in Critically Ill Patients   221

Amanda Cheung and Steven Flamm

Critically ill patients frequently present with the systemic inflammatory response syndrome, which is largely a reflection of the liver's response to injury. Underlying hepatic congestion is a major risk factor for hypoxic liver injury, the most common cause for hepatocellular injury. Cholestatic liver injury often occurs in critically ill patients due to inhibition of farnesoid X receptor (FXR), the main regulator of bile acid handling, particularly in the liver and intestines. Additional injury to the liver occurs due to alterations in the bile acid pool with increased cytotoxic forms and disturbance in the typical processing of xenobiotics in the liver.

Endocrine Diseases and the Liver: An Update   233

Miguel Malespin and Ammar Nassri

The endocrine system is a complex interconnected system of organs that control corporeal processes and function. Primary endocrine organs are involved in hormonal production and secretion but rely on a bevy of signals from the hypothalamic-pituitary axis and secondary endocrine organs, such as the liver. In turn, proper hepatic function is maintained through hormonal signaling. Thus, the endocrine system and liver are codependent, and diseases affecting either organs can lead to alterations in function within their counterparts. This article explores the hepato–endocrine relationship, including the effects on endocrine diseases on the liver.

Rheumatologic Diseases and the Liver   247

Agazi Gebreselassie, Farshad Aduli, and Charles D. Howell

A variety of rheumatologic disorders may affect the liver. There is a significant epidemiologic, genetic, and immunologic overlap between immune-mediated rheumatologic disorders and autoimmune liver diseases. There is an increased frequency of autoimmune liver diseases, such as primary biliary cholangitis, autoimmune hepatitis, primary sclerosing cholangitis, or overlap syndrome, in patients with systemic lupus erythematosus, rheumatoid arthritis, Sjögren syndrome, systemic sclerosis, vasculitis, and other immune-related diseases. Non-immune-mediated rheumatologic diseases such as gouty arthritis may also have hepatic manifestations. Furthermore, medications used to treat rheumatologic diseases occasionally cause liver dysfunction. Conversely, primary immune-mediated and non-immune-mediated liver disorders may present with rheumatologic manifestations.

Hepatic Manifestations of Cystic Fibrosis   263

Sasan Sakiani, David E. Kleiner, Theo Heller, and Christopher Koh

Cystic fibrosis liver disease (CFLD) remains the third leading cause of death in patients with cystic fibrosis. Although most patients with CFLD present in childhood, recent studies suggest a second wave of liver disease in adulthood. There are no clear guidelines for diagnosing CFLD. Treatment options for CFLD remain limited, and while UDCA is widely used, its long-term benefit is unclear. Those who develop hepatic decompensation or uncontrolled variceal bleeding may benefit from liver transplant, either alone, or in combination with lung transplant.

Intestinal Failure-Associated Liver Disease   279

Loris Pironi and Anna Simona Sasdelli

Intestinal failure-associated liver disease (IFALD) is characterized by either liver steatosis or cholestasis and may develop in patients on long-term home parenteral nutrition for chronic intestinal failure. The pathogenesis of IFALD is multifactorial and includes gastrointestinal disease-related, parenteral nutrition-related, and systemic-related factors. Alteration of bile acid enterohepatic circulation, gut microbiome, and intestinal permeability, seem to be the main mechanisms. Patients forced to a total oral fasting regimen are at greater risk. Parenteral nutrition overfeeding and/or of soybean-based lipid emulsion may be contributing factors. Prevention and treatment are based on avoiding and promptly treating all the risk factors.

Hepatic Manifestations of Lymphoproliferative Disorders   293

Chalermrat Bunchorntavakul and K. Rajender Reddy

Hepatic abnormalities in patients with lymphoproliferative disorders are common and can occur from direct infiltration by abnormal cells, bile duct obstruction, paraneoplastic syndrome, hemophagocytic syndrome, drug-induced liver injury, opportunistic infections, and reactivation of viral hepatitis. Hepatic involvement by lymphoma is often in association with systemic disease and rarely seen as a primary hepatic lymphoma. Vanishing bile duct syndrome is a well-known complication of Hodgkin disease. Antiviral prophylaxis for hepatitis B virus (HBV) reactivation is recommended for all HBsAg+ patients undergoing chemotherapy and all resolved HBV patients undergoing rituximab therapy and stem cell transplantation.

Liver Disease in Human Immunodeficiency Virus Infection   309

Katerina G. Oikonomou, Eugenia Tsai, Dost Sarpel, and Douglas T. Dieterich

Liver disease in human immunodeficiency virus (HIV) remains a main cause of morbidity and mortality. Liver-related morbidity and mortality can be caused by multiple etiologic factors, including opportunistic infections, direct and indirect effects of antiretrovirals, direct and indirect effects of HIV, and viral hepatitides. These factors present with varied liver pathophysiologic mechanisms that lead to abnormalities in liver enzymes and synthetic function test, followed by distinct clinical presentations. This article elucidates the direct effects on HIV in the liver and explores the diagnostic and management challenges in patients with HIV in the era of highly active antiretroviral treatment.

Sarcoidosis and the Liver   331

Manoj Kumar and Jorge L. Herrera

Hepatic granulomas are a common finding in systemic sarcoidosis, but most patients remain asymptomatic. Elevated alkaline phosphatase is the most common sign of hepatic sarcoidosis (HS). Lacking a specific diagnostic test, the diagnosis of HS is one of exclusion. Therapy may be indicated in a minority of patients to control symptoms, but the effects of therapy in the natural history of HS are unknown.

Liver Diseases During Pregnancy   345

Karen Ma, Daniel Berger, and Nancy Reau

Liver diseases during pregnancy pose a unique clinical challenge because they can affect the lives of both the mother and unborn child. Although severe liver disease is rare, pregnancy-related liver disease affects approximately 3% of pregnancies and can be fatal. Timely recognition and diagnosis are essential in order to institute appropriate management strategies. This article provides an overview of liver diseases during pregnancy and is divided into 2 sections: (1) liver diseases specific to pregnancy, and (2) preexisting or coincident liver diseases during pregnancy.

Obstructive Sleep Apnea and the Liver   363

Malav P. Parikh, Niyati M. Gupta, and Arthur J. McCullough

Nonalcoholic fatty liver disease (NAFLD), a disorder of altered metabolic pathways, is increasing worldwide. Recent studies established obstructive sleep apnea (OSA) and chronic intermittent hypoxia (CIH) as NAFLD risk factors. Studies have ascertained that CIH is independently related to NAFLD. Continuous positive airway pressure (CPAP) shows inconsistent results regarding its efficacy in improving NAFLD. Observational, longer duration CPAP therapy studies have shown positive outcomes, whereas shorter duration, randomized controlled trials have shown no benefit. A multifaceted approach to NAFLD management with sufficiently longer duration of CPAP therapy may be beneficial in patients with moderate to severe OSA.

CLINICS IN LIVER DISEASE

FORTHCOMING ISSUES

August 2019
Hepatitis B Virus
Tarek Hassanein, *Editor*

November 2019
Portal Hypertension
Sammy Saab, *Editor*

February 2020
Drug Hepatotoxicity
Pierre Gholam, *Editor*

RECENT ISSUES

February 2019
Alcoholic Liver Disease
Norman L. Sussman and
Michael R. Lucey, *Editors*

November 2018
Pediatric Liver Disease
Philip Rosenthal, *Editor*

August 2018
Primary Biliary Cholangitis
Cynthia Levy and Elizabeth J. Carey,
Editors

THE CLINICS ARE AVAILABLE ONLINE!
Access your subscription at:
www.theclinics.com

Preface

The Liver in Systemic Disease

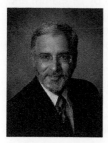

Jorge L. Herrera, MD
Editor

The liver, being the largest internal organ in humans, is often involved in systemic diseases either as an innocent bystander or as part of the pathologic process itself. Elevated liver tests may be the first manifestation of a systemic condition unrelated to the liver, may develop as a result of a known systemic illness, or may be caused by a primary, unrelated liver disease. Differentiating primary liver disease from manifestations of systemic illness is often a difficult task faced by gastroenterologists and hepatologists. This issue of the *Clinics in Liver Disease* reviews the latest developments on the diagnosis and management of a range of disorders that directly or indirectly affect the liver.

Drs Murray and Rubio-Tapia elegantly discuss the hepatic manifestations of celiac disease, a common scenario where the liver may be an "innocent bystander," and elevated liver tests may be the first and only sign of underlying celiac disease. In contrast, the liver is directly involved in other conditions, such as sickle cell disease, sarcoidosis, HIV infection, pregnancy, cystic fibrosis, cardiac disease, and lymphoproliferative disorders, all of which are discussed in various articles of this issue.

Advances in the therapy of inflammatory bowel disease (IBD) and rheumatologic disorders have resulted in improved outcomes for patients with these conditions, but also in new liver complications related to therapy. Drs Martin, Howell, and colleagues discuss the well-known liver disorders associated with IBD and rheumatologic disorders as well as the recently described hepatic complications of the biologics and immunomodulators used to treat these patients. Advice on the best practice for monitoring and managing these patients is provided.

The remainder of the issue focuses on hepatic complications of systemic issues, such as endocrine disorders, obstructive sleep apnea, and prolonged total parental nutrition; conditions that are increasing in prevalence, such as obesity, small bowel disorders, and small bowel transplantation, are becoming increasingly common. The

Clin Liver Dis 23 (2019) xiii–xiv
https://doi.org/10.1016/j.cld.2019.02.001
1089-3261/19/© 2019 Published by Elsevier Inc.

articles emphasize clinically relevant diagnostic and therapeutic approaches to these disorders.

Over the last decades, the complexity of illness affecting our patients has significantly increased, and with it, the likelihood that the liver will be directly or indirectly involved in the pathologic process. This is best exemplified by the myriad of liver-related disorders that can affect critically ill patients, as discussed by Dr Flamm and colleagues. Recognition of the various hepatic manifestations of systemic disease is of paramount importance in the management of these complex patients. I hope that this issue will provide you with a useful resource in your daily practice.

Jorge L. Herrera, MD
Division of Gastroenterology
University of South Alabama
College of Medicine
Mobile, AL 36688, USA

E-mail address:
jherrera18@gmail.com

The Liver and Celiac Disease

Alberto Rubio-Tapia, MD, Joseph A. Murray, MD*

KEYWORDS

- Hepatitis • Cirrhosis • Alanine aminotransferase

KEY POINTS

- Abnormal liver blood tests are common in celiac disease.
- Celiac hepatitis is the most common liver disorder in patients with celiac disease and respond to a gluten-free diet.
- Celiac disease may be associated to other chronic liver conditions.

INTRODUCTION

Celiac disease (CD) is a multisystem disorder characterized by permanent intolerance to gluten (wheat, barley, and rye).[1,2] Although the hallmark of CD is enteropathy, other organs, including the liver, may also be affected. Liver abnormalities in untreated CD are common.[3] CD can cause direct liver damage (celiac hepatitis) but also may be associated with other liver conditions.[4] Abnormal liver blood tests (especially hypertransaminasemia) may be the sole manifestation of hitherto unrecognized CD. The pathophysiology of liver injury in CD remains poorly understood. The aim of this study is to review the full spectrum of liver injury related to CD.

INITIAL WORKUP

A complete liver test panel is strongly recommended in patients with newly diagnosed CD.[3] Mild elevation of transaminases (3–5 times the upper limit of normal) in the absence of clinical manifestations of chronic liver disease is characteristic of celiac hepatitis. Resolution of the abnormal liver tests after strict adherence to a gluten-free diet (GFD) confirms the diagnosis.[3] Thus, if liver tests were abnormal at the time of diagnosis, it should be rechecked after 6 to 12 months on a strict GFD.[3,5] In patients with typical findings for celiac hepatitis, it is reasonable to treat with a GFD first and plan for further investigation in the subset of patients (10%–25%) with persistent liver test abnormalities after 1 year on strict adherence to GFD. However, an initial

---

The authors have nothing to disclose.
Division of Gastroenterology and Hepatology, Department of Medicine, Mayo Clinic College of Medicine, 200 First Street Southwest, Rochester, MN 55905, USA
* Corresponding author.
E-mail address: murray.joseph@mayo.edu

evaluation is strongly recommended for coexistent liver disorder in patients with symptoms or physical signs that suggest chronic liver disorder and/or transaminases levels greater than 5 times the upper limit of normal (**Fig. 1**).[6–8]

Isolated elevation of alkaline phosphatase is not characteristic of celiac hepatitis. Metabolic bone disease may be the most common explanation for an isolated alkaline phosphatase in patients with CD.[2,9] Check calcium, phosphate, 25-(OH) vitamin D, and parathyroid hormone for evaluation for osteomalacia.[10] A very low 25-(OH) vitamin D, low calcium and phosphate, and elevated parathyroid hormone levels strongly support the diagnosis of malabsorption-related osteomalacia. Dual energy x-ray absorptiometry is suggested for all patients with newly diagnosed CD.[10] Thyroid stimulant hormone measurement is also useful.[10] Chronic cholestatic liver disorders should be considered after exclusion of nonliver causes for isolated elevation of alkaline phosphatase.

Liver biopsy is not necessary in most patients with newly diagnosed CD who have isolated hypertransaminasemia.[6,11] Liver biopsy may be useful in selected patients with suspicion of chronic cholestatic liver disease with negative noninvasive tests, unexplained persistent hypertransaminasemia (after 1 year on strict adherence to GFD), and coexistent liver disease in which the liver biopsy has therapeutic or prognostic significance.[3]

CELIAC HEPATITIS

Celiac hepatitis is a gluten-dependent injury and liver abnormality resolved on a GFD, typically after 12 months of strict adherence.[5–7,12,13] Histologic changes also improve after a GFD.[14]

Hypertransaminasemia is frequent in untreated CD (13%–60%) (**Table 1**).[6,7,12] Conversely, CD is present in as many as 9% of persons with unexplained

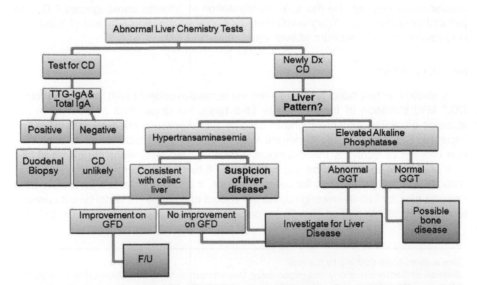

Fig. 1. Suggested approach to abnormal liver test and CD. [a]Clues for suspicion of concurrent liver disease include hyperbilirubinemia, hypertransaminasemia greater than 5 times upper limit of normal, aspartate aminotransferase (AST):alanine aminotransferase (ALT) ratio greater than 1.0, and abnormal physical examination. CD, celiac disease; F/U, follow-up; GFD, gluten-free diet; GGT, gamma-glutamyl transferase; TTG, tissue transglutaminase antibody.

Table 1
Frequency of abnormal liver chemistry test and the effect of a gluten-free diet in patients with celiac disease

Reference	Cases	Female (n, %)	Age, y (range)	Abnormal Liver Test (n, %)	Response to GFD (n, %)	Time on GFD
Bardella et al,[6] 1995	158	127, 80	18–68	67, 42	60/67, 90	6 mo
Hagander et al,[7] 1977	74	43, 58	14–73	29/53, 55	N/A[a]	N/A
Bonamico et al,[12] 1986	65	43, 66	0.5–18	37, 60	N/A	N/A
Jacobsen et al,[13] 1990	132	64, 48	25–86	62, 47	24/32, 75	2 y
Dickey et al,[5] 1995	129	88, 68	17–88	17, 13	15/17, 88	6–12 mo
Castillo et al,[57] 2015	463	328,71	44 (+/–14)[b]	190, 41	150, 79	18 mo
Lee et al,[58] 2016	388	235,61	10 (+/–4.4)	185, 48	15/21, 71	N/A
Aarela et al,[22] 2016	150	103, 69	4.3–11.8[b]	22, 15	18, 80	12 mo

Abbreviation: N/A, not available.
[a] Transaminase levels dropped significantly 2.5 to 8 weeks after starting a GFD.
[b] +/– standard deviation.

hypertransaminasemia.[15,16] Celiac patients have both an increased risk of subsequent liver disease and risk of death from liver cirrhosis than the general population.[3,15,17,18]

The mechanisms underlying celiac hepatitis are poorly understood.[19] Intestinal permeability was quantitatively higher in patients with CD and hypertransaminasemia than in those with CD and normal liver tests.[11] The phenomenon is gluten dependent as demonstrated by normalization of both intestinal permeability and elevation of transaminases with a GFD.[11] It has been speculated that increased intestinal permeability may facilitate the entry to the portal circulation (and then to the liver) of toxins, microbial and other antigens, cytokines, and/or other mediators of liver injury (**Fig. 2**).[7,16,20,21] However, liver injury is not commonly seen in other intestinal disorders associated with increased intestinal permeability.

Most patients with celiac hepatitis have no symptoms or signs of liver disease.[6,7,15] Thus, the presence of palmar erythema, jaundice, ascites, splenomegaly, encephalopathy, coagulopathy, or portal hypertension suggests advanced liver disease or the coexistence with other chronic liver disease.[3,6] Mild to moderate (less than 5 times the upper limit of normal) levels of aspartate aminotransferase and/or alanine aminotransferase are typical.[6,7,12,16] The ratio of aspartate to alanine aminotransferase is usually less than 1.[3] Elevated alanine aminotransferase is associated with poor growth and severe villous atrophy in children.[22]

Conjugated hyperbilirubinemia is not expected in the absence of advanced cirrhosis.[6,10,23] Abdominal ultrasound is not necessary during the initial workup, and findings on the liver vary according to the degree of liver injury, from normal (most common) to coarse echo texture.[23] Other nonspecific abdominal ultrasound findings suggestive of CD include dilated small bowel loops, enlarged mesenteric lymph nodes, nonocclusive intussusception, abnormal jejunum folds, and increased fasting gallbladder volume.[24,25]

Liver biopsy is rarely needed for celiac hepatitis. Mild and/or nonspecific histologic changes are seen.[13,26] Extensive fibrosis and cirrhosis are rare (**Box 1**).[23]

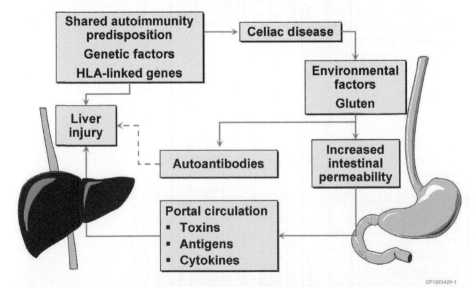

Fig. 2. Potential mechanisms of liver injury in CD. (*From* Rubio-Tapia A, Murray JA. The liver in celiac disease. Hepatology 2007;46(5):1651; with permission.)

Box 1
Liver pathology of patients with celiac disease

- Periportal inflammation[a]
- Mononuclear infiltration on the parenchyma[a]
- Steatosis
- Bile duct obstruction
- Hyperplasia of Kupffer cells
- Fibrosis (all stages)
- Granuloma
- Cirrhosis

[a] Most common findings.

Finally, there is considerable evidence and expert opinion support for testing for CD in patients with unexplained abnormal liver tests.[27] Advanced liver disease is associated with false positive results of the tissue transglutaminase antibody (especially if titer is <3 times upper limit of normal).[3] Endomysial antibodies are more specific in this context and may be helpful in the diagnostic evaluation of patients with advanced liver disease. Biopsy confirmation of CD is strongly recommended.[3]

CELIAC DISEASE AND SELECTED LIVER DISORDERS
Autoimmune Liver Disorders

Primary biliary cholangitis and autoimmune hepatitis may be associated with CD.[3,28,29] The frequency of CD in patients with primary biliary cholangitis (1%–7%) and primary biliary cholangitis in patients with CD (0.1%–3%) is variable between studies (**Tables 2** and **3**).[8,30–37] CD is present in 4% to 6% of patients with both type 1 and type 2 autoimmune hepatitis.[3,28–30] There are also case reports of primary sclerosing cholangitis and CD.[38]

The reasons for the association between CD and autoimmune liver disorders are unknown. Shared genetic susceptibility to autoimmunity and perhaps vulnerability of both biliary and small intestine epithelium to immune-mediated damage may play a role.[32] CD and primary sclerosing cholangitis share the at-risk gene risk HLA-DQ2. The presence of HLA-DQ2 is associated with an increased rapid

---

Table 2
Selected studies on screening of celiac disease with biopsy confirmation in primary biliary cholangitis

Reference	Cases with Primary Biliary Cholangitis	Cases Identified with CD, n (%)
Volta et al,[30] 2002	173	7 (4)
Dickey et al,[31] 1997	57	4 (7)
Kingham and Parker,[32] 1998	67	4 (6)
Niveloni et al,[33] 1998	10	2
Floreani et al,[34] 2002	87	3 (3.4)
Gillett et al,[35] 2000	378	5 (1.3)

Table 3
Selected studies on the prevalence of primary biliary cholangitis in patients with celiac disease

Reference	Cases with CD	Cases Identified with Primary Biliary Cholangitis, n (%)
Lawson et al,[8] 2005	4732	9 (0.1)
Kingham and Parker,[32] 1998	143	4 (3)
Bardella et al,[36] 1997	336	1 (0.3)
Sorensen et al,[37] 1999	896	2 (0.2)

progression of the liver disease in primary sclerosing cholangitis.[39] Likewise, homozygosity for DQ2 increases CD risk and perhaps severity.[40,41] A GFD appears to have little effect on coexistent liver disease outcome because it may not improve liver tests or symptoms.[29,31]

Viral Hepatitis and Vaccines

There is no association between CD and chronic hepatitis C.[42] Most patients with concurrent CD and hepatitis C have a well-defined route of transmission for hepatitis C.[43] Hepatitis C treatment with interferon-α and/or ribavirin may activate silent or latent CD.[3,44,45] The clinical relevance of this observation has decreased with the newly available direct active antiviral drugs. Nonresponse to hepatitis B vaccine given before diagnosis of CD is frequent (54%–68%).[46,47] Rate of seroconversion correlated with the amount of gluten ingestion, and greater than 95% of CD patients vaccinated after treatment with a GFD may respond.[48] HLA-DQ2 may play a role in vaccine nonresponse.[46,49]

Nonalcoholic Fatty Liver

The frequency of CD in patients with nonalcoholic fatty liver disease is 3% to 7%.[50,51] Screening all patients with nonalcoholic fatty liver disease for CD is controversial. However, a high index of suspicion may result in early diagnosis. Active screening is reasonable in patients with nonalcoholic fatty liver disease with unexplained anemia, nutritional deficiencies, and recurrent abdominal symptoms.[51] The GFD may improve liver tests in patients with nonalcoholic fatty liver disease and CD, but it is unclear if this effect is independent of nutritional factors.[50] Moreover, there is an increased risk of nonalcoholic fatty liver disease (hazard ratio = 2.8) following a GFD, and close monitoring of weight is recommended after GFD.[52] Increased risk was higher in children and nonoverweight CD patients.[52,53] Nonalcoholic fatty liver disease risk remains elevated even beyond 15 years after the diagnosis of CD.[52]

Liver Transplantation

The prevalence of CD in liver transplant patients with end-stage liver disease of multiple causes varied from 3% to 4.3%.[23,54] Strict adherence for 6 months to a GFD in a small group of enlisted patients with CD and end-stage liver disease improved liver function to the point that made liver transplant unnecessary.[23,54,55] A large Swedish study showed no increased risk of liver transplantation in diagnosed CD despite increased risk of acute hepatitis, chronic hepatitis, primary sclerosing cholangitis, fatty liver disease, liver failure, liver cirrhosis/fibrosis, and primary biliary cholangitis.[17]

Mortality of Liver Cause in Celiac Disease

Mortality of liver cause is increased in patients with CD (standardized mortality ratio 3.10), although the absolute risk of liver-related mortality is modest.[56]

SUMMARY

Liver blood test abnormalities are common in patients with CD. Conversely, abnormal liver blood tests (especially hypertransaminasemia) may be the sole manifestation of unrecognized CD. Celiac hepatitis is the most common liver manifestation of CD and responsive to GFD. Finally, CD may be associated with selected liver conditions, especially immune-mediated, and the effect of GFD on the progression of coexistent liver disease is unclear.

REFERENCES

1. Catassi C. The world map of celiac disease. Acta Gastroenterol Latinoam 2005; 35(1):37–55.
2. Green PH, Cellier C. Celiac disease. N Engl J Med 2007;357(17):1731–43.
3. Rubio-Tapia A, Murray JA. The liver in celiac disease. Hepatology 2007;46(5): 1650–8.
4. Sood A, Khurana MS, Mahajan R, et al. Prevalence and clinical significance of IgA anti-tissue transglutaminase antibodies in patients with chronic liver disease. J Gastroenterol Hepatol 2017;32(2):446–50.
5. Dickey W, McMillan SA, Collins JS, et al. Liver abnormalities associated with celiac sprue. How common are they, what is their significance, and what do we do about them? J Clin Gastroenterol 1995;20(4):290–2.
6. Bardella MT, Fraquelli M, Quatrini M, et al. Prevalence of hypertransaminasemia in adult celiac patients and effect of gluten-free diet. Hepatology 1995;22(3): 833–6.
7. Hagander B, Berg NO, Brandt L, et al. Hepatic injury in adult coeliac disease. Lancet 1977;2(8032):270–2.
8. Lawson A, West J, Aithal GP, et al. Autoimmune cholestatic liver disease in people with coeliac disease: a population-based study of their association. Aliment Pharmacol Ther 2005;21(4):401–5.
9. Buess M, Steuerwald M, Wegmann W, et al. Obstructive jaundice caused by enteropathy-associated T-cell lymphoma in a patient with celiac sprue. J Gastroenterol 2004;39(11):1110–3.
10. Rostom A, Murray JA, Kagnoff MF. American Gastroenterological Association (AGA) Institute technical review on the diagnosis and management of celiac disease. Gastroenterology 2006;131(6):1981–2002.
11. Novacek G, Miehsler W, Wrba F, et al. Prevalence and clinical importance of hypertransaminasaemia in coeliac disease. Eur J Gastroenterol Hepatol 1999;11(3): 283–8.
12. Bonamico M, Pitzalis G, Culasso F, et al. Hepatic damage in celiac disease in children. Minerva Pediatr 1986;38(21):959–62 [in Italian].
13. Jacobsen MB, Fausa O, Elgjo K, et al. Hepatic lesions in adult coeliac disease. Scand J Gastroenterol 1990;25(7):656–62.
14. Majumdar K, Sakhuja P, Puri AS, et al. Coeliac disease and the liver: spectrum of liver histology, serology and treatment response at a tertiary referral centre. J Clin Pathol 2018;71(5):412–9.

15. Bardella MT, Vecchi M, Conte D, et al. Chronic unexplained hypertransaminasemia may be caused by occult celiac disease. Hepatology 1999;29(3):654–7.

16. Volta U, De Franceschi L, Lari F, et al. Coeliac disease hidden by cryptogenic hypertransaminasaemia. Lancet 1998;352(9121):26–9.

17. Ludvigsson JF, Elfstrom P, Broome U, et al. Celiac disease and risk of liver disease: a general population-based study. Clin Gastroenterol Hepatol 2007;5(1): 63–9.e61.

18. Peters U, Askling J, Gridley G, et al. Causes of death in patients with celiac disease in a population-based Swedish cohort. Arch Intern Med 2003;163(13): 1566–72.

19. Hoffmanova I, Sanchez D, Tuckova L, et al. Celiac disease and liver disorders: from putative pathogenesis to clinical implications. Nutrients 2018;10(7) [pii: E892].

20. Pelaez-Luna M, Schmulson M, Robles-Diaz G. Intestinal involvement is not sufficient to explain hypertransaminasemia in celiac disease? Med Hypotheses 2005; 65(5):937–41.

21. Korponay-Szabo IR, Halttunen T, Szalai Z, et al. In vivo targeting of intestinal and extraintestinal transglutaminase 2 by coeliac autoantibodies. Gut 2004;53(5): 641–8.

22. Aarela L, Nurminen S, Kivela L, et al. Prevalence and associated factors of abnormal liver values in children with celiac disease. Dig Liver Dis 2016;48(9): 1023–9.

23. Kaukinen K, Halme L, Collin P, et al. Celiac disease in patients with severe liver disease: gluten-free diet may reverse hepatic failure. Gastroenterology 2002; 122(4):881–8.

24. Fraquelli M, Colli A, Colucci A, et al. Accuracy of ultrasonography in predicting celiac disease. Arch Intern Med 2004;164(2):169–74.

25. Rettenbacher T, Hollerweger A, Macheiner P, et al. Adult celiac disease: US signs. Radiology 1999;211(2):389–94.

26. Pollock DJ. The liver in coeliac disease. Histopathology 1977;1(6):421–30.

27. Kwo PY, Cohen SM, Lim JK. ACG clinical guideline: evaluation of abnormal liver chemistries. Am J Gastroenterol 2017;112(1):18–35.

28. Volta U, De Franceschi L, Molinaro N, et al. Frequency and significance of antigliadin and anti-endomysial antibodies in autoimmune hepatitis. Dig Dis Sci 1998;43(10):2190–5.

29. Villalta D, Girolami D, Bidoli E, et al. High prevalence of celiac disease in autoimmune hepatitis detected by anti-tissue tranglutaminase autoantibodies. J Clin Lab Anal 2005;19(1):6–10.

30. Volta U, Rodrigo L, Granito A, et al. Celiac disease in autoimmune cholestatic liver disorders. Am J Gastroenterol 2002;97(10):2609–13.

31. Dickey W, McMillan SA, Callender ME. High prevalence of celiac sprue among patients with primary biliary cirrhosis. J Clin Gastroenterol 1997;25(1):328–9.

32. Kingham JG, Parker DR. The association between primary biliary cirrhosis and coeliac disease: a study of relative prevalences. Gut 1998;42(1):120–2.

33. Niveloni S, Dezi R, Pedreira S, et al. Gluten sensitivity in patients with primary biliary cirrhosis. Am J Gastroenterol 1998;93(3):404–8.

34. Floreani A, Betterle C, Baragiotta A, et al. Prevalence of coeliac disease in primary biliary cirrhosis and of antimitochondrial antibodies in adult coeliac disease patients in Italy. Dig Liver Dis 2002;34(4):258–61.

35. Gillett HR, Cauch-Dudek K, Jenny E, et al. Prevalence of IgA antibodies to endomysium and tissue transglutaminase in primary biliary cirrhosis. Can J Gastroenterol 2000;14(8):672–5.
36. Bardella MT, Quatrini M, Zuin M, et al. Screening patients with celiac disease for primary biliary cirrhosis and vice versa. Am J Gastroenterol 1997;92(9):1524–6.
37. Sorensen HT, Thulstrup AM, Blomqvist P, et al. Risk of primary biliary liver cirrhosis in patients with coeliac disease: Danish and Swedish cohort data. Gut 1999;44(5):736–8.
38. Hay JE, Wiesner RH, Shorter RG, et al. Primary sclerosing cholangitis and celiac disease. A novel association. Ann Intern Med 1988;109(9):713–7.
39. Boberg KM, Spurkland A, Rocca G, et al. The HLA-DR3,DQ2 heterozygous genotype is associated with an accelerated progression of primary sclerosing cholangitis. Scand J Gastroenterol 2001;36(8):886–90.
40. Murray JA, Moore SB, Van Dyke CT, et al. HLA DQ gene dosage and risk and severity of celiac disease. Clin Gastroenterol Hepatol 2007;5(12):1406–12.
41. Al-Toma A, Goerres MS, Meijer JW, et al. Human leukocyte antigen-DQ2 homozygosity and the development of refractory celiac disease and enteropathy-associated T-cell lymphoma. Clin Gastroenterol Hepatol 2006;4(3):315–9.
42. Fine KD, Ogunji F, Saloum Y, et al. Celiac sprue: another autoimmune syndrome associated with hepatitis C. Am J Gastroenterol 2001;96(1):138–45.
43. Thevenot T, Boruchowicz A, Henrion J, et al. Celiac disease is not associated with chronic hepatitis C. Dig Dis Sci 2007;52(5):1310–2.
44. Bardella MT, Marino R, Meroni PL. Celiac disease during interferon treatment. Ann Intern Med 1999;131(2):157–8.
45. Adinolfi LE, Durante Mangoni E, Andreana A. Interferon and ribavirin treatment for chronic hepatitis C may activate celiac disease. Am J Gastroenterol 2001;96(2):607–8.
46. Noh KW, Poland GA, Murray JA. Hepatitis B vaccine nonresponse and celiac disease. Am J Gastroenterol 2003;98(10):2289–92.
47. Park SD, Markowitz J, Pettei M, et al. Failure to respond to hepatitis B vaccine in children with celiac disease. J Pediatr Gastroenterol Nutr 2007;44(4):431–5.
48. Nemes E, Lefler E, Szegedi L, et al. Gluten intake interferes with the humoral immune response to recombinant hepatitis B vaccine in patients with celiac disease. Pediatrics 2008;121(6):e1570–6.
49. Craven DE, Awdeh ZL, Kunches LM, et al. Nonresponsiveness to hepatitis B vaccine in health care workers. Results of revaccination and genetic typings. Ann Intern Med 1986;105(3):356–60.
50. Bardella MT, Valenti L, Pagliari C, et al. Searching for coeliac disease in patients with non-alcoholic fatty liver disease. Dig Liver Dis 2004;36(5):333–6.
51. Kamal S, Aldossari KK, Ghoraba D, et al. Clinicopathological and immunological characteristics and outcome of concomitant coeliac disease and non-alcoholic fatty liver disease in adults: a large prospective longitudinal study. BMJ Open Gastroenterol 2018;5(1):e000150.
52. Reilly NR, Lebwohl B, Hultcrantz R, et al. Increased risk of non-alcoholic fatty liver disease after diagnosis of celiac disease. J Hepatol 2015;62(6):1405–11.
53. Tovoli F, Negrini G, Fari R, et al. Increased risk of nonalcoholic fatty liver disease in patients with coeliac disease on a gluten-free diet: beyond traditional metabolic factors. Aliment Pharmacol Ther 2018;48(5):538–46.
54. Rubio-Tapia A, Abdulkarim AS, Wiesner RH, et al. Celiac disease autoantibodies in severe autoimmune liver disease and the effect of liver transplantation. Liver Int 2008;28(4):467–76.

55. Dalekos GN, Bogdanos DP, Neuberger J. Celiac disease-related autoantibodies in end-stage autoimmune liver diseases: what is the message? Liver Int 2008; 28(4):426–8.

56. Holmes GKT, Muirhead A. Mortality in coeliac disease: a population-based cohort study from a single centre in Southern Derbyshire, UK. BMJ Open Gastroenterol 2018;5(1):e000201.

57. Castillo NE, Vanga RR, Theethira TG, et al. Prevalence of abnormal liver function tests in celiac disease and the effect of a gluten-free diet in the US population. Am J Gastroenterol 2015;110(8):1216–22.

58. Lee GJ, Boyle B, Ediger T, et al. Hypertransaminasemia in newly diagnosed pediatric patients with celiac disease. J Pediatr Gastroenterol Nutr 2016;63(3): 340–3.

The Liver in Sickle Cell Disease

Eleni Theocharidou, PhD, Abid R. Suddle, MD, FRCP*

KEYWORDS

- Sickle cell hepatopathy • Intrahepatic cholestasis • Sickle hepatic crisis
- Iron overload • Viral hepatitis • Cholelithiasis

KEY POINTS

- Liver involvement in sickle cell disease (SCD) is not uncommon, and it can occur as the result of multiple liver insults.
- Sickle hepatopathy is an "umbrella" term encompassing a diverse range and sometimes mixed pattern of hepatic pathology that occurs in patients with SCD.
- The range of hepatic pathology seen includes ischemic injury as a result of sickling within the liver, the consequences of multiple blood transfusions, including viral hepatitis and iron overload, and (pigment) gallstones.
- The clinical spectrum of liver disease encountered is wide and often multifactorial.
- Limited evidence exists for medical treatments. Exchange blood transfusions can be effective in acute liver syndromes; evidence for this is mainly based on case reports. Liver transplantation may have a role for end-stage liver disease.

INTRODUCTION

Sickle cell disease (SCD) or homozygous sickle cell anemia is the most common inherited disorder of erythrocytes, characterized by the presence of pathologic hemoglobin S (HbS). A substitution of a single amino acid (glutamic acid to valine) in the sixth position of the beta-globin chain results in formation of HbS. HbS polymerizes in deoxygenated conditions, precipitating changes in the red cell membrane and dehydration of red cells leading to formation of sickle cells.[1] Intravascular sickling of erythrocytes results in vaso-occlusive crises and hemolysis, which are the hallmarks of SCD. Vaso-occlusive crises result in tissue and end-organ damage, with common manifestations including acute chest syndrome, stroke, osteonecrosis, sickle nephropathy, and hyposplenism.

The authors have nothing to disclose.
Institute of Liver Studies, King's College Hospital NHS Foundation Trust, Denmark Hill, London SE5 9RS, UK
* Corresponding author.
E-mail address: abid.suddle@nhs.net

Clin Liver Dis 23 (2019) 177–189
https://doi.org/10.1016/j.cld.2018.12.002
1089-3261/19/Crown Copyright © 2018 Published by Elsevier Inc. All rights reserved.
liver.theclinics.com

The prevalence of SCD is high in populations of Black African and African Caribbean origin, and to a lesser extent in South Asian, Middle Eastern, and Mediterranean populations.[2] The disease is inherited in an autosomal recessive pattern. Compound heterozygotes (SC or S beta thalassemia) typically have milder disease expression.

Sickle cell hepatopathy is an "umbrella" term encompassing the different kinds of liver disease encountered in patients with SCD. As such, a diverse range of hepatic pathology, resulting in diverse clinical phenotypes of liver disease, is included: intrahepatic sickling, multiple blood transfusions with the consequent risks of viral hepatitis and iron overload, and gallstones (**Table 1**). The incidence of sickle hepatopathy is difficult to determine, as abnormalities in liver function tests are common in patients with SCD. Increases in bilirubin (predominantly unconjugated), aspartate aminotransferase (AST), and lactate dehydrogenase are common in SCD, often reflecting hemolysis rather than liver damage per se. The direct manifestations of SCD in the liver are predominantly related to vascular occlusion from sickling with resultant acute ischemia, sequestration, and cholestasis. Liver complications of multiple transfusions include viral hepatitis and iron overload. A consequence of chronic hemolysis is the development of pigment gallstones. The clinical spectrum of sickle hepatopathy ranges from mild liver function test abnormalities in asymptomatic patients, to dramatic clinical crises with marked hyperbilirubinemia and liver failure (**Fig. 1**).

MANIFESTATIONS SECONDARY TO INTRAHEPATIC SICKLING OF ERYTHROCYTES
Acute Sickle Hepatic Crisis

Acute sickle hepatic crisis is estimated to occur in 10% of patients with SCD, resulting in transient hepatic ischemic injury. The clinical presentation is typically within the clinical context of a vaso-occlusive crisis with right upper quadrant pain, tender hepatomegaly, low-grade fever, and jaundice. There is usually a moderate elevation in liver function tests with alanine transaminase (ALT) and AST elevation less than 10-fold the upper limit of normal (rarely exceeding 1000 IU/L) and bilirubin elevation less than 15 mg/dL (predominantly conjugated). Symptoms and biochemical abnormalities usually respond to intravenous fluid administration and analgesia, but rarely may require exchange blood transfusions (EBT).[3] An acute sickle hepatic crisis typically resolves within 2 weeks, although recurrences can occur in a small proportion of patients.[3]

A liver biopsy is very rarely required to confirm the diagnosis, and can be associated with increased risk of complications in the acute sickling setting. In a series of 14

Table 1 Classification of hepatobiliary disease in sickle cell disease	
Acute Liver Disease	**Chronic Liver Disease**
Related to sickling process • Acute sickle hepatic crisis • Acute sickle intrahepatic cholestasis • Acute hepatic sequestration	Related to sickling process • Chronic cholestasis • Biliary-type cirrhosis
Complications of treatment • Viral hepatitis B and C	Complications of treatment • Iron overload • Chronic viral hepatitis B and C
Miscellaneous • Cholelithiasis • Budd-Chiari syndrome • Hepatic abscess/biloma	Miscellaneous • Cholelithiasis • Coexistent liver disease (eg, autoimmune hepatitis)

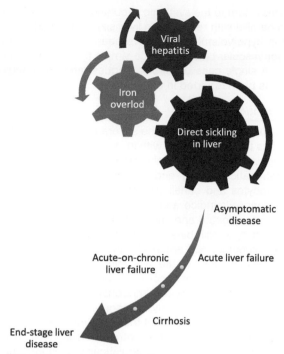

Fig. 1. Evolution of liver disease in sickle cell disease.

patients with SCD who underwent percutaneous liver biopsy, 5 patients (36%) developed severe bleeding complications and 4 (28%) died.[4] Most patients (4 of 5) who developed complications were in acute sickle crisis at the time of the biopsy. Histologic data from older series consistently showed sinusoidal dilatation, Kupffer cell hyperplasia, and erythrophagocytosis.[5,6] The more recent series confirmed these histologic findings, but also demonstrated that patients with features of chronic venous outflow obstruction (sinusoidal dilatation with centrilobular fibrosis and parenchymal loss) were more likely to develop complications.[4] Importantly, the investigators did not feel that the histologic data significantly changed the management of these patients. In view of the high risk of hemorrhage and low-level clinical impact, SCD particularly in the setting of an acute sickle crisis, could be considered a relative contraindication to liver biopsy.

Acute Sickle Hepatic Sequestration

Sequestration of large numbers of sickled erythrocytes most commonly occurs in the pulmonary vasculature and the spleen in early life before the development of hyposplenism. Less commonly, sequestration can occur within the liver. Published experience is very limited in the form of case reports. Clinical presentation is similar to acute sickle hepatic crisis with right upper quadrant pain, fever, and jaundice.[7] There is a significant rapid increase in the size of the organ due to the volume of trapped erythrocytes, with concurrent rapid decrease in hemoglobin levels, which can result in hypovolemic shock.[8] Elevated conjugated bilirubin and Alkaline Phosphotase usually reflect biliary compression, although the derangement in liver function tests can be mild.[9,10] Acute sequestration resolves in 3 to 4 days with supportive management and simple blood transfusions or EBT.[11] On resolution of sequestration, part of the trapped erythrocytes return to the systemic circulation, resulting in an increase in hemoglobin levels in parallel with reduction in liver size. This rapid reversion of sequestration can result in hypervolemia, congestive heart failure, and also hyperviscosity with implications for vascular patency, hence simple transfusions should be administered cautiously.[12] A single case of chronic sequestration responding to treatment with hydroxyurea has been reported in the literature.[13]

Acute Sickle Intrahepatic Cholestasis

Acute intrahepatic cholestasis stands in the severe end of the spectrum of sickle cell hepatopathy, and has been associated with increased mortality. It mainly affects patients with homozygous HbSS disease, and rarely those with HbSC or HBS beta thalassemia.[14–17] Intrahepatic sickling and hypoxic hepatocellular damage lead to ballooning of hepatocytes and canalicular cholestasis. The clinical presentation is more severe, with deeper jaundice and marked hyperbilirubinemia typically greater than 15 mg/dL. Both conjugated and unconjugated bilirubin secondary to hemolysis contribute to profound hyperbilirubinemia, with the conjugated fraction usually being higher than the unconjugated. ALT and AST can be markedly elevated (>1000 IU/L), reflecting severe ischemic injury. Acute liver injury with coagulopathy (international normalized ratio prolongation) is not uncommon, and can evolve rapidly to acute liver failure (ALF), with development of hepatic encephalopathy and multiorgan failure.[18] It should be noted that the term ALF is likely not accurate, as the insult rarely occurs in a previously healthy liver. It is more likely that the acute insult secondary to intrahepatic sickling of erythrocytes is superimposed on other various insults (viral hepatitis, iron overload, previous ischemic injury) that synergistically result in significant liver injury and liver failure.[19] Acute kidney injury is commonly observed in this context, and can be the direct result of sickle cell nephropathy or the result of the circulatory changes secondary to liver failure.[20] This usually recovers with the improvement in liver function.[18] Recurrent and continuing/chronic intrahepatic cholestasis also has been described.[21,22]

Liver biopsy is rarely indicated, and can be associated with high risk of bleeding, as previously outlined. Histologic data from 13 patients with intrahepatic cholestasis who had no concomitant liver disease and either had liver biopsy or postmortem examination showed canalicular dilatation with bile plugs, erythrophagocytosis with Kupffer cell hyperplasia in all cases.[3] Other findings were parenchymal necrosis and variable stages of fibrosis in half of the patients.

Experience with management of this severe manifestation of SCD derives mainly from case reports and small case series. Reversal of acute intrahepatic cholestasis can rarely occur only with supportive measures and simple blood transfusions.[17,23] An aggressive EBT strategy may reverse acute liver injury and improve survival.[3] Cases of reversal of ALF have been reported.[17,24–26] The target of this strategy is to maintain an HbS fraction less than 20% to 30% and hemoglobin greater than 100 g/L, aiming to restore and maintain adequate tissue oxygenation. Nonresponders to EBT, in particular those with advanced underlying chronic liver disease, have poor prognosis.[15] The role of hydroxyurea in this context is unknown. The experience with liver transplantation (LT) in cases presenting with ALF is limited and with variable outcomes.[3,16,27–30]

Ahn and colleagues[3] reviewed 22 cases of acute intrahepatic cholestasis presenting with severe hepatic dysfunction. Nine patients were treated with EBT, 8 of whom responded. The patient who did not respond died post-LT. Two of the 8 responders experienced recurrence, requiring repeat EBT. The remaining 13 patients received supportive treatment that did not include EBT. Eleven of 13 patients died during their initial hospitalization. The 2 patients who survived had recurrence that was treated with EBT. The overall mortality rate was 50% during initial hospitalization, and was significantly higher among patients who did not receive EBT. These data support a potential therapeutic benefit with EBT in patients presenting with acute sickle cell intrahepatic cholestasis, even in the advent of ALF. Patients who do not respond to EBT are likely to have worse prognosis.

Chronic Liver Disease and Cirrhosis

Recurrent ischemic insults with parenchymal necrosis can result in hepatic fibrosis, chronic liver disease, and cirrhosis.[31] In the presence of coexistent liver pathologies, such as iron overload or viral hepatitis, progression of fibrosis can be accelerated. Cirrhosis has been reported in 16% to 29% of patients with SCD in autopsy studies.[3,32] Decompensation with ascites, hepatic encephalopathy, or variceal bleeding can develop in patients with advanced disease.[33] Acute intrahepatic cholestasis when superimposed on a cirrhotic liver can present as acute-on-chronic liver failure.[19,32] There have been case reports of patients diagnosed with SCD following their presentation with decompensated cirrhosis.[34,35] These reports may suggest that even low-grade intrahepatic sickling of erythrocytes can result in progressive liver damage and cirrhosis. The management of complications of cirrhosis is similar to any other etiology.

Sickle cholangiopathy is a reported complication of SCD.[28,36,37] The bile ducts are more susceptible to ischemic insults, as their blood supply is exclusively arterial. Biliary ischemia results in necrosis of the biliary epithelium with subsequent development of fibrosis and strictures. Ascending cholangitis is a known complication of cholangiopathy, and bilomas and biliary abscesses also have been described in the context of ischemic cholangiopathy in patients with SCD.[38] Magnetic resonance cholangiopancreatography (MRCP) is the most sensitive noninvasive modality for the assessment of the biliary tree. Endoscopic retrograde cholangiopancreatography (ERCP) is indicated only in cases in which biliary drainage/treatment of dominant strictures is required. Although the efficacy of ursodeoxycholic acid in this setting is unknown, it likely represents a reasonable option in the absence of other effective treatment. There are very few case reports of LT for sclerosing cholangitis in SCD.[28]

Other Complications

Vascular disorders of the liver can develop as a result of vascular occlusion in SCD. There have been case reports of Budd-Chiari syndrome secondary to hepatic vein occlusion, portal vein thrombosis, and veno-occlusive disease with nodular regenerative hyperplasia.[39,40]

TRANSFUSION-RELATED LIVER DISORDERS
Viral Hepatitis

Patients with SCD are likely to receive multiple blood transfusions throughout their lifetime. These patients historically acquired hepatitis B or C via blood transfusions in the era before universal screening of blood products for blood-borne viruses. New infections are unlikely to occur via this route of transmission, but there is a burden of chronic viral hepatitis secondary to previous infections. In a cohort of 150 multitransfused patients with SCD from the United Stated (1983–2001), hepatitis C virus (HCV) antibodies were positive in 35.3%, with the prevalence being much higher in patients transfused before 1992 (58%) compared with after 1992 (21%) when screening of blood donors for HCV was introduced in the United States.[41] In subsequent cohorts, the prevalence of HCV ranged between 10.1% and 23.0%,[42–45] and was significantly lower (2.38%) in a more recent cohort (1996–2005) from Turkey.[46] A consistent finding in all studies was that the risk of HCV infection increased in parallel with the number of blood transfusions, with more than 10 transfusions being associated with significantly higher risk (23.3%–30.3%) compared with less than 10 (7.9%–8.6%).

With regard to hepatitis B virus (HBV) infection, an initial report demonstrated HBV positivity in 28.6% children with SCD at the age of 4 years.[47] In a series of 170 patients with SCD from Egypt, the prevalence of HBV was 10.6%.[45] In the more recent cohort from Turkey, only 2 (0.99%) among 210 patients with SCD were HBV positive.[46]

The assessment of necro-inflammatory activity and fibrosis in this population is problematic due to the risks associated with liver biopsy. In the series from Egypt, 10 patients with HCV and 12 patients with HBV underwent liver biopsies.[45] Although all patients were stable from the SCD perspective, histologic features of sickle hepatopathy (sinusoidal dilatation, erythrophagocytosis, and Kupffer cell hyperplasia, and variable degrees of parenchymal necrosis) were present in all cases, along with the histologic features of chronic viral hepatitis and hepatic siderosis. None of the patients with HCV and 3 of the patients with HBV had cirrhosis on histology. The utility of noninvasive markers of hepatic fibrosis has not been evaluated in this population. Noninvasive markers and in particular transient elastography (FibroScan) are extensively used in patients with chronic hepatitis B and C. The lack of histologic data to validate against and the multiple synergistic pathologies render the use and interpretation of these markers problematic.[48]

Treatment of chronic hepatitis B should be with nucleot(s)ide analogues according to guidelines. The indications for commencing antiviral therapy are based on HBV viral load, ALT activity, and the severity of the underlying liver disease. In patients with SCD, the extent of hepatic fibrosis is often difficult to assess, and ALT elevations can be multifactorial. In this context, and given the multiple synergistic liver insults, the threshold for commencing antiviral therapy may need to be lower.

With regard to treatment for HCV, before the advent of oral direct-acting antiviral (DAA) agents, there was reluctance in using interferon and ribavirin in patients with SCD due to the risk of anemia. However, there were reports of good tolerability of both normal-dose and low-dose ribavirin among patients with HCV. Sustained virological response (SVR) rates were similar to patients without SCD. The novel DAA therapies have changed the landscape in HCV treatment demonstrating very good safety profile and excellent SVR rates. Sofosbuvir/ledipasvir[49] and elbasvir/grazoprevir[50] have been tested in HCV-infected SCD cohorts. Ten patients with genotype 1 and 4 were treated with sofosbuvir/ledipasvir for 12 or 24 weeks, with SVR rate 90% (9/10). Nineteen patients were treated with elbasvir/grazoprevir for 12 weeks with 94.17% (18/19) SVR. There were no concerns regarding safety in either study. Some of the DAA regimens may still require concomitant ribavirin, especially in patients with decompensated cirrhosis. Patients with SCD may need lower starting dose or reduction in the dose of ribavirin in case of significant anemia.

With universal screening of blood and blood-derived products for HBV and HCV, the anticipated HCV elimination with DAA therapies and the effective suppression strategies for HBV, the burden of viral hepatitis in patients with SCD is expected to decrease significantly in the coming decades.

Iron Overload

Iron overload has been considered a major cause of end-organ damage in multitransfused patients with hemoglobinopathies. The heart, liver, and endocrine glands can be affected, with heart failure being a major driver of mortality in patients with thalassemia major. The source of excessive iron burden in SCD is primarily blood transfusions but also intravascular hemolysis. Hepatic iron deposition secondary to multiple blood transfusions predominantly occurs in the reticuloendothelial system and to a lesser extent in the hepatocytes, as opposed to predominantly hepatocellular iron deposition in hereditary hemochromatosis.[51] Hemosiderosis can precipitate inflammation and fibrosis, and can eventually lead to cirrhosis.

Hepatic iron content (HIC) can be measured invasively on liver biopsy specimens or noninvasively with novel MRI techniques (FerriScan).[52,53] There is very close correlation between the 2 methods,[53] as a result of which MRI has largely eliminated the need for liver biopsies.

In a study of 27 children with SCD, liver biopsies were performed before commencing iron chelation therapy.[54] HIC was associated with the number of transfusions. Presence of hepatic fibrosis was associated with higher HIC. In a study of 40 adult patients with SCD who underwent liver biopsy, fibrosis was present in 28% and was associated with HIC, although there were patients with high HIC that did not have any fibrosis.[55] Ferritin levels correlated with HIC in this study, although not in a linear manner. Despite the use of potent iron chelation agents, iron overload can still occur. A study included 30 children with SCD and 7 with thalassemia major who received multiple blood transfusions and chelation therapy.[56] HIC was measured with FerriScan, and was found to be elevated ($\geq$14 mg/g of dry weight) in 38.3%. HIC correlated with serum ferritin levels. Although serum ferritin levels correlate with HIC, they are not considered an adequately sensitive surrogate of hepatic iron overload. In a study of 28 patients with SCD, 30.4% had an HIC greater than 7 mg/g of dry weight and a serum ferritin of less than 2000 μg/L. Of note, although cardiac overload is a major cause of mortality in patients with thalassemia, it is rarely so in patients with SCD,[52,56] and patients with SCD may be less susceptible to hepatic injury/fibrosis secondary to iron overload.[51]

It should be taken into consideration that hepatic deposition also can occur in patients who are not transfusion dependent,[57] and there have been reports of iron overload in patients with SCD who never received blood transfusions.[58] These reports indicate that chronic hemolysis might be an important source of iron in these patients.

To investigate the contribution of chronic liver disease to mortality in SCD, a large cohort of 247 patients was followed for 30 months.[55] Mortality rate was 9%. Direct bilirubin and ferritin were independent predictors of mortality. Ferritin levels correlated with HIC and blood transfusion burden. All patients with advanced fibrosis had iron overload, although there were patients with high HIC who did not have fibrosis. These data suggest that hepatic iron deposition is an important cofactor to the development of chronic liver disease, but the latter usually occurs as a result of multiple hepatic insults.

Patients with SCD should undergo screening for iron overload. Parameters that should be taken into consideration when screening these patients include the number of blood transfusions, spot ferritin levels. and mean ferritin levels. Patients at high risk should undergo periodic assessments of iron overload with MRI being the preferred method. The main strategies to prevent or minimize iron overload in multitransfused patients include EBT as opposed to conventional transfusions, and iron chelation that facilitates renal and biliary iron excretion. The main chelation agents include deferoxamine via intravenous or subcutaneous administration, and deferiprone or deferasirox via oral administration.[59]

HEMOLYSIS-RELATED HEPATOBILIARY DISORDERS
Cholelithiasis and Choledocholithiasis

Cholelithiasis is a common finding among patients with SCD, in particular those with homozygous (SS) disease. The lysis of sickled erythrocytes and breakdown of heme results in significant increases in unconjugated bilirubin. The bile becomes saturated with bilirubin, leading to precipitation and formation of pigment gallstones. Gallstones in SCD are usually multiple and small in size.

Gallstones are detected in 15% of patients with SCD younger than 10 years, 50% by the age of 22 years, and 58% by the age of 65 years.[60,61] Concomitant choledocholithiasis is found in 18%. Contrary to the general population in whom cholelithiasis remains asymptomatic in most affected individuals, patients with SCD are at higher risk of developing complications. These include biliary colic, cholecystitis, ascending cholangitis, and pancreatitis. In a cohort of 107 patients with SCD, 27 (25.2%) had cholelithiasis, 16 of whom required cholecystectomy for symptomatic disease.[62]

The clinical presentation of biliary complications is often similar to acute sickle hepatic crisis with right upper quadrant pain and fever. Ultrasonography can accurately detect the presence of gallstones, but is less sensitive for the diagnosis of cholecystitis or pancreatitis. MRCP is a more accurate imaging modality for the diagnosis of choledocholithiasis. Computed tomography (CT) is the modality of choice for the diagnosis of cholecystitis and pancreatitis. Radionuclide biliary imaging is rarely required, as CT imaging has become widely available.

In the general population, laparoscopic cholecystectomy (LC) is the treatment of choice for symptomatic cholelithiasis. LC is also the treatment of choice in patients with SCD, as it is associated with lower risk of complications and faster postoperative recovery compared with open cholecystectomy.[63] Although there is no consensus, prophylactic LC is advocated by several experts in SCD.[64–66] The main concern with this approach is that any surgical intervention in SCD is associated with increased risk of developing an acute sickle crisis perioperatively, although acute cholecystitis per se can also precipitate acute sickle crises. The rationale for prophylactic LC in asymptomatic patients incorporates the significant risk of developing complications throughout the lifetime, and the higher perioperative risk with emergency as opposed to elective procedures. In series of 191 LCs in children with SCD, 51 procedures were performed electively in asymptomatic patients, 110 electively for symptomatic disease, and 30 procedures were emergent.[65] Emergent LCs were associated with longer hospital stay compared with elective procedures. The complication rate was low and similar across the 3 groups. In another series of 103 LCs in patients with SCD, 52 were performed prophylactically and 51 for symptomatic cholelithiasis. The total complication rate (25.5% vs 5.0%), the incidence of acute sickle crises, and the length of hospital stay were significantly higher in the symptomatic group.[66] ERCP with clearance of the common bile duct before LC is required in patients with concomitant choledocholithiasis.[63,67,68] All patients require prophylactic antibiotics perioperatively because of the increased risk of infections. An important issue is the perioperative optimization in an effort to prevent acute sickle crises. This usually includes simple or exchange transfusions aiming for HbSS fraction less than 30% and hemoglobin level greater than 100 g/L.

MANAGEMENT OF LIVER DISEASE IN SICKLE CELL DISEASE

The management of sickle hepatopathy depends on the etiology, although very often multiple insults and pathophysiological mechanisms contribute to the development of liver disease (Table 2). As discussed in more detail in the previous sections, acute or chronic liver disease as a result of intrahepatic sickling of erythrocytes is managed with supportive measures, simple or EBT, with the latter being the treatment of choice in severe presentations. Whether hydroxyurea has a role in sickle hepatopathy remains unclear. Chronic hepatitis B is treated with nucleot(s)ide analogue, and hepatitis

Table 2	
Management of hepatobiliary disease in sickle cell disease	
Liver Pathology	**Treatment**
Acute sickle hepatic crisis	Supportive measures, occasionally EBT[1]
Hepatic sequestration	Supportive measures, EBT
Acute intrahepatic cholestasis	Supportive measures, aggressive EBT
Chronic cholestatic liver disease/sickle cholangiopathy	Regular EBT, UDCA,[2] ERCP[3] (dominant biliary strictures)
Hepatic hemosiderosis	Chelation therapy (HIC[4] >7 mg/g dry weight)
Chronic hepatitis B	Nucleot(s)ide analogues
Chronic hepatitis C	DAA[5] therapy (ribavirin-free or low-ribavirin regimens)
Cirrhosis/End-stage liver disease	Management of complications of cirrhosis Potential role of liver transplantation in highly selected cases
Cholelithiasis Choledocholithiasis	Cholecystectomy for symptomatic disease, potentially prophylactic cholecystectomy for asymptomatic disease ERCP

Abbreviations: DAA, direct-acting antiviral; EBT, exchange blood transfusion; ERCP, endoscopic retrograde cholangiopancreatography; HIC, hepatic iron content; UDCA, ursodeoxycholic acid.

C with DAA therapy according to genotype. EBT and chelation therapy can improve iron overload. LC is the treatment of choice for symptomatic cholelithiasis, although prophylactic LC in asymptomatic patients has an emerging role. ERCP is usually effective in the management of choledocholithiasis.

Of particular interest is the role of LT in patients with SCD presenting with ALF, acute-on-chronic liver failure, or end-stage chronic liver disease. The experience is very limited, with only 20 reported cases, 15 in adults and 5 in children.[16,27–30,32,69–72] The indication for LT in most cases was liver failure secondary to acute intrahepatic cholestasis. Two patients received LT for sclerosing cholangitis (likely sickle cholangiopathy).[28,72] Five patients had coexistent chronic hepatitis C, but HCV was not the primary indication for LT. The reported outcomes of LT have been variable, with initial reports demonstrating high risk of vascular (mainly thrombotic) and infectious complications. An important limitation in interpreting these results is the lack of long-term follow-up in most cases. The most comprehensive report included 6 adult patients, 5 of whom received LT for liver failure in the context of acute intrahepatic cholestasis and one for ALF secondary to autoimmune hepatitis.[28] Three patients had concomitant HCV. Only one patient died in the immediate post-LT period secondary to severe rejection. The 1-year survival rate was 83.3% and the actuarial 5-year survival 44.4%. The peri-transplant hematological management included EBT aiming for HbS less than 30% and hemoglobin 80 to 100 g/L for at least 6 months post-LT. The target after the first 6 months was HbS less than 40%. Two patients were able to stop EBT at 1 year, and continued with hydroxyurea. An interesting observation was that all patients had underlying cirrhosis on explant histology, with siderosis and features of sickle cell hepatopathy. These observations are encouraging, as LT seems to be feasible in patients with SCD, with acceptable outcomes. The eligibility of patients with SCD might be limited by SCD-related cardiac and pulmonary comorbidities. The perioperative hematological management is paramount in an effort to reduce complications. LT, unfortunately, does not alter the natural history of SCD, and these patients will continue to suffer the sequelae of SCD following LT.

SUMMARY

Liver involvement in SCD is not uncommon, and can develop as a result of multiple liver insults. Ischemic injury can be transient, as in acute sickle crisis, or can be more severe in the form of acute intrahepatic cholestasis. Other potential cofactors for liver disease in SCD include viral hepatitis and iron overload secondary to multiple blood transfusions. Liver disease can progress to cirrhosis in a proportion of patients. Clinical presentation can be variable, ranging from mild disease to ALF, acute-on-chronic liver failure or end-stage liver disease. Aggressive EBT has improved outcomes in SCD, and can even reverse liver failure. Iron overload is managed with chelation therapy, and viral hepatitis with potent antiviral therapy similar to non-SCD populations. Recent encouraging results with LT provide a potential option for patients who progress despite EBT, although more research in this direction is required.

REFERENCES

1. De Franceschi L, Cappellini MD, Olivieri O. Thrombosis and sickle cell disease. Semin Thromb Hemost 2011;37(3):226–36.
2. Ware RE, de Montalembert M, Tshilolo L, et al. Sickle cell disease. Lancet 2017; 390(10091):311–23.
3. Ahn H, Li CS, Wang W. Sickle cell hepatopathy: clinical presentation, treatment, and outcome in pediatric and adult patients. Pediatr Blood Cancer 2005;45(2): 184–90.
4. Zakaria N, Knisely A, Portmann B, et al. Acute sickle cell hepatopathy represents a potential contraindication for percutaneous liver biopsy. Blood 2003;101(1): 101–3.
5. Rosenblate HJ, Eisenstein R, Holmes AW. The liver in sickle cell anemia. A clinical-pathologic study. Arch Pathol 1970;90(3):235–45.
6. Omata M, Johnson CS, Tong M, et al. Pathological spectrum of liver diseases in sickle cell disease. Dig Dis Sci 1986;31(3):247–56.
7. Sarma PS. Hepatic sequestration of red cells in sickle cell anaemia. J Assoc Physicians India 1987;35(5):384–6.
8. Hatton CS, Bunch C, Weatherall DJ. Hepatic sequestration in sickle cell anaemia. Br Med J (Clin Res Ed) 1985;290(6470):744–5.
9. Gutteridge C, Newland AC, Sequeira J. Hepatic sequestration in sickle cell anemia. Br Med J (Clin Res Ed) 1985;290(6476):1214–5.
10. Singh NK, el-Mangoush M. Hepatic sequestration crisis presenting with severe intrahepatic cholestatic jaundice. J Assoc Physicians India 1996;44(4):283–4.
11. Norris WE. Acute hepatic sequestration in sickle cell disease. J Natl Med Assoc 2004;96(9):1235–9.
12. Lee ES, Chu PC. Reverse sequestration in a case of sickle crisis. Postgrad Med J 1996;72(850):487–8.
13. Jeng MR, Rieman MD, Naidu PE, et al. Resolution of chronic hepatic sequestration in a patient with homozygous sickle cell disease receiving hydroxyurea. J Pediatr Hematol Oncol 2003;25(3):257–60.
14. Vlachaki E, Andreadis P, Neokleous N, et al. Successful outcome of chronic intrahepatic cholestasis in an adult patient with sickle cell/beta (+) thalassemia. Case Rep Hematol 2014;2014:213631.
15. Costa DB, Miksad RA, Buff MS, et al. Case of fatal sickle cell intrahepatic cholestasis despite use of exchange transfusion in an African-American patient. J Natl Med Assoc 2006;98(7):1183–7.

16. Gilli SC, Boin IF, Sergio Leonardi L, et al. Liver transplantation in a patient with S(beta)o-thalassemia. Transplantation 2002;74(6):896–8.
17. Betrosian A, Balla M, Kafiri G, et al. Reversal of liver failure in sickle cell vaso-occlusive crisis. Am J Med Sci 1996;311(6):292–5.
18. Malik A, Merchant C, Rao M, et al. Rare but lethal hepatopathy-sickle cell intra-hepatic cholestasis and management strategies. Am J Case Rep 2015;16:840–3.
19. Im DD, Essien U, DePasse JW, et al. Acute on chronic liver failure in a patient with sickle cell anaemia (HbSS). BMJ Case Rep 2015;2015 [pii:bcr2015210166].
20. Chitturi S, George J, Ranjitkumar S, et al. Exchange transfusion for severe intra-hepatic cholestasis associated with sickle cell disease? J Clin Gastroenterol 2002;35(4):362–3.
21. O'Callaghan A, O'Brien SG, Ninkovic M, et al. Chronic intrahepatic cholestasis in sickle cell disease requiring exchange transfusion. Gut 1995;37(1):144–7.
22. Altintas E, Tiftik EN, Ucbilek E, et al. Sickle cell anemia connected with chronic intrahepatic cholestasis: a case report. Turk J Gastroenterol 2003;14(3):215–8.
23. Hosiriluck N, Rassameehiran S, Argueta E, et al. Reversal of liver function without exchange transfusion in sickle cell intrahepatic cholestasis. Proc (Bayl Univ Med Cent) 2014;27(4):361–3.
24. Papafragkakis H, Ona MA, Changela K, et al. Acute liver function decompensa-tion in a patient with sickle cell disease managed with exchange transfusion and endoscopic retrograde cholangiography. Therap Adv Gastroenterol 2014;7(5): 217–23.
25. Brunetta DM, Silva-Pinto AC, do Carmo Favarin de Macedo M, et al. Intrahepatic cholestasis in sickle cell disease: a case report. Anemia 2011;2011:975731.
26. Shao SH, Orringer EP. Sickle cell intrahepatic cholestasis: approach to a difficult problem. Am J Gastroenterol 1995;90(11):2048–50.
27. Blinder MA, Geng B, Lisker-Melman M, et al. Successful orthotopic liver trans-plantation in an adult patient with sickle cell disease and review of the literature. Hematol Rep 2013;5(1):1–4.
28. Baichi MM, Arifuddin RM, Mantry PS, et al. Liver transplantation in sickle cell ane-mia: a case of acute sickle cell intrahepatic cholestasis and a case of sclerosing cholangitis. Transplantation 2005;80(11):1630–2.
29. Ross AS, Graeme-Cook F, Cosimi AB, et al. Combined liver and kidney transplan-tation in a patient with sickle cell disease. Transplantation 2002;73(4):605–8.
30. Emre S, Kitibayashi K, Schwartz ME, et al. Liver transplantation in a patient with acute liver failure due to sickle cell intrahepatic cholestasis. Transplantation 2000; 69(4):675–6.
31. D'Ambrosio R, Maggioni M, Graziadei G. Chronic cholestasis in a patient with sickle-cell anemia: histological findings. Dig Liver Dis 2016;48(11):1402.
32. Hurtova M, Bachir D, Lee K, et al. Transplantation for liver failure in patients with sickle cell disease: challenging but feasible. Liver Transpl 2011;17(4):381–92.
33. D'Ambrosio R, Maggioni M, Donato MF, et al. Decompensated cirrhosis and sickle cell disease: case reports and review of the literature. Hemoglobin 2017; 41(2):131–3.
34. Cross TJ, Berry PA, Akbar N, et al. Sickle liver disease—an unusual presentation in a compound heterozygote for HbS and a novel beta-thalassemia mutation. Am J Hematol 2007;82(9):852–4.
35. Dosi R, Patell R, Jariwala P, et al. Cirrhosis: an unusual presentation of sickle cell disease. J Clin Diagn Res 2015;9(2):OD03–4.
36. Ahmed M, Dick M, Mieli-Vergani G, et al. Ischaemic cholangiopathy and sickle cell disease. Eur J Pediatr 2006;165(2):112–3.

37. Hillaire S, Gardin C, Attar A, et al. Cholangiopathy and intrahepatic stones in sickle cell disease: coincidence or ischemic cholangiopathy? Am J Gastroenterol 2000;95(1):300–1.

38. Middleton JP, Wolper JC. Hepatic biloma complicating sickle cell disease. A case report and a review of the literature. Gastroenterology 1984;86(4):743–4.

39. Attal HC, Gupta VL, Salkar HR. Budd-Chiari syndrome due to inferior vena cava obstruction in sickle cell trait. J Assoc Physicians India 1984;32(6):526–7.

40. Arnold KE, Char G, Serjeant GR. Portal vein thrombosis in a child with homozygous sickle-cell disease. West Indian Med J 1993;42(1):27–8.

41. Hassan M, Hasan S, Giday S, et al. Hepatitis C virus in sickle cell disease. J Natl Med Assoc 2003;95(10):939–42.

42. Hasan MF, Marsh F, Posner G, et al. Chronic hepatitis C in patients with sickle cell disease. Am J Gastroenterol 1996;91(6):1204–6.

43. Torres MC, Pereira LM, Ximenes RA, et al. Hepatitis C virus infection in a Brazilian population with sickle-cell anemia. Braz J Med Biol Res 2003;36(3):323–9.

44. DeVault KR, Friedman LS, Westerberg S, et al. Hepatitis C in sickle cell anemia. J Clin Gastroenterol 1994;18(3):206–9.

45. Maher MM, Mansour AH. Study of chronic hepatopathy in patients with sickle cell disease. Gastroenterology Res 2009;2(6):338–43.

46. Ocak S, Kaya H, Cetin M, et al. Seroprevalence of hepatitis B and hepatitis C in patients with thalassemia and sickle cell anemia in a long-term follow-up. Arch Med Res 2006;37(7):895–8.

47. Miller ST, Jensen D, Rao SP. Hepatitis B vaccine in sickle-cell anemia. J Pediatr 1988;113(5):955–6.

48. Drasar E, Fitzpatrick E, Gardner K, et al. Interim assessment of liver damage in patients with sickle cell disease using new non-invasive techniques. Br J Haematol 2017;176(4):643–50.

49. Moon J, Hyland RH, Zhang F, et al. Efficacy and safety of ledipasvir/sofosbuvir for the treatment of chronic hepatitis C in persons with sickle cell disease. Clin Infect Dis 2017;65(5):864–6.

50. Hezode C, Colombo M, Bourliere M, et al. Elbasvir/grazoprevir for patients with hepatitis C virus infection and inherited blood disorders: a phase III study. Hepatology 2017;66(3):736–45.

51. Hankins JS, Smeltzer MP, McCarville MB, et al. Patterns of liver iron accumulation in patients with sickle cell disease and thalassemia with iron overload. Eur J Haematol 2010;85(1):51–7.

52. Badawy SM, Liem RI, Rigsby CK, et al. Assessing cardiac and liver iron overload in chronically transfused patients with sickle cell disease. Br J Haematol 2016;175(4):705–13.

53. Wood JC, Enriquez C, Ghugre N, et al. MRI R2 and R2 mapping accurately estimates hepatic iron concentration in transfusion-dependent thalassemia and sickle cell disease patients. Blood 2005;106(4):1460–5.

54. Brown K, Subramony C, May W, et al. Hepatic iron overload in children with sickle cell anemia on chronic transfusion therapy. J Pediatr Hematol Oncol 2009;31(5):309–12.

55. Feld JJ, Kato GJ, Koh C, et al. Liver injury is associated with mortality in sickle cell disease. Aliment Pharmacol Ther 2015;42(7):912–21.

56. Aubart M, Ou P, Elie C, et al. Longitudinal MRI and ferritin monitoring of iron overload in chronically transfused and chelated children with sickle cell anemia and thalassemia major. J Pediatr Hematol Oncol 2016;38(7):497–502.

57. Yassin M, Soliman A, De Sanctis V, et al. Liver iron content (LIC) in adults with sickle cell disease (SCD): correlation with serum ferritin and liver enzymes concentrations in transfusion dependent (TD-SCD) and non-transfusion dependent (NT-SCD) patients. Mediterr J Hematol Infect Dis 2017;9(1):e2017037.

58. Demosthenous C, Rizos G, Vlachaki E, et al. Hemosiderosis causing liver cirrhosis in a patient with Hb S/beta thalassemia and no other known causes of hepatic disease. Hippokratia 2017;21(1):43–5.

59. Allali S, de Montalembert M, Brousse V, et al. Management of iron overload in hemoglobinopathies. Transfus Clin Biol 2017;24(3):223–6.

60. Al Talhi Y, Shirah BH, Altowairqi M, et al. Laparoscopic cholecystectomy for cholelithiasis in children with sickle cell disease. Clin J Gastroenterol 2017; 10(4):320–6.

61. Billa RF, Biwole MS, Juimo AG, et al. Gall stone disease in African patients with sickle cell anaemia: a preliminary report from Yaounde, Cameroon. Gut 1991; 32(5):539–41.

62. Martins RA, Soares RS, Vito FB, et al. Cholelithiasis and its complications in sickle cell disease in a university hospital. Rev Bras Hematol Hemoter 2017;39(1): 28–31.

63. Al-Salem AH, Issa H. Laparoscopic cholecystectomy in children with sickle cell anemia and the role of ERCP. Surg Laparosc Endosc Percutan Tech 2012; 22(2):139–42.

64. Curro G, Meo A, Ippolito D, et al. Asymptomatic cholelithiasis in children with sickle cell disease: early or delayed cholecystectomy? Ann Surg 2007;245(1): 126–9.

65. Goodwin EF, Partain PI, Lebensburger JD, et al. Elective cholecystectomy reduces morbidity of cholelithiasis in pediatric sickle cell disease. Pediatr Blood Cancer 2017;64(1):113–20.

66. Muroni M, Loi V, Lionnet F, et al. Prophylactic laparoscopic cholecystectomy in adult sickle cell disease patients with cholelithiasis: a prospective cohort study. Int J Surg 2015;22:62–6.

67. Amoako MO, Casella JF, Strouse JJ. High rates of recurrent biliary tract obstruction in children with sickle cell disease. Pediatr Blood Cancer 2013;60(4):650–2.

68. Issa H, Al-Salem AH. Role of ERCP in the era of laparoscopic cholecystectomy for the evaluation of choledocholithiasis in sickle cell anemia. World J Gastroenterol 2011;17(14):1844–7.

69. Kindscher JD, Laurin J, Delcore R, et al. Liver transplantation in a patient with sickle cell anemia. Transplantation 1995;60(7):762–4.

70. van den Hazel SJ, Metselaar HJ, Tilanus HW, et al. Successful liver transplantation in a patient with sickle-cell anaemia. Transpl Int 2003;16(6):434–6.

71. Mekeel KL, Langham MR Jr, Gonzalez-Peralta R, et al. Liver transplantation in children with sickle-cell disease. Liver Transpl 2007;13(4):505–8.

72. Gardner K, Suddle A, Kane P, et al. How we treat sickle hepatopathy and liver transplantation in adults. Blood 2014;123(15):2302–7.

Hepatic Complications of Inflammatory Bowel Disease

Mahmoud Mahfouz, MD[a], Paul Martin, MD, FRCP, FRCPI[b],*, Andres F. Carrion, MD[b]

KEYWORDS

- Inflammatory bowel disease • Hepatobiliary disorders
- Primary sclerosing cholangitis • Autoimmune hepatitis
- Nonalcoholic fatty liver disease • Drug-induced liver injury • Hepatitis B reactivation

KEY POINTS

- Various hepatobiliary disorders are associated with inflammatory bowel disease (IBD) and they may occur at any time throughout the course of the disease.
- Abnormal liver chemistries in patients with IBD should prompt investigation for disorders, such as primary sclerosing cholangitis, autoimmune hepatitis, nonalcoholic fatty liver disease, cholelithiasis, drug-induced liver injury, and others.
- Most agents used for treatment of IBD have the potential to cause drug-induced liver injury, which ranges from transient asymptomatic elevation of liver enzymes to severe hepatotoxicity and even acute liver failure.
- Reactivation of hepatitis B in patients with IBD treated with systemic corticosteroids or biologic agents is a major concern. Antiviral prophylaxis is recommended prior to therapy with biological agents.
- Less common but important hepatobiliary disorders encountered in patients with IBD include portal vein thrombosis, granulomatous hepatitis, IgG 4 cholangiopathy, and hepatic amyloidosis.

A variety of hepatobiliary disorders are associated with inflammatory bowel disease (IBD), with abnormal liver biochemical tests recognized in up to 30% of patients during long-term follow-up.[1,2] Although primary sclerosing cholangitis (PSC) is the stereotypical hepatobiliary disorder associated with IBD, other diseases, such as autoimmune hepatitis (AIH), drug-induced liver injury (DILI), nonalcoholic fatty liver disease (NAFLD), cholangiocarcinoma (CCA), and others, are encountered in this population (**Table 1**).

---

[a] Department of Internal Medicine, Mount Sinai Medical Center, 4300 Alton Road, Suite 301, Miami Beach, FL 33140, USA; [b] Division of Gastroenterology and Hepatology, University of Miami Miller School of Medicine, 1120 Northwest 14 Street #1115, Miami, FL 33136, USA
* Corresponding author.
E-mail address: pmartin2@med.miami.edu

Clin Liver Dis 23 (2019) 191–208
https://doi.org/10.1016/j.cld.2018.12.003
1089-3261/19/© 2018 Elsevier Inc. All rights reserved.

Table 1	
Hepatic complications of inflammatory bowel disease	
Common	PSC
	Small-duct PSC
	AIH
	PSC/AIH overlap syndrome
	Cholelithiasis
	NAFLD
	DILI
	Reactivation of HBV
Less common	Portal vein thrombosis
	Liver abscess
	Hepatic amyloidosis
	Primary biliary cholangitis
	Granulomatous hepatitis

PRIMARY SCLEROSING CHOLANGITIS

Approximately 75% of patients with PSC have concomitant IBD, most frequently ulcerative colitis (UC); however, only 5% of patients with IBD develop PSC.[3] Some studies suggest that recognition of IBD in PSC is higher when random colonic biopsies are routinely obtained (approximately 90%).[4] PSC is more prevalent in men and young to middle-aged adults.[5] Patients with PSC-IBD usually develop clinical symptoms earlier than those with PSC without IBD. The presence of IBD also may affect outcomes of PSC. For instance, the incidence of CCA, hepatocellular carcinoma, and colorectal cancer is higher and the need for liver transplantation (LT) and overall mortality are greater in patients with PSC and concomitant IBD compared with patients with PSC but without IBD.[6,7] Furthermore, PSC may continue to progress or even present initially after total colectomy is performed for treatment of IBD.[8]

In a study of 1500 patients with UC, 5% were noted to have elevated serum alkaline phosphatase levels (most of them asymptomatic), and 85% of these patients had evidence of PSC on endoscopic retrograde cholangiopancreatography.[9] Similarly, when magnetic resonance cholangiopancreatography (MRCP) was performed in more than 300 patients with IBD after the initial diagnosis of bowel disease, 8% had PSC-like lesions despite prior recognition of PSC in only 2.2%. IBD is commonly asymptomatic in patients with PSC, particularly early in the disease process; thus, colonoscopy with random biopsies is indicated in all newly diagnosed patients with PSC without prior diagnosis of IBD. Extensive UC and more clinically severe colitis were more common in patients with PSC compared with those without PSC.[10] Isolated colitis is the most common phenotype of Crohn disease (CD) in patients with PSC, followed by ileocolitis, and the disease activity is milder with lower frequency of stricturing and penetrating disease compared to patients with CD without PSC.[11]

Although the exact mechanisms responsible for the association between PSC and IBD remain undetermined, several hypotheses have been proposed.

Portal Bacteremia

Chronic or recurrent entry of bacteria into the portal circulation from the affected bowel may induce an inflammatory reaction in the hepatobiliary system.[12] The absence of features of portal phlebitis (a typical feature of portal bacteremia), however, in patients with PSC and IBD has raised important questions regarding this hypothesis.[13]

Chronic Viral Infections

Unrecognized infections, such as cytomegalovirus, have been proposed as a potential etiology for PSC. Biliary tract abnormalities with cholangiographic features similar to PSC have been reported in patients with AIDS and cytomegalovirus infection.[14] Cytomegalovirus replication and reactivation, however, have not been implicated in progression of PSC.[15]

Ischemic Cholangiopathy

Ischemic changes of the biliary tract result in cholangiopathy similar to PSC.[16] Histologic evidence of vascular injury, however, is typically absent in liver explants from patients with PSC undergoing LT.[17]

Alteration in the Intestinal Microbiota and Endotoxemia

Recent studies have suggested a role for the intestinal microbiota in the pathophysiology of PSC. Increased enterohepatic circulation of gut-derived microbial metabolites or derivatives, such as lipopolysaccharide, lipoteichoic acid, and peptidoglycan, may play a pathogenic role.[18] N-formyl L-methionine L-leucine L-tyrosine, a peptide produced by enteric flora, has been associated with histologic changes in murine models similar to those seen in PSC.[19] Injection of nonpathogenic *Escherichia coli* into the portal venous circulation produced portal vein fibrosis and pericholangitis in rabbits.[20] Furthermore, rats with experimentally induced small intestinal bacterial overgrowth developed similar inflammatory changes, which are believed related to bacterial byproducts.[21] Finally, reports suggesting that oral vancomycin could have a therapeutic role in PSC, particularly in pediatric populations, support a role for intestinal microbiota in the pathogenesis of PSC.[22,23]

Genetic Predisposition

A genetic component is strongly suspected in the pathogenesis of PSC, although specific patterns of inheritance have not been identified.[24] Multiple genetic factors of susceptibility have been reported, including HLA-DRB1*0301 (DR3), HLA-B8, and HLA-DRB3*0101 (DRw52a).[25] The association of PSC with other autoimmune disorders, including thyroiditis and type 1 diabetes mellitus, also suggests a role for genetic abnormalities of immunoregulation or bile transport in its pathophysiology. For instance, inhibition of leukocyte migration in the presence of biliary antigens could play a role in PSC.[26]

Large-duct PSC is male predominant and usually coexists with IBD. The associated bowel disease typically can have features of either UC or CD, with pancolitis and backwash ileitis in UC being common findings. Patients are usually younger and are at higher risk of colorectal cancer compared with those with IBD but without PSC.[10] In contrast, patients with PSC but without IBD typically are older and have better prognosis.[5] Patients who have IBD with abnormal liver chemistries but normal cholangiogram require a liver biopsy to exclude small-duct PSC (previously referred to as pericholangitis). Small-duct PSC possibly represents an early stage of the more typical large-duct PSC and is associated with significantly better long-term prognosis; however, up to 25% of patients with small-duct PSC at the time of diagnosis may progress to large-duct PSC (**Table 2**).[27,28]

Primary Sclerosing Cholangitis/Autoimmune Hepatitis Overlap Syndrome

The term, PSC/AIH overlap syndrome, has been used to describe liver disease that meets the diagnostic criteria for AIH (based on those of the International Autoimmune Hepatitis Group) but that also has cholangiographic (large-duct) or histologic

Table 2
Large-duct primary sclerosing cholangitis versus small-duct primary sclerosing cholangitis

	Large-duct Primary Sclerosing Cholangitis	Small-duct Primary Sclerosing Cholangitis
Association with IBD	Lower	Higher
Age at diagnosis	Older	Younger
Cholangiographic changes	Yes	No
Respond to steroids	No	No
Risk of CCA	High	Low
Need for LT	More	Less
Long-term prognosis	Worse	Better

(small-duct) features of PSC. This syndrome appears to be more common in children, and sometimes described as autoimmune sclerosing cholangitis.[29] Patients with PSC/AIH overlap may benefit from immunosuppressive therapy in conjunction with urso-deoxycholic acid (UDCA). Commonly used immunosuppressants, such as thiopurines and corticosteroids, for treatment of AIH also have therapeutic efficacy in IBD. Long-term prognosis of patients with PSC/AIH is in general better compared with that of patients with isolated PSC.[30]

Evolution from AIH to PSC after years of well-controlled AIH has been reported in both pediatric and adult populations. It has been suggested that the 2 diseases may be sequential in their occurrence, whereby patients have features of AIH and then after few years develop features of PSC. Thus, cholangiogram is recommended to rule out PSC in patients with AIH refractory to immunosuppressive therapy or in those with significant cholestasis.[31]

Diagnosis of Primary Sclerosing Cholangitis

PSC should always be suspected in patients with IBD and abnormal liver chemistries, particularly in those with a cholestatic pattern (elevated alkaline phosphatase). Most patients are asymptomatic at the time of diagnosis, with fatigue and pruritus the most common symptoms. A large study of approximately 1500 pediatric patients with IBD showed that 1.8% were diagnosed with liver disease (21 had PSC, 6 had PSC/AIH overlap syndrome, and 2 had AIH) within 30 days of their diagnosis of IBD. Most of these patients had elevated levels of both alanine aminotransferase (ALT) and γ-glutamyl transpeptidase (GGT) within 3 months of their IBD diagnosis, which led to the conclusion that elevated ALT and GGT levels could predict patients who are more likely to develop IBD-related liver disease.[32]

Cholangiogram is essential for establishing the diagnosis of PSC. Cholangiographic features include multifocal segmental strictures with saccular dilatations of the normal areas between them, which produce a classic beads-on-a-string appearance.[33] MRCP is the preferred initial diagnostic test for PSC because of its noninvasive nature and high sensitivity and specificity.[34] Liver biopsy is recommended only when other studies are inconclusive or small-duct PSC is suspected.[35]

Treatment

The management of PSC in the presence or absence of IBD is similar. No pharmacologic therapy has proved efficacy in slowing the progression of cholangiopathy and associated liver disease. Treatment goals are to control the symptoms and to manage the complications. UDCA, at a dose of 13 mg/kg/d to 23 mg/kg/d, has been shown to improve liver biochemical tests but has no beneficial effect on liver histology, requirements for LT, or overall mortality.[36] Higher doses of UDCA (28–30 mg/kg d) were studied in a large randomized controlled study, which had to be terminated prematurely because of excess mortality and increased need for LT in the group treated with UDCA compared with placebo; thus, high-dose UDCA is not recommended.[37] Currently, the role for low-dose UDCA in slowing the progression of PSC is controversial, and the American Association for the Study of Liver Diseases recommends against the use of this agent for treatment of PSC.[38] If liver function tests improve on low-dose ursodiol, however, it may be reasonable to continue it.[39] Treatment with UDCA in patients with PSC and UC does not decrease the risk of adenomas or colon cancer.[40] Current biological therapies used for treatment of IBD, including anti–tumor necrosis factor (TNF) agents (such as infliximab and adalimumab) and integrin antagonists (such as natalizumab and vedolizumab), have no proved therapeutic efficacy in PSC.[41] LT remains the only definitive therapy for PSC, with survival rates at 5 years and 10 years of 85% and 70%, respectively.[42] Severe hepatic dysfunction is a common and well-established indication for LT in patients with PSC (with or without IBD).[43] Other indications for LT in patients with PSC include intractable pruritus, recurrent bacterial cholangitis, and perihilar CCA eligible for neoadjuvant protocols.[38]

Patients with PSC are at high risk of developing CCA. Although intrahepatic CCA is generally regarded as a contraindication to LT due to poor outcomes, a subset of patients with perihilar CCA may be considered candidates for this intervention using the following criteria: radial dimension of mass lesion less than 3 cm, no intrahepatic or extrahepatic metastasis, no prior abdominal radiation therapy, without prior transperitoneal biopsy of the tumor, and after neoadjuvant therapy with external beam and bile duct luminal radiation therapy plus capecitabine for 2 weeks to 3 weeks prior to LT.[44,45]

Recurrent PSC in the liver graft has been reported in 20% to 25% of patients transplanted for complications of this disease.[46] Studies suggested that colectomy performed before LT may lower rates of recurrent PSC, which highlights an important—albeit unclear—role of the colon in the pathophysiology of PSC.[47] Prophylactic colectomy is not advocated, however, in LT recipients with IBD until long-term benefit of this intervention is confirmed.

IgG4-RELATED SCLEROSING CHOLANGITIS

The IgG4-related sclerosing form of cholangitis characterized by massive infiltration of IgG-4 positive plasma cells, severe interstitial fibrosis, and obliterative phlebitis. IgG4-related sclerosing cholangitis is considered a biliary manifestation of IgG4-related disease and is frequently associated with autoimmune pancreatitis. Although case reports have described cases of IgG4-related sclerosing cholangitis and IBD, a clear association is unproved. A diagnosis of IgG4-related sclerosing cholangitis can be challenging and is supported by cholangiographic features similar to those seen on PSC, serum IgG4 concentration greater than 135 mg/dL, and presence of IgG4-positive plasma cells on immunohistochemistry.[48,49] Cholangioscopy may be useful in differentiating IgG4-related sclerosing cholangitis from PSC.[50] The distinction between these 2 diseases is important because IgG4-related sclerosing cholangitis is highly responsive to corticosteroids and immunomodulators and seems less progressive than PSC.[51]

AUTOIMMUNE HEPATITIS

The prevalence of AIH in patients with IBD ranges from 0.6% to 1.6%.[52] Patients with IBD and AIH are more likely to fail therapy for IBD, relapse, and ultimately require proctocolectomy compared with those without AIH. Similarly, patients with IBD and AIH are also more likely to be refractory to AIH treatment, are at higher risk for progressing to cirrhosis, and exhibit higher mortality and need for LT compared with those without IBD.[53,54]

Infliximab-induced AIH has been reported in patients with IBD. In most cases, AIH resolved after discontinuation of infliximab and initiation of corticosteroids. In other cases, AIH resolved after substitution of infliximab for adalimumab, suggesting an absence of cross-reactivity between these agents.[52] Infliximab has been successfully used to treat difficult cases of AIH in some reports, resulting in normalization of liver chemistries, and some patients achieved full remission.[55]

CHOLANGIOCARCINOMA

PSC is a major risk factor for CCA. A recent case series of young adults (ages 18–25 years) with CCA indicated that a majority had long-standing IBD (mean 11 years) in addition to PSC, with a higher prevalence of CD (colitis) than UC.[56] Approximately half of patients were diagnosed with CCA within the first year after recognition of PSC, and the 10-year cumulative incidence reached 9%.[57] The distinction between a benign dominant stricture and CCA in PSC can be challenging. Use of serum CA 19-9 alone as a screening modality is not recommended because of its poor sensitivity and specificity (it can be spuriously high in patients with bacterial cholangitis or normal in patients with CCA who are negative for the Lewis antigen).[58]

MRI with gadolinium and MRCP sequences has overall high sensitivity and specificity, particularly when specific contrast-enhancement patterns are seen; however, these are less common in early stages of CCA. Currently, screening with MRI/MRCP plus CA 19-9 annually is often used in the absence of alternatives.[59] Endoscopic retrograde cholangiopancreatography with conventional brush cytology has almost (100%) specificity for the diagnosis of CCA but unfortunately has low sensitivity (18%-40%).[60] New modalities, such as fluorescence in situ hybridization, cholangioscopy, and intraductal ultrasonography, improve the diagnostic yield for CCA in PSC.[61]

Noncirrhotic patients with CCA can be evaluated for surgical resection. Patients with advanced hepatic fibrosis or nonremediable cholestasis with jaundice, however, are unlikely to benefit from surgical or chemotherapeutic options. As discussed previously, patients with early-stage perihilar CCA can be considered for LT under specific protocols.[62]

GALLSTONE DISEASE

The incidence of gallstones in patients with CD is significantly higher compared with controls without IBD. In contrast, no excess risk was reported for patients with UC.[63] Cholelithiasis in CD reflects malabsorption of bile acids with impaired enterohepatic circulation, depletion of bile salts, and formation of cholesterol gallstones. Prolonged fasting state or the use of total parenteral nutrition diminishes gallbladder emptying and predisposes to sludge or gallstone formation.[63]

Predictors of cholelithiasis include age (4-fold higher risk for patients older than 50 years of age compared with those younger than 30 years of age), location of CD at diagnosis (ileocecal or ileocolonic involvement is associated with 2-fold higher risk of developing gallstones compared with small bowel involvement alone), history of bowel resection, more extensive ileal resection (>30 cm), length of hospital stay, number of hospitalizations, frequency of IBD flares, and use of total parenteral nutrition.[63] Prevention strategies have been proposed to reduce the risk of gallstones formation in high-risk patients, such as those expected to undergo an extensive ileal resection. These interventions include stimulation of cholecystokinin secretion or reducing cholesterol crystallization with UDCA during the period of parenteral nutrition.[63] Cholecystectomy is indicated for symptomatic cholelithiasis. Prophylactic cholecystectomy during ileocolonic resection for CD, however, is not recommended.[64]

NONALCOHOLIC FATTY LIVER DISEASE

NAFLD is a clinical syndrome with a histologic spectrum ranging from steatosis without hepatocellular injury (nonalcoholic fatty liver) to nonalcoholic steatohepatitis (NASH), the latter characterized by hepatocyte ballooning and lobular inflammatory infiltrate. Sonographic evidence of hepatic steatosis has been reported in up to 35% of patients with IBD and severe steatosis in 12% of patients according to a recent study.[65] Steatosis was present in up to 50% of liver biopsies in patients with IBD and elevated liver chemistries.[66] Despite the high prevalence of NAFLD in patients with IBD, some reports suggest lower frequency of metabolic risk factors in this population compared with controls with NAFLD but without IBD. In a multivariate analysis, a history of small bowel surgeries (odds ratio [OR] 3.7), use of corticosteroids at the time of imaging (OR 3.7), hypertension (OR 3.5), and obesity (OR 2.1) were independent factors associated with NAFLD.[67] Small bowel resection results in increased plasma levels of free fatty acids and decreased carnitine levels, which may be associated with hepatic fat deposition.[68] In a recent cohort study of 380 IBD patients screened using transient elastography, the prevalence of NAFLD was 33% and significant hepatic fibrosis was present in 12.2%.[69] Similar to the non-IBD population, most patients with NAFLD and IBD have no symptoms attributable to liver disease; however, a correlation between the severity of colitis and hepatic steatosis has been reported in this population.[70] Elevated levels of serum TNF-α as well as messenger RNA expression in hepatocytes have been demonstrated in patients with NASH compared with healthy controls. Therefore, anti-TNF agents, such as infliximab, may lead to reduction of steatosis, improvement of insulin action, and potentially decreased fibrosis and may have a therapeutic role in NAFLD.[71]

DRUG-INDUCED LIVER INJURY

Hepatic side effects and DILI have been ascribed to several medications used for treatment of IBD.[72]

Aminosalicylates

Sulfasalazine has a low incidence of hepatotoxicity. Hypersensitivity to its sulfa component is rare but manifests as elevation of liver enzymes (most commonly aminotransferases and less often hyperbilirubinemia) with or without fever and lymphadenopathy.[73] Granulomatous hepatitis has also been reported in patients with IBD treated with sulfasalazine.[74] Sulfasalazine has been largely replaced in the United States for newer aminosalicylates, such as mesalamine, which does not seem to have an increased risk for hepatotoxicity. Liver injury from mesalamine is rare and can manifest as asymptomatic transient elevation of liver chemistries or mild hypersensitivity reaction within a few days or weeks.[75] Cholestatic or hepatocellular injury typically arises after 1 month to 6 months, and most cases with jaundice resolve rapidly on stopping this agent.[76]

Thiopurines

The thiopurines class of medications includes azathioprine (AZA) and 6-mercapto-purine (6-MP), which are immunomodulators typically prescribed for maintenance of remission and to reduce steroid use in IBD. Both agents are known to cause DILI, which is mediated by the hepatotoxic metabolite 6-methylmercaptopurine (6-MMP). Metabolism of thiopurines results in several metabolites. The active metabolite, 6-thioguanine (6-TG), is responsible for the immunomodulatory effects. Although high levels of 6-TG may result in liver injury, in particular the development of nodular regenerative hyperplasia (NRH), hepatotoxicity is primarily related to 6-MMP.[77,78]

Different patterns of liver injury associated with thiopurines have been identified: asymptomatic transient elevation of aminotransferases, cholestatic hepatitis, peliosis hepatis, sinusoidal obstruction syndrome (SOS), and NRH. Both hypersensitivity and cholestatic reactions are idiosyncratic reactions (dose independent) and typically occur within 3 months of exposure.[79] In contrast, NRH, peliosis hepatitis, fibrosis, and SOS are dose dependent and most often occur between 3 months and 3 years after initiation of treatment.[80] Cholestatic hepatitis associated with thiopurines may present with low or normal serum alkaline phosphatase levels at the onset of jaundice.[81]

Mild transient elevation of aminotransferases (<5 times the upper limit of normal) may occur shortly after starting therapy with thiopurines but usually resolves spontaneously without dose adjustments. Dose reduction by 50% is recommended for patients with higher elevations of aminotransferase levels ($\geq$5 times the upper limit of normal), and the dose can be increased once liver chemistries have normalized. Liver biopsy is recommended in cases in which liver chemistries do not improve after discontinuation of thiopurines.[80] Thiopurines should be discontinued immediately if severe cholestatic jaundice occurs, because progression to acute liver failure may occur.

Idiosyncratic reactions can occur in patients with IBD treated with thiopurines resulting in endothelial injury presenting with features of SOS, NRH, or peliosis hepatis. These reactions can occur at any time during treatment with thiopurines and may ultimately lead to noncirrhotic portal hypertension.[82,83] The mechanism of SOS induced by AZA involves the depletion of glutathione in sinusoidal endothelial cells. Cases of peliosis hepatis have been described in young patients treated with AZA after binge alcohol use. Acute SOS has been reported after 14 months of thiopurines initiation.[84,85]

The use of 6-TG as a therapeutic agent had been suggested as an alternative agent for 2 groups of patients with IBD: those with intolerance/allergy and those with inadequate respond due to suboptimal production of the active metabolite (6-TG). Elevation of liver chemistries, however, occurred in 26% of patients treated with 6-TG and idiopathic noncirrhotic portal hypertension was found in 76% of these patients. Histology demonstrated NRH concomitantly with small portal tract fibrosis in most cases, suggesting obliterative portal venopathy caused by this agent.[86] Splitting the normal daily dose of 6-TG may diminish the its hepatotoxicity.[87]

Although DILI associated with thiopurines can be severe, the prognosis is in general favorable except in patients with preexisting liver disease. Rarely, severe cholestatic injury may persist.

Methotrexate

Prolonged administration of methotrexate (MTX) is associated with risk of hepatotoxicity, primarily caused by its metabolite polyglutamate.[88] The histologic features of MTX-induced liver injury may resemble those seen in NASH or alcoholic steatohepatitis. Cirrhosis and end-stage liver disease secondary to MTX-induced liver injury is rare. In a large retrospective study of patients listed for LT over 24 years in the United States, only 0.07% had MTX-induced liver disease.[89] Risk factors for MTX-induced hepatotoxicity were identified, and these include alcohol use, obesity, diabetes mellitus, abnormal liver chemistries at baseline, and a cumulative dose greater than 1.5 g.[90]

Close monitoring of liver biochemical tests during treatment with MTX is recommended and liver biopsy is indicated in specific cases. The American College of Gastroenterology guidelines recommend consideration of a biopsy prior to initiation of MTX in patients with elevated liver chemistries at baseline, patients with 1 or more risk factors for hepatotoxicity, and patients with suspected chronic liver disease.[91] Noninvasive assessment of hepatic fibrosis with transient elastography has been proposed as an additional tool to liver chemistries to evaluate for liver fibrosis in patients with IBD on long-term therapy with MTX, particularly those with risk factors for NAFLD or excessive alcohol intake.[92] Supplementation with either folic acid or folinic acid is recommended because it may lower rates of abnormal liver biochemistries.

Biologic Agents

A variety of hepatic events have been linked to use of these medications. In a large cohort study, including 1753 patients with IBD treated with anti-TNF agents, 6% developed new-onset elevations of aminotransferases after initiation of therapy, but half of them had another cause identifiable, and it was difficult to determine a cause-and-effect association between liver damage and these drugs. The elevation occurred within the first 5 months of initiation the therapy, was transient, and resolved in most cases without the need to stop therapy or reduce the dose of the anti-TNF agent. Few patients developed cholestatic or an AIH-like pattern. A vast majority of patients received infliximab and cross-reactivity was not reported among different anti-TNF agents. Furthermore, switching to another biological agent in cases of infliximab-induced hepatotoxicity was shown to be safe.[93]

Reactivation of chronic hepatitis B (HBV) as a result of immunosuppression from biologic agents has been recognized.[94] Thus, guidelines recommend routine screenings for HBV before starting biologic agents. Prophylactic antiviral therapy to prevent reactivation of HBV is indicated.[95]

Liver enzymes should be monitored during use of biologics. In patients with ALT elevation (<3 times UNL), anti-TNF may be continued with close monitoring until resolution. Patients with persistent elevation (>3 times UNL) or jaundice should be considered for treatment with systemic corticosteroids. A liver biopsy may be helpful.[96,97]

Hepatosplenic T-cell lymphoma is a rare extranodal form of non-Hodgkin lymphoma that has been associated, although rarely, with long-term use of infliximab in combination with thiopurines.[98]

The risk of DILI from adalimumab seems significantly lower than that of infliximab based on data from a population-based study from Iceland: 0.4%, versus 0.83%, respectively.[99] Similarly, drug-induced AIH or cholestatic injury occurs less often with adalimumab compared with infliximab.[100–102]

Golimumab and certolizumab pegol can cause asymptomatic mild to moderate elevations of aminotransferases, usually not accompanied by jaundice.[103]

Vedolizumab is a humanized monoclonal antibody with specificity to the intestinal α4β7 integrin used for treatment of CD and UC.[104,105] Cholestatic liver injury due to vedolizumab has been recently reported.[106]

Natalizumab is a nonselective monoclonal antibody that prevents leukocyte trafficking. Similar to vedolizumab, clinically significant DILI related to this agent usually manifests as cholestatic injury but liver failure has not been reported.[107]

Elevation of liver chemistries is expected in approximately one-third of patients with IBD treated with tofacitinib; however, these are usually mild and transient and typically do not require dose adjustments (**Table 3**).[108]

VIRAL HEPATITIS

Older epidemiologic studies showed that patients with IBD had higher prevalence of HBV infection and hepatitis C virus (HCV) infection compared with the general population, which was mainly related to multiple surgical interventions and blood transfusions before the use of viral screening for blood donors.[109] More recent data, however, have identified similar HBV and HCV rates in patients with IBD compared with the general population.

HBV reactivation during treatment of IBD with specific agents is a concern because it may lead to acute liver failure.[110] High-dose corticosteroids, anti-TNF agents, and anti-integrins potentially lead to HBV reactivation. A multicenter retrospective Spanish study described HBV reactivation in 36% in patients with hepatitis B surface antigen (HBsAg) positivity, with high risk for progression into acute liver failure. The combination of 2 or more immunosuppressive drugs was an independent predictor of HBV reactivation.[111] HBV reactivation associated with anti-TNF agents may occur at any time within 2 years after starting treatment.[112] As a preventive measure, all IBD patients should be screened with HBsAg, hepatitis B surface antibody (anti-HBs), and hepatitis B core antibody (anti-HBc) at the time of diagnosis regardless if anti-TNF therapy is considered for treatment.[113,114]

Patients with IBD who are HBsAg positive should prophylactically initiate antiviral therapy with tenofovir or entecavir between 1 week and 3 weeks prior to anti-TNF

Table 3
Drug-induced liver injury manifestations in inflammatory bowel disease

Injury Type	Medication
Elevation of liver function tests	Aminosalicylates Thiopurines (AZT and 6-MP) MTX Anti-TNF
Cholestatic liver disease	Thiopurines (AZT and 6-MP) Anti-TNF
NAFLD	Corticosteroids
Hepatic fibrosis	MTX
Reactivation of HBV	Anti-TNF therapy Corticosteroids Anti-integrins
Venoocclusive disease	Thiopurines (AZT and 6-MP)
Granulomatous hepatitis	Sulfasalazine
Hepatosplenic T-cell lymphoma	Anti-TNF combined with immunosuppressive therapy

therapy. Antivirals should be continued for 6 months to 12 months after cessation of anti-TNF therapy.[115] Tenofovir or entecavir is preferred to lamivudine or other older nucleos(t)ide analogs for long-term antiviral prophylaxis due to higher barrier to resistance. Antiviral prophylaxis has been associated with an 87% relative risk reduction of reactivation and an 84% relative risk reduction of HBV-associated hepatitis flares.[113]

All HBV-seronegative patients should be vaccinated, and postvaccination immune response should be documented to ensure immunity (anti-HBs >10 mIU/mL). Vaccination ideally should be performed prior to initiation of immunosuppression, because it results in increased immunogenicity. Patients with IBD typically have lower response rates to vaccines and may not be protected completely against HBV.[116,117] An accelerated vaccination course with double vaccine doses at 0 months, 1 month, and 2 months has been suggested to improve HBV immunity.[118] Other studies, however, did not support this intervention, and the routine 3-dose regimen is recommended.[119]

PORTAL VEIN THROMBOSIS/HEPATIC VEIN THROMBOSIS

Patients with IBD are at high risk for thromboembolism, portal and systemic. IBD, in particular active disease, is associated with a procoagulant state due to elevated platelets count (reactive), increased factor V and factor VIII levels, and concomitantly low antithrombin III levels.[120,121] Even though portal vein thrombosis is a not a common complication in patients with IBD in the absence of chronic liver disease, its incidence is higher than the general population.[122] There are also reports of Budd-Chiari syndrome occurring in patients with IBD.[123]

LIVER ABSCESS

Hepatic abscess can be an initial manifestation of CD or can occur during the course of the disease, particularly in patients with fistulizing or fibrostenotic phenotypes. Direct extension of an intra-abdominal infection or portal bacteremia with secondary seeding of the liver is involved in the pathophysiology of hepatic abscess in IBD.[124] In contrast to the general population, patients with IBD are usually younger and usually present with multiple liver abscesses.[125]

HEPATIC AMYLOIDOSIS

Secondary amyloidosis can be identified in up to 1% of patients with IBD. Chronic intestinal inflammation contributes to amyloid deposition in the liver, resulting in asymptomatic hepatomegaly during initial stages of the disease. Hepatic amyloidosis occurs more commonly in men with colonic disease and is associated more frequently with CD than UC.[126] Treatment is based on decreasing the acute-phase reactant serum amyloid A by controlling intestinal inflammation. Treatment with colchicine or anti-TNF agents has shown some benefit.[127]

SUMMARY

Multiple hepatobiliary disorders are commonly recognized in patients with IBD. These disorders vary with regard to severity from mild asymptomatic elevations of liver chemistries due to DILI from agents used for treatment of IBD to complex diseases, such as PSC and CCA. Prompt identification of hepatic disorders in patients with IBD permits instituting specific interventions to ameliorate hepatic injury or to establish surveillance programs to recognize complications.

REFERENCES

1. Mendes FD, Levy C, Enders FB, et al. Abnormal hepatic biochemistries in patients with inflammatory bowel disease. Am J Gastroenterol 2007;102(2):344–50.
2. Gisbert JP, Luna M, Gonzalez-Lama Y, et al. Liver injury in inflammatory bowel disease: long-term follow-up study of 786 patients. Inflamm Bowel Dis 2007; 13(9):1106–14.
3. Broome U, Bergquist A. Primary sclerosing cholangitis, inflammatory bowel disease, and colon cancer. Semin Liver Dis 2006;26(1):31–41.
4. Rojas-Feria M, Castro M, Suarez E, et al. Hepatobiliary manifestations in inflammatory bowel disease: the gut, the drugs and the liver. World J Gastroenterol 2013;19(42):7327–40.
5. Wiesner RH, Grambsch PM, Dickson ER, et al. Primary sclerosing cholangitis: natural history, prognostic factors and survival analysis. Hepatology 1989; 10(4):430–6.
6. Ngu JH, Gearry RB, Wright AJ, et al. Inflammatory bowel disease is associated with poor outcomes of patients with primary sclerosing cholangitis. Clin Gastroenterol Hepatol 2011;9(12):1092–7 [quiz: e1135].
7. Martin P, Lindor KD. Heterogeneity of outcomes following liver transplantation for primary sclerosing cholangitis: age matters. Dig Dis Sci 2017;62(11):3210–1.
8. Cangemi JR, Wiesner RH, Beaver SJ, et al. Effect of proctocolectomy for chronic ulcerative colitis on the natural history of primary sclerosing cholangitis. Gastroenterology 1989;96(3):790–4.
9. Olsson R, Danielsson A, Jarnerot G, et al. Prevalence of primary sclerosing cholangitis in patients with ulcerative colitis. Gastroenterology 1991;100(5 Pt 1): 1319–23.
10. Lunder AK, Hov JR, Borthne A, et al. Prevalence of sclerosing cholangitis detected by magnetic resonance cholangiography in patients with long-term inflammatory bowel disease. Gastroenterology 2016;151(4):660–9.e4.
11. de Vries AB, Janse M, Blokzijl H, et al. Distinctive inflammatory bowel disease phenotype in primary sclerosing cholangitis. World J Gastroenterol 2015; 21(6):1956–71.
12. Brooke BN, Dykes PW, Walker FC. A study of liver disorder in ulcerative colitis. Postgrad Med J 1961;37(427):245–51.
13. Palmer KR, Duerden BI, Holdsworth CD. Bacteriological and endotoxin studies in cases of ulcerative colitis submitted to surgery. Gut 1980;21(10):851–4.
14. Cello JP. Acquired immunodeficiency syndrome cholangiopathy: spectrum of disease. Am J Med 1989;86(5):539–46.
15. Mehal WZ, Hattersley AT, Chapman RW, et al. A survey of cytomegalovirus (CMV) DNA in primary sclerosing cholangitis (PSC) liver tissues using a sensitive polymerase chain reaction (PCR) based assay. J Hepatol 1992;15(3):396–9.
16. Ludwig J, Kim CH, Wiesner RH, et al. Floxuridine-induced sclerosing cholangitis: an ischemic cholangiopathy? Hepatology 1989;9(2):215–8.
17. Ludwig J, LaRusso NF, Wiesner RH. The syndrome of primary sclerosing cholangitis. Prog Liver Dis 1990;9:555–66.
18. O'Mahony CA, Vierling JM. Etiopathogenesis of primary sclerosing cholangitis. Semin Liver Dis 2006;26(1):3–21.
19. Hobson CH, Butt TJ, Ferry DM, et al. Enterohepatic circulation of bacterial chemotactic peptide in rats with experimental colitis. Gastroenterology 1988; 94(4):1006–13.

20. Kono K, Ohnishi K, Omata M, et al. Experimental portal fibrosis produced by intraportal injection of killed nonpathogenic Escherichia coli in rabbits. Gastroenterology 1988;94(3):787–96.
21. Lichtman SN, Sartor RB, Keku J, et al. Hepatic inflammation in rats with experimental small intestinal bacterial overgrowth. Gastroenterology 1990;98(2): 414–23.
22. Davies YK, Cox KM, Abdullah BA, et al. Long-term treatment of primary sclerosing cholangitis in children with oral vancomycin: an immunomodulating antibiotic. J Pediatr Gastroenterol Nutr 2008;47(1):61–7.
23. Damman JL, Rodriguez EA, Ali AH, et al. Review article: the evidence that vancomycin is a therapeutic option for primary sclerosing cholangitis. Aliment Pharmacol Ther 2018;47(7):886–95.
24. Bergquist A, Montgomery SM, Bahmanyar S, et al. Increased risk of primary sclerosing cholangitis and ulcerative colitis in first-degree relatives of patients with primary sclerosing cholangitis. Clin Gastroenterol Hepatol 2008;6(8): 939–43.
25. Karlsen TH, Schrumpf E, Boberg KM. Genetic epidemiology of primary sclerosing cholangitis. World J Gastroenterol 2007;13(41):5421–31.
26. McFarlane IG, Wojcicka BM, Tsantoulas DC, et al. Leukocyte migration inhibition in response to biliary antigens in primary biliary cirrhosis, sclerosing cholangitis, and other chronic liver diseases. Gastroenterology 1979;76(6):1333–40.
27. Bjornsson E, Olsson R, Bergquist A, et al. The natural history of small-duct primary sclerosing cholangitis. Gastroenterology 2008;134(4):975–80.
28. Bjornsson E. Small-duct primary sclerosing cholangitis. Curr Gastroenterol Rep 2009;11(1):37–41.
29. Gregorio GV, Portmann B, Karani J, et al. Autoimmune hepatitis/sclerosing cholangitis overlap syndrome in childhood: a 16-year prospective study. Hepatology 2001;33(3):544–53.
30. Floreani A, Rizzotto ER, Ferrara F, et al. Clinical course and outcome of autoimmune hepatitis/primary sclerosing cholangitis overlap syndrome. Am J Gastroenterol 2005;100(7):1516–22.
31. Abdo AA, Bain VG, Kichian K, et al. Evolution of autoimmune hepatitis to primary sclerosing cholangitis: a sequential syndrome. Hepatology 2002;36(6):1393–9.
32. Goyal A, Hyams JS, Lerer T, et al. Liver enzyme elevations within 3 months of diagnosis of inflammatory bowel disease and likelihood of liver disease. J Pediatr Gastroenterol Nutr 2014;59(3):321–3.
33. Lee YM, Kaplan MM. Primary sclerosing cholangitis. N Engl J Med 1995; 332(14):924–33.
34. Dave M, Elmunzer BJ, Dwamena BA, et al. Primary sclerosing cholangitis: meta-analysis of diagnostic performance of MR cholangiopancreatography. Radiology 2010;256(2):387–96.
35. Jeffrey GP, Reed WD, Carrello S, et al. Histological and immunohistochemical study of the gall bladder lesion in primary sclerosing cholangitis. Gut 1991; 32(4):424–9.
36. Lindor KD. Ursodiol for primary sclerosing cholangitis. Mayo primary sclerosing cholangitis-ursodeoxycholic acid study group. N Engl J Med 1997;336(10): 691–5.
37. Lindor KD, Kowdley KV, Luketic VA, et al. High-dose ursodeoxycholic acid for the treatment of primary sclerosing cholangitis. Hepatology 2009;50(3):808–14.
38. Chapman R, Fevery J, Kalloo A, et al. Diagnosis and management of primary sclerosing cholangitis. Hepatology 2010;51(2):660–78.

39. Tabibian JH, Lindor KD. Ursodeoxycholic acid in primary sclerosing cholangitis: if withdrawal is bad, then administration is good (right?). Hepatology 2014;60(3): 785–8.
40. Ashraf I, Choudhary A, Arif M, et al. Ursodeoxycholic acid in patients with ulcerative colitis and primary sclerosing cholangitis for prevention of colon cancer: a meta-analysis. Indian J Gastroenterol 2012;31(2):69–74.
41. Tse CS, Loftus EV Jr, Raffals LE, et al. Effects of vedolizumab, adalimumab and infliximab on biliary inflammation in individuals with primary sclerosing cholangitis and inflammatory bowel disease. Aliment Pharmacol Ther 2018;48(2):190–5.
42. Graziadei IW, Wiesner RH, Marotta PJ, et al. Long-term results of patients undergoing liver transplantation for primary sclerosing cholangitis. Hepatology 1999; 30(5):1121–7.
43. Leidenius M, Höckerstedt K, Broomé U, et al. Hepatobiliary carcinoma in primary sclerosing cholangitis: a case control study. J Hepatol 2001;34(6):792–8.
44. Kaya M, de Groen PC, Angulo P, et al. Treatment of cholangiocarcinoma complicating primary sclerosing cholangitis: the Mayo Clinic experience. Am J Gastroenterol 2001;96(4):1164–9.
45. Carbone M, Neuberger J. Liver transplantation in PBC and PSC: indications and disease recurrence. Clin Res Hepatol Gastroenterol 2011;35(6–7):446–54.
46. Graziadei IW, Wiesner RH, Batts KP, et al. Recurrence of primary sclerosing cholangitis following liver transplantation. Hepatology 1999;29(4):1050–6.
47. Alabraba E, Nightingale P, Gunson B, et al. A re-evaluation of the risk factors for the recurrence of primary sclerosing cholangitis in liver allografts. Liver Transplant 2009;15(3):330–40.
48. Bjornsson E, Chari ST, Smyrk TC, et al. Immunoglobulin G4 associated cholangitis: description of an emerging clinical entity based on review of the literature. Hepatology 2007;45(6):1547–54.
49. Kalaitzakis E, Levy M, Kamisawa T, et al. Endoscopic retrograde cholangiography does not reliably distinguish IgG4-associated cholangitis from primary sclerosing cholangitis or cholangiocarcinoma. Clin Gastroenterol Hepatol 2011;9(9):800–3.e2.
50. Itoi T, Kamisawa T, Igarashi Y, et al. The role of peroral video cholangioscopy in patients with IgG4-related sclerosing cholangitis. J Gastroenterol 2013;48(4): 504–14.
51. Culver EL, Chapman RW. Systematic review: management options for primary sclerosing cholangitis and its variant forms - IgG4-associated cholangitis and overlap with autoimmune hepatitis. Aliment Pharmacol Ther 2011;33(12): 1273–91.
52. Dotson JL, Hyams JS, Markowitz J, et al. Extraintestinal manifestations of pediatric inflammatory bowel disease and their relation to disease type and severity. J Pediatr Gastroenterol Nutr 2010;51(2):140–5.
53. DeFilippis EM, Kumar S. Clinical presentation and outcomes of autoimmune hepatitis in inflammatory bowel disease. Dig Dis Sci 2015;60(10):2873–80.
54. Perdigoto R, Carpenter HA, Czaja AJ. Frequency and significance of chronic ulcerative colitis in severe corticosteroid-treated autoimmune hepatitis. J Hepatol 1992;14(2–3):325–31.
55. Weiler-Normann C, Schramm C, Quaas A, et al. Infliximab as a rescue treatment in difficult-to-treat autoimmune hepatitis. J Hepatol 2013;58(3):529–34.
56. Bjornsson E, Angulo P. Cholangiocarcinoma in young individuals with and without primary sclerosing cholangitis. Am J Gastroenterol 2007;102(8): 1677–82.

57. Burak K, Angulo P, Pasha TM, et al. Incidence and risk factors for cholangiocarcinoma in primary sclerosing cholangitis. Am J Gastroenterol 2004;99(3):523–6.
58. Steinberg W. The clinical utility of the CA 19-9 tumor-associated antigen. Am J Gastroenterol 1990;85(4):350–5.
59. Charatcharoenwitthaya P, Enders FB, Halling KC, et al. Utility of serum tumor markers, imaging, and biliary cytology for detecting cholangiocarcinoma in primary sclerosing cholangitis. Hepatology 2008;48(4):1106–17.
60. Boberg KM, Jebsen P, Clausen OP, et al. Diagnostic benefit of biliary brush cytology in cholangiocarcinoma in primary sclerosing cholangitis. J Hepatol 2006;45(4):568–74.
61. Tischendorf JJ, Kruger M, Trautwein C, et al. Cholangioscopic characterization of dominant bile duct stenoses in patients with primary sclerosing cholangitis. Endoscopy 2006;38(7):665–9.
62. Khan SA, Miras A, Pelling M, et al. Cholangiocarcinoma and its management. Gut 2007;56(12):1755–6.
63. Parente F, Pastore L, Bargiggia S, et al. Incidence and risk factors for gallstones in patients with inflammatory bowel disease: a large case-control study. Hepatology 2007;45(5):1267–74.
64. Chew SS, Ngo TQ, Douglas PR, et al. Cholecystectomy in patients with Crohn's ileitis. Dis colon rectum 2003;46(11):1484–8.
65. Bargiggia S, Maconi G, Elli M, et al. Sonographic prevalence of liver steatosis and biliary tract stones in patients with inflammatory bowel disease: study of 511 subjects at a single center. J Clin Gastroenterol 2003;36(5):417–20.
66. McGowan CE, Jones P, Long MD, et al. Changing shape of disease: nonalcoholic fatty liver disease in Crohn's disease-a case series and review of the literature. Inflamm Bowel Dis 2012;18(1):49–54.
67. Sourianarayanane A, Garg G, Smith TH, et al. Risk factors of non-alcoholic fatty liver disease in patients with inflammatory bowel disease. J Crohns Colitis 2013; 7(8):e279–85.
68. Allard JP. Other disease associations with non-alcoholic fatty liver disease (NAFLD). Best Pract Res Clin Gastroenterol 2002;16(5):783–95.
69. Saroli Palumbo C, Restellini S, Chao CY, et al. Screening for nonalcoholic fatty liver disease in inflammatory bowel diseases: a cohort study using transient elastography. Inflamm Bowel Dis 2019;25(1):124–33.
70. Riegler G, D'Inca R, Sturniolo GC, et al. Hepatobiliary alterations in patients with inflammatory bowel disease: a multicenter study. Caprilli & Gruppo Italiano Studio Colon-Retto. Scand J Gastroenterol 1998;33(1):93–8.
71. Barbuio R, Milanski M, Bertolo MB, et al. Infliximab reverses steatosis and improves insulin signal transduction in liver of rats fed a high-fat diet. J Endocrinol 2007;194(3):539–50.
72. Shamberg L, Vaziri H. Hepatotoxicity of inflammatory bowel disease medications. J Clin Gastroenterol 2018;52(8):674–84.
73. Candelli M, Nista EC, Pignataro G, et al. Steatohepatitis during methylprednisolone therapy for ulcerative colitis exacerbation. J Intern Med 2003;253(3): 391–2.
74. Callen JP, Soderstrom RM. Granulomatous hepatitis associated with salicylazosulfapyridine therapy. South Med J 1978;71(9):1159–60.
75. Khokhar OS, Lewis JH. Hepatotoxicity of agents used in the management of inflammatory bowel disease. Dig Dis 2010;28(3):508–18.
76. Sandborn WJ, Korzenik J, Lashner B, et al. Once-daily dosing of delayed-release oral mesalamine (400-mg tablet) is as effective as twice-daily dosing

for maintenance of remission of ulcerative colitis. Gastroenterology 2010;138(4): 1286–96, 1296.e1-3.

77. Cuffari C, Theoret Y, Latour S, et al. 6-Mercaptopurine metabolism in Crohn's disease: correlation with efficacy and toxicity. Gut 1996;39(3):401–6.

78. de Boer NK, Mulder CJ, van Bodegraven AA. Nodular regenerative hyperplasia and thiopurines: the case for level-dependent toxicity. Liver Transplant 2005; 11(10):1300–1.

79. Bastida G, Nos P, Aguas M, et al. Incidence, risk factors and clinical course of thiopurine-induced liver injury in patients with inflammatory bowel disease. Aliment Pharmacol Ther 2005;22(9):775–82.

80. Gisbert JP, Gonzalez-Lama Y, Mate J. Thiopurine-induced liver injury in patients with inflammatory bowel disease: a systematic review. Am J Gastroenterol 2007; 102(7):1518–27.

81. Zimmerman HJ. Hepatotoxicity: the adverse effects of drugs and other chemicals on the liver. Philadelphia: Lippincott Williams & Wilkins; 1999.

82. Russmann S, Zimmermann A, Krahenbuhl S, et al. Veno-occlusive disease, nodular regenerative hyperplasia and hepatocellular carcinoma after azathioprine treatment in a patient with ulcerative colitis. Eur J Gastroenterol Hepatol 2001;13(3):287–90.

83. Haboubi NY, Ali HH, Whitwell HL, et al. Role of endothelial cell injury in the spectrum of azathioprine-induced liver disease after renal transplant: light microscopy and ultrastructural observations. Am J Gastroenterol 1988;83(3):256–61.

84. DeLeve LD, Wang X, Kuhlenkamp JF, et al. Toxicity of azathioprine and monocrotaline in murine sinusoidal endothelial cells and hepatocytes: the role of glutathione and relevance to hepatic venoocclusive disease. Hepatology 1996;23(3):589–99.

85. Larrey D, Freneaux E, Berson A, et al. Peliosis hepatis induced by 6-thioguanine administration. Gut 1988;29(9):1265–9.

86. Dubinsky MC, Vasiliauskas EA, Singh H, et al. 6-thioguanine can cause serious liver injury in inflammatory bowel disease patients. Gastroenterology 2003; 125(2):298–303.

87. Pavlidis P, Ansari A, Duley J, et al. P342 Splitting the normal daily dose of thioguanine may be efficacious treatment for IBD and avoid hepatic toxicity. J Crohns Colitis 2014;8:S207.

88. Kremer JM, Galivan J, Streckfuss A, et al. Methotrexate metabolism analysis in blood and liver of rheumatoid arthritis patients. Association with hepatic folate deficiency and formation of polyglutamates. Arthritis Rheum 1986;29(7):832–5.

89. Dawwas MF, Aithal GP. End-stage methotrexate-related liver disease is rare and associated with features of the metabolic syndrome. Aliment Pharmacol Ther 2014;40(8):938–48.

90. Sandborn WJ. A review of immune modifier therapy for inflammatory bowel disease: azathioprine, 6-mercaptopurine, cyclosporine, and methotrexate. Am J Gastroenterol 1996;91(3):423–33.

91. Lichtenstein GR, Hanauer SB, Sandborn WJ. Management of Crohn's disease in adults. Am J Gastroenterol 2009;104(2):465–83 [quiz 464, 484].

92. Barbero-Villares A, Mendoza J, Trapero-Marugan M, et al. Evaluation of liver fibrosis by transient elastography in methotrexate treated patients. Med Clin (Barc) 2011;137(14):637–9.

93. Khanna R, Feagan BG. Safety of infliximab for the treatment of inflammatory bowel disease: current understanding of the potential for serious adverse events. Expert Opin Drug Saf 2015;14(6):987–97.

94. Esteve M, Saro C, Gonzalez-Huix F, et al. Chronic hepatitis B reactivation following infliximab therapy in Crohn's disease patients: need for primary prophylaxis. Gut 2004;53(9):1363–5.
95. Perrillo RP, Martin P, Lok AS. Preventing hepatitis B reactivation due to immunosuppressive drug treatments. JAMA 2015;313(16):1617–8.
96. Tobon GJ, Canas C, Jaller JJ, et al. Serious liver disease induced by infliximab. Clin Rheumatol 2007;26(4):578–81.
97. Menghini VV, Arora AS. Infliximab-associated reversible cholestatic liver disease. Mayo Clin Proc 2001;76(1):84–6.
98. Kotlyar DS, Osterman MT, Diamond RH, et al. A systematic review of factors that contribute to hepatosplenic T-cell lymphoma in patients with inflammatory bowel disease. Clin Gastroenterol Hepatol 2011;9(1):36–41.e1.
99. Bjornsson ES, Gunnarsson BI, Grondal G, et al. Risk of drug-induced liver injury from tumor necrosis factor antagonists. Clin Gastroenterol Hepatol 2015;13(3): 602–8.
100. Adar T, Mizrahi M, Pappo O, et al. Adalimumab-induced autoimmune hepatitis. J Clin Gastroenterol 2010;44(1):e20–2.
101. Grasland A, Sterpu R, Boussoukaya S, et al. Autoimmune hepatitis induced by adalimumab with successful switch to abatacept. Eur J Clin Pharmacol 2012; 68(5):895–8.
102. Kim E, Bressler B, Schaeffer DF, et al. Severe cholestasis due to adalimumab in a Crohn's disease patient. World J Hepatol 2013;5(10):592–5.
103. Shelton E, Chaudrey K, Sauk J, et al. New onset idiosyncratic liver enzyme elevations with biological therapy in inflammatory bowel disease. Aliment Pharmacol Ther 2015;41(10):972–9.
104. Feagan BG, Rutgeerts P, Sands BE, et al. Vedolizumab as induction and maintenance therapy for ulcerative colitis. N Engl J Med 2013;369(8):699–710.
105. Sandborn WJ, Feagan BG, Rutgeerts P, et al. Vedolizumab as induction and maintenance therapy for Crohn's disease. N Engl J Med 2013;369(8):711–21.
106. Stine JG, Wang J, Behm BW. Chronic cholestatic liver injury attributable to vedolizumab. J Clin Transl Hepatol 2016;4(3):277–80.
107. Bezabeh S, Flowers CM, Kortepeter C, et al. Clinically significant liver injury in patients treated with natalizumab. Aliment Pharmacol Ther 2010;31(9):1028–35.
108. van Vollenhoven RF, Fleischmann R, Cohen S, et al. Tofacitinib or adalimumab versus placebo in rheumatoid arthritis. N Engl J Med 2012;367(6):508–19.
109. Biancone L, Pavia M, Del Vecchio Blanco G, et al. Hepatitis B and C virus infection in Crohn's disease. Inflamm Bowel Dis 2001;7(4):287–94.
110. Zeitz J, Mullhaupt B, Fruehauf H, et al. Hepatic failure due to hepatitis B reactivation in a patient with ulcerative colitis treated with prednisone. Hepatology 2009;50(2):653–4.
111. Loras C, Gisbert JP, Minguez M, et al. Liver dysfunction related to hepatitis B and C in patients with inflammatory bowel disease treated with immunosuppressive therapy. Gut 2010;59(10):1340–6.
112. Tanaka E, Urata Y. Risk of hepatitis B reactivation in patients treated with tumor necrosis factor-alpha inhibitors. Hepatol Res 2012;42(4):333–9.
113. Reddy KR, Beavers KL, Hammond SP, et al. American Gastroenterological Association Institute guideline on the prevention and treatment of hepatitis B virus reactivation during immunosuppressive drug therapy. Gastroenterology 2015; 148(1):215–9 [quiz: e16-7].
114. Lok AS, McMahon BJ. Chronic hepatitis B: update 2009. Hepatology 2009; 50(3):661–2.

115. Gisbert JP, Chaparro M, Esteve M. Review article: prevention and management of hepatitis B and C infection in patients with inflammatory bowel disease. Aliment Pharmacol Ther 2011;33(6):619–33.

116. Rahier JF, Moutschen M, Van Gompel A, et al. Vaccinations in patients with immune-mediated inflammatory diseases. Rheumatology (Oxford) 2010; 49(10):1815–27.

117. Pratt PK Jr, David N, Weber HC, et al. Antibody response to hepatitis b virus vaccine is impaired in patients with inflammatory bowel disease on infliximab therapy. Inflamm Bowel Dis 2018;24(2):380–6.

118. Gisbert JP, Menchen L, Garcia-Sanchez V, et al. Comparison of the effectiveness of two protocols for vaccination (standard and double dosage) against hepatitis B virus in patients with inflammatory bowel disease. Aliment Pharmacol Ther 2012;35(12):1379–85.

119. Gisbert JP, Villagrasa JR, Rodriguez-Nogueiras A, et al. Efficacy of hepatitis B vaccination and revaccination and factors impacting on response in patients with inflammatory bowel disease. Am J Gastroenterol 2012;107(10):1460–6.

120. Danese S, Papa A, Saibeni S, et al. Inflammation and coagulation in inflammatory bowel disease: the clot thickens. Am J Gastroenterol 2007;102(1):174–86.

121. Solem CA, Loftus EV, Tremaine WJ, et al. Venous thromboembolism in inflammatory bowel disease. Am J Gastroenterol 2004;99(1):97–101.

122. Miehsler W, Reinisch W, Valic E, et al. Is inflammatory bowel disease an independent and disease specific risk factor for thromboembolism? Gut 2004; 53(4):542–8.

123. Vassiliadis T, Mpoumponaris A, Giouleme O, et al. Late onset ulcerative colitis complicating a patient with Budd-Chiari syndrome: a case report and review of the literature. Eur J Gastroenterol Hepatol 2009;21(1):109–13.

124. Rickes S, von Arnim U, Peitz U, et al. Sonographic diagnosis of a liver abscess caused by an enterohepatic fistula in a patient with Crohn's disease. Ultraschall Med 2006;27(6):572–6 [in German].

125. Mir-Madjlessi SH, McHenry MC, Farmer RG. Liver abscess in Crohn's disease. Report of four cases and review of the literature. Gastroenterology 1986;91(4): 987–93.

126. Greenstein AJ, Sachar DB, Panday AK, et al. Amyloidosis and inflammatory bowel disease. A 50-year experience with 25 patients. Medicine 1992;71(5): 261–70.

127. Serra I, Oller B, Manosa M, et al. Systemic amyloidosis in inflammatory bowel disease: retrospective study on its prevalence, clinical presentation, and outcome. J Crohns Colitis 2010;4(3):269–74.

The Liver in Circulatory Disturbances

Moira B. Hilscher, MD, Patrick S. Kamath, MD*

KEYWORDS

- Ischemia • Congenital heart disease • Cirrhosis • Fontan procedure
- Liver transplantation • Hepatopulmonary syndrome • Portopulmonary hypertension

KEY POINTS

- Liver disease may coexist with heart disease and may be secondary to cardiac dysfunction or of a distinct cause.
- Cardiac dysfunction may promote liver injury through congestion or ischemia.
- It is important to determine the cause of coexistent cardiac and liver disease when considering heart or liver transplantation.

Liver diseases frequently coexist with heart disease. The causes of coexistent heart and liver disease are categorized into four groups: (1) heart disease affecting the liver, (2) liver disease affecting the heart, (3) cardiac and hepatic manifestations of a common cause, and (4) coexistent heart and liver disease with distinct causes.[1] Discerning the cause of cardiac and liver dysfunction is important in the management of these conditions, particularly when considering surgical intervention or heart or liver transplantation.

HEART DISEASE AFFECTING THE LIVER

The liver is a highly vascular organ that receives approximately 25% of cardiac output and is prone to circulatory disturbances and vascular insult.[2] Cardiac dysfunction may promote liver injury through congestion or ischemia. In addition, patients with chronic heart disease may experience liver dysfunction related to therapies used for management of cardiac disease, such as drug toxicity and transfusion-related iron overload.

Overview of Hepatic Circulation

The liver receives approximately 25% of cardiac output from a dual blood supply of oxygenated blood from the hepatic artery and deoxygenated blood from the portal

---

Division of Gastroenterology and Hepatology, Mayo Clinic, 200 First Street Southwest, Rochester, MN 55905, USA
* Corresponding author.
E-mail address: Kamath.patrick@mayo.edu

Clin Liver Dis 23 (2019) 209–220
https://doi.org/10.1016/j.cld.2018.12.004
1089-3261/19/© 2018 Elsevier Inc. All rights reserved.

liver.theclinics.com

vein (**Fig. 1**). The liver is therefore susceptible to hemodynamic changes in the arterial and portal venous circulations. Well-oxygenated arterial blood comprises approximately 25% of total hepatic blood flow. The remaining 75% of hepatic blood flow consists of deoxygenated blood from the portal vein when post-prandial, but with higher oxygen concentrations during fasting.[3] The arterial and venous blood supplies converge in hepatic sinusoids, which are high-compliance, hepatic microvascular channels (**Fig. 2**).[4] A dynamic and compensatory communication exists between the hepatic arterial and portal venous blood supplies.[5] The hepatic artery autoregulates blood flow via the hepatic arterial buffer response, whereby decreased portal flow instigates compensatory upregulation of hepatic arterial flow and vice versa.[6] This regulatory response maintains hepatic oxygenation and preserves a constant level of total hepatic blood flow.[7,8] It is estimated that the hepatic arterial buffer response can compensate for a 25% to 60% decrease in portal blood flow.[6,9] However, portal venous flow is not autoregulated and is therefore dependent on mesenteric circulation and the gradient between portal and hepatic venous pressures. The liver circulation can also increase oxygen extraction from blood to maintain normal oxygen uptake.[10]

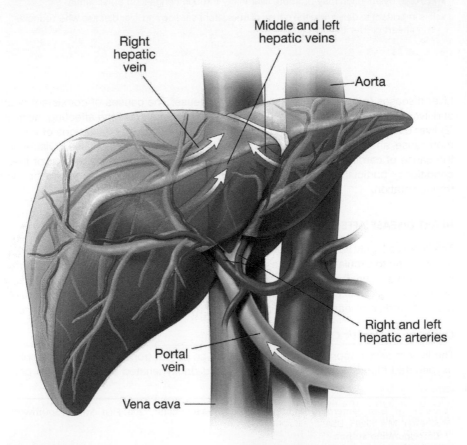

Fig. 1. Hepatic circulation. The liver receives a dual blood supply of oxygenated blood from the hepatic artery and deoxygenated blood from the portal vein and mesenteric circulation. (*Used with permission of* Mayo Foundation for Medical Education and Research, all rights reserved.)

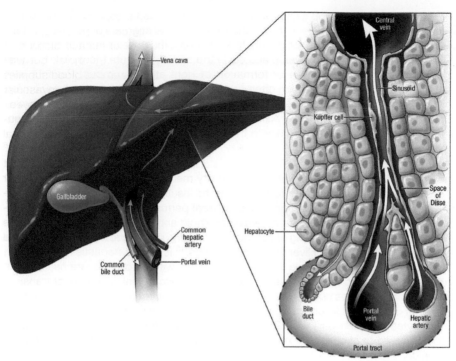

Fig. 2. Liver sinusoids. Arterial and venous blood converge in high-compliance sinusoids. (*Used with permission of* Mayo Foundation for Medical Education and Research, all rights reserved.)

Congestive Hepatopathy

Congestive hepatopathy can occur in the setting of right ventricular heart failure of several etiologies, including constrictive pericarditis, tricuspid regurgitation, cardiomyopathy, and cor pulmonale. Congestion predisposes to hepatic injury through three major pathogenic mechanisms: (1) insufficient hepatic blood flow, (2) decreased arterial oxygen saturation, and (3) increased hepatic venous pressures.[11] Elevated central venous pressure transmits to the hepatic veins and sinusoids and further decreases portal venous inflow.[11,12] Increased hepatic venous pressure also causes sinusoidal congestion, dilation of sinusoidal fenestrae, and exudation of protein and fluid into the space of Disse. Accumulation of exudate into the space of Disse impairs diffusion of oxygen and nutrients to hepatocytes.[11,13]

Many patients with chronic hepatic congestion remain asymptomatic from their liver disease and present with signs and symptoms of right-sided heart failure. Liver test abnormalities are often identified during routine laboratory evaluation. Characteristic laboratory abnormalities include mild elevations of serum aminotransferase levels to two to five times the upper limit of normal.[14] Unconjugated hyperbilirubinemia may be present although the total bilirubin level rarely exceeds 3 mg/dL. Hypoalbuminemia is present in 30% to 50% of patients and is generally mild. Patients may also develop prolongation of the prothrombin time, which is out of proportion to other markers of liver dysfunction. When symptomatic, patients may experience dull right upper quadrant pain secondary to stretching of the liver capsule or, uncommonly, jaundice. Physical examination may reveal pulsatile hepatomegaly. Up to 25% of patients with chronic congestion develop high protein ascites (ascitic total protein >2.5 g/dL) with a serum albumin-ascites gradient greater than 1.1.[2] Clinical stigmata of portal hypertension or portosystemic shunts are generally absent until the development of cirrhosis.[15]

Hepatic congestion may develop acutely in the setting of acute tricuspid regurgitation, right ventricular infarction, or formation of right atrial thrombus. Patients with acute onset of hepatic congestion often present with right upper quadrant discomfort and ascites. Physical examination may reveal hepatojugular reflux. Laboratory evaluation is often remarkable for hyperbilirubinemia with elevation in aspartate aminotransferase and alanine aminotransferase to five to eight times the upper limit of normal.

Ischemic Hepatitis

The hepatic circulation has robust compensatory mechanisms to maintain blood flow and oxygenation. However, the liver is prone to insult in the setting of severe, prolonged hypotension, which compromises visceral perfusion and predisposes to hypoxemia. Ischemic hepatitis is characterized by rapid and transient increases in serum aminotransferases in the setting of cardiac, circulatory, or respiratory failure and in the absence of other causes of liver test abnormalities.[16] Ischemic hepatitis may occur in the setting of acute cardiogenic shock or in patients with chronic severe heart failure and a drop in cardiac output caused by arrhythmia, myocardial infarction, or transient hypotension.[15] Studies suggest that most patients diagnosed with ischemic hepatitis have right-sided heart failure, suggesting that chronic passive congestion predisposes hepatocytes to ischemic injury.[17] Reduction in flow of well-oxygenated hepatic arterial blood can lead to centrilobular necrosis of zone 3, which is most susceptible to hypoxic injury.

Ischemic hepatitis is frequently diagnosed with the detection of elevated liver tests following hypotension or a cardiac event. Patients may present with symptoms of acute hepatitis including nausea, anorexia, malaise, and right upper quadrant pain. Characteristic laboratory abnormalities include a dramatic and rapid elevation in serum aminotransferase levels to 25 to 250 times the upper limit of normal within 24 to 48 hours of an inciting event.[18] Profound elevations in serum lactate dehydrogenase often occur early and to a greater extent than aminotransferase elevation. As a result, an alanine aminotransferase/lactate dehydrogenase ratio less than 1.5 is helpful in distinguishing ischemic hepatitis from viral hepatitis and drug-induced liver injury.[2,19] In the absence of ongoing hemodynamic insult, serum aspartate aminotransferase and alanine aminotransferase levels typically decrease by 50% within 72 hours and normalize within 7 to 10 days. Serum bilirubin levels often increase later and have more prolonged recovery.[2]

Management of ischemic hepatitis relies on stabilization of cardiac function and hemodynamics to optimize end-organ perfusion and oxygenation. Inotropic or circulatory support is sometimes needed. Although ischemic hepatitis is usually a self-limiting event, the prognosis remains poor and is mainly related to the severity of the underlying systemic disease. Acute liver failure secondary to ischemic hepatitis can rarely occur and is more often reported in patients with chronic congestive heart failure or underlying cirrhosis.[20]

Chronic Hepatic Congestion Secondary to Fontan Procedure

The Fontan procedure is considered the definitive palliation for patients with single-ventricle physiology.[21] The procedure results in an anastomosis between the vena cava or right atrium and the pulmonary arteries, whereby systemic venous blood is returned to the lungs without using a pumping chamber (**Fig. 3**).[21,22] Several of the physiologic derangements inherent to the Fontan circulation compromise the liver,

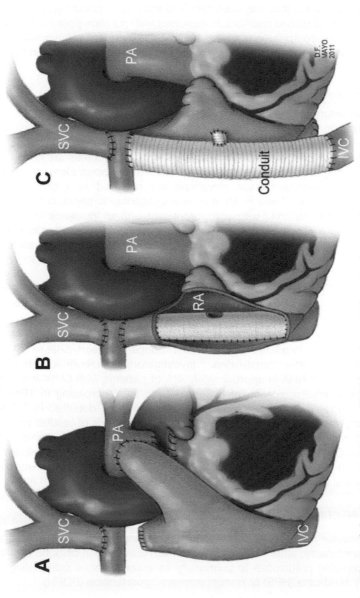

Fig. 3. Anatomic variants of the Fontan circulation. (A) This depicts a bidirectional cavopulmonary shunt. In this variant, the superior vena cava is ligated to the right pulmonary artery, and the inferior vena cava is anastomosed to the pulmonary artery to supply blood to the lungs. (B) Fontan with an intra-atrial conduit, which channels blood from the inferior vena cava to the pulmonary artery through the right atrium. (C) An extracardiac Fontan uses a conduit from the inferior vena cava to the right pulmonary artery with anastomosis of the superior vena cava to the pulmonary artery. IVC, inferior vena cava; PA, pulmonary artery; RA, right atrium; SVC, superior vena cava. (*Used with permission of Mayo Foundation for Medical Education and Research, all rights reserved.*)

including hypoxemia in the setting of chronic low cardiac output state, chronic eleva-tion of central venous pressure, and increased mesenteric vascular resistance. The physiologic consequences of the operation place individuals with a Fontan circulation at risk for long-term complications related to passive venous congestion of the liver.[23,24] Chronic vascular shear-stress and injury in the setting of Fontan physiology instigate fibrogenic pathways that may culminate in cirrhosis and portal hypertension. The risk of hepatic complications and fibrosis increases with duration post-Fontan; in-creases in risk of hepatic complications have been noted 10 years following creation of the Fontan circulation.[25] Hepatocellular carcinoma is a feared late complication of the Fontan procedure,[26–29] which may occur even in the absence of cirrhosis.

Drug-Induced Liver Injury

Patients with heart failure are susceptible to other forms of liver injury, including hep-atotoxicity related to drug use. Amiodarone is an antiarrhythmic drug used in manage-ment of life-threatening recurrent ventricular arrhythmias that has a high incidence of side effects, including hepatotoxicity. Amiodarone and its metabolites are lipophilic and thus readily accumulate in the liver and other tissues, including skin, lung, and fat.[30] Asymptomatic aminotransferase elevations are reported in approximately 25% of patients taking amiodarone.[31] More severe symptomatic hepatitis and fatal hepatotoxicity have been reported with amiodarone use with an incidence less than 3%.[31,32] As a result, guidelines caution use of amiodarone in patients with advanced liver disease or cirrhosis.[30] Liver tests should be monitored at 6-month intervals and amiodarone discontinued if there is concern for amiodarone hepatotoxicity.

Liver Disease Secondary to Transfusion

Anemia is common among patients with heart failure and is an independent risk factor for adverse outcomes.[33] Thus, transfusions are commonly recommended to support a hemoglobin level greater than 7 to 8 g/dL in patients with congestive heart failure or coronary artery disease.[34] In addition, patients with congenital heart disease (CHD) frequently receive perioperative transfusions.[35] Investigators have reported detection of hepatitis C virus (HCV) RNA in approximately 4% of patients with CHD who had heart surgery before implementation of high-sensitivity HCV screening in 1992.[36] HCV antibodies suggestive of prior exposure or infection were detected in 8% of this patient cohort, and in 5% in another cohort.[36,37] Performance of cardiac opera-tions before 1992 has been directly related to risk of HCV infection in patients with CHD. Patients with CHD who had cardiac surgery before initiation of routine hepatitis C screening have a five-fold increased prevalence of HCV infection compared with the age-matched general population.[36,38,39]

LIVER DISEASE AFFECTING THE HEART

Advanced liver disease is associated with changes in systemic vascular resistance and a resting hyperdynamic state.[40] These changes can culminate in cirrhotic cardio-myopathy and can also predispose to pulmonary vascular changes culminating in hepatopulmonary syndrome (HPS) or portopulmonary hypertension (POPH).

Hepatopulmonary Syndrome

HPS is a clinical syndrome characterized by pulmonary vascular dilation and abnormal arterial oxygenation in the setting of liver disease.[41] HPS is diagnosed in patients with a triad of liver disease, pulmonary vascular dilation, and oxygenation defect as demonstrated by a partial pressure of oxygen less than 80 mm Hg or an alveolar-arterial oxygen gradient greater than or equal to 15 mm Hg while breathing ambient air. Pulmonary vascular dilation is demonstrated by contrast-enhanced echocardiography or lung radionuclide perfusion scanning. The exact cause of HPS is unclear but is thought to be caused by impaired pulmonary vascular reactivity, vascular remodeling, and decreased clearance of pulmonary vasodilators from the circulation by the liver.[42] The prevalence of HPS reported in transplant centers ranges from 5% to 32%.[43] The severity of HPS is categorized according to the alveolar-arterial oxygen gradient and partial pressure of oxygen (**Table 1**) and is an important predictor of survival and risk of liver transplantation.[44] Patients with hypoxemia may require long-term supplemental oxygen therapy. Liver transplantation is currently the only effective therapy for HPS.[45] Studies report complete or near complete resolution of HPS within the first 6 to 12 months after liver transplantation.[46–50]

Portopulmonary Hypertension

POPH is defined as pulmonary arterial hypertension in the setting of portal hypertension without an alternate cause of pulmonary hypertension. It is diagnosed if right heart catheterization shows mean pulmonary artery pressure greater than 25 mm Hg at rest and pulmonary capillary wedge pressure less than 15 mm Hg in patients with pulmonary hypertension.[51] The prevalence of POPH is estimated as 5% in patients evaluated for liver transplantation.[52–54] Patients with POPH are treated with pulmonary vasomotor pharmacologic therapies, which have vasodilatory, antiplatelet, and antiproliferative effects.[55] Post-transplant mortality is higher in patients with POPH, particularly those with mean pulmonary arterial pressures greater than or equal to 35 mm Hg.[48,56]

DISEASES THAT AFFECT THE LIVER AND THE HEART

The liver and heart may be conjointly impacted by an underlying pathogenic, systemic process. A series of 32 patients who underwent both endomyocardial and liver biopsies identified hemochromatosis, chronic alcoholism, and amyloidosis as the most common causes of coexistent heart and liver disease.[1] Other more rare causes of concurrent heart and liver disease include sepsis,[57] glycogen storage diseases, sarcoidosis, AIDS,[58] and acetaminophen toxicity.[59]

Chronic Alcohol Use Disorder

Alcohol-associated liver disease is among the leading causes of chronic liver disease worldwide. Alcohol use can also accelerate fibrogenesis in other forms of liver disease, such as viral hepatitis or hemochromatosis.[60] Alcoholic cardiomyopathy is a consequence of chronic heavy alcohol use, which is characterized by dilation of the left ventricle (LV), normal or reduced LV wall thickness, and increased LV mass.[61] A

Table 1		
Classification of severity of hepatopulmonary syndrome		
Stage	**Alveolar-Arterial Oxygen Gradient**	**Arterial Oxygen Tension**
Mild	$\geq$15 mm Hg	$\geq$80 mm Hg
Moderate	$\geq$15 mm Hg	$\geq$60 and <80 mm Hg
Severe	>15 mm Hg	<60 and $\geq$50 mm Hg
Very severe	$\geq$15 mm Hg	<50 (<300 on 100% O_2)

diagnosis of alcoholic cardiomyopathy is suspected in patients with signs and symptoms of heart failure and a history of chronic, heavy alcohol use. It may be difficult to distinguish alcoholic cardiomyopathy from cirrhotic cardiomyopathy, which is defined as chronic cardiac dysfunction characterized by blunted contractile responses and/or diastolic dysfunction and electrophysiologic abnormalities in patients with cirrhosis and no other known cardiac disease.[62] Management of alcoholic cardiomyopathy and alcohol-associated liver disease consists of complete abstinence from alcohol and correction of nutritional deficiencies. Heart failure with low ejection fraction may require pharmacotherapy, such as β-blockers, diuretics, digoxin, and angiotensin-converting enzyme inhibitors.

Amyloidosis

Amyloidosis is a disorder characterized by tissue deposition of low-molecular-weight subunits of serum proteins. Although amyloid commonly presents with symptoms secondary to infiltration of the kidney, heart, and peripheral nervous system, hepatic infiltration with amyloid deposits has been found in approximately 70% of patients with amyloidosis.[63,64] Amyloid deposits have been observed within the hepatic parenchyma, stroma, and vasculature.[65] Most patients with hepatic involvement of amyloidosis present with hepatomegaly and elevated alkaline phosphatase.[66] Cardiac involvement with amyloidosis can present with systolic or diastolic heart failure, conduction defects, or myocardial infarction if coronary arteries are involved.[67] Heart failure with preserved ejection fraction is a common presentation of amyloid cardiomyopathy. A series of 32 patients with endomyocardial and liver biopsies included five patients with amyloidosis. All five patients had diastolic dysfunction, but only one patient had hepatic involvement with amyloid. Hepatic dysfunction in three patients was caused by congestion as opposed to primary involvement with amyloid, whereas one patient had heart disease secondary to senile amyloidosis and liver disease caused by granulomatous hepatitis.[1] This series suggests that liver disease in the setting of amyloid with cardiac involvement is often multifactorial.

Hemochromatosis

Hemochromatosis is characterized by increased intestinal iron absorption, which leads to excess accumulation of iron. Iron deposition within the liver can lead to fibrosis and cirrhosis. Within the heart, excess iron initially accumulates in the epicardium and progresses to involve the myocardium and endocardium.[68] The cardiac manifestations of hemochromatosis include diastolic dysfunction that progresses to LV systolic dysfunction with dilated cardiomyopathy. Deposition of iron within the conduction system can result in cardiac arrhythmias necessitating pacemaker placement.

HEART AND LIVER DISEASE WITH INDEPENDENT CAUSES

A series of 32 patients who underwent endomyocardial and liver biopsies revealed that 50% had coexistent heart and liver diseases with distinct causes. One-half of these patients had hepatitis of varying etiologies, including viral, drug-induced, and granulomatous hepatitis. Cardiac biopsies among these patients revealed idiopathic dilated cardiomyopathy, restrictive cardiomyopathy, and myocarditis.[1]

TRANSPLANTATION IN PATIENTS WITH HEART AND LIVER DISEASE

Among patients with liver or cardiac dysfunction, evaluation for transplantation requires assessment of the functional capacity of other organ systems to estimate likelihood of postoperative dysfunction of nontransplanted organs and to determine need for combined transplantation. This is particularly true among Fontan patients with cardiac and hepatic dysfunction. Combined heart-liver transplant has been performed in patients with CHD and systemic amyloidosis.

REFERENCES

1. Ocel JJ, Edwards WD, Tazelaar HD, et al. Heart and liver disease in 32 patients undergoing biopsy of both organs, with implications for heart or liver transplantation. Mayo Clin Proc 2004;79(4):492–501.
2. Ford RM, Book W, Spivey JR. Liver disease related to the heart. Transplant Rev (Orlando) 2015;29(1):33–7.
3. Lautt WW. Hepatic circulation: physiology and pathophysiology. San Rafael (CA): Morgan and Claypool publishers; 2009.
4. Greuter T, Shah VH. Hepatic sinusoids in liver injury, inflammation, and fibrosis: new pathophysiological insights. J Gastroenterol 2016;51(6):511–9.
5. Feldman M, Friedman LS, Brandt LJ. Sleisenger and Fordtran's gastrointestinal and liver disease E-book: pathophysiology, diagnosis, management. Philadelphia: Elsevier Health Sciences; 2015.
6. Lautt WW. Mechanism and role of intrinsic regulation of hepatic arterial blood flow: hepatic arterial buffer response. Am J Physiol 1985;249(5 Pt 1):G549–56.
7. Lautt WW. The hepatic artery: subservient to hepatic metabolism or guardian of normal hepatic clearance rates of humoral substances. Gen Pharmacol 1977; 8(2):73–8.
8. Eipel C, Abshagen K, Vollmar B. Regulation of hepatic blood flow: the hepatic arterial buffer response revisited. World J Gastroenterol 2010;16(48):6046–57.
9. Lautt WW. Relationship between hepatic blood flow and overall metabolism: the hepatic arterial buffer response. Fed Proc 1983;42(6):1662–6.
10. Bacon B, Joshi S, Granger D. Ischemia, congestive failure, Budd-Chiari syndrome, and veno-occlusive disease. In: Kaplowitz N, editor. Liver and biliary diseases. Baltimore (MD): Williams and Wilkins; 1992. p. 421–31.
11. Giallourakis CC, Rosenberg PM, Friedman LS. The liver in heart failure. Clin Liver Dis 2002;6(4):947–67, viii-ix.
12. Asrani SK, Asrani NS, Freese DK, et al. Congenital heart disease and the liver. Hepatology 2012;56(3):1160–9.
13. Safran AP, Schaffner F. Chronic passive congestion of the liver in man. Electron microscopic study of cell atrophy and intralobular fibrosis. Am J Pathol 1967; 50(3):447–63.
14. Weisberg IS, Jacobson IM. Cardiovascular diseases and the liver. Clin Liver Dis 2011;15(1):1–20.
15. Naschitz JE, Slobodin G, Lewis RJ, et al. Heart diseases affecting the liver and liver diseases affecting the heart. Am Heart J 2000;140(1):111–20.
16. Taylor RM, Tujios S, Jinjuvadia K, et al. Short and long-term outcomes in patients with acute liver failure due to ischemic hepatitis. Dig Dis Sci 2012;57(3):777–85.
17. Seeto RK, Fenn B, Rockey DC. Ischemic hepatitis: clinical presentation and pathogenesis. Am J Med 2000;109(2):109–13.
18. Lightsey JM, Rockey DC. Current concepts in ischemic hepatitis. Curr Opin Gastroenterol 2017;33(3):158–63.
19. Cassidy WM, Reynolds TB. Serum lactic dehydrogenase in the differential diagnosis of acute hepatocellular injury. J Clin Gastroenterol 1994;19(2):118–21.

20. Nouel O, Henrion J, Bernuau J, et al. Fulminant hepatic failure due to transient circulatory failure in patients with chronic heart disease. Dig Dis Sci 1980; 25(1):49–52.

21. Driscoll DJ. Long-term results of the Fontan operation. Pediatr Cardiol 2007;28(6): 438–42.

22. Gewillig M, Goldberg DJ. Failure of the Fontan circulation. Heart Fail Clin 2014; 10(1):105–16.

23. Burkhart HM, Dearani JA, Mair DD, et al. The modified Fontan procedure: early and late results in 132 adult patients. J Thorac Cardiovasc Surg 2003;125(6): 1252–9.

24. Khairy P, Fernandes SM, Mayer JE Jr, et al. Long-term survival, modes of death, and predictors of mortality in patients with Fontan surgery. Circulation 2008; 117(1):85–92.

25. Baek JS, Bae EJ, Ko JS, et al. Late hepatic complications after Fontan operation: non-invasive markers of hepatic fibrosis and risk factors. Heart 2010;96(21): 1750–5.

26. Saliba T, Dorkhom S, O'Reilly EM, et al. Hepatocellular carcinoma in two patients with cardiac cirrhosis. Eur J Gastroenterol Hepatol 2010;22(7):889–91.

27. Asrani SK, Warnes CA, Kamath PS. Hepatocellular carcinoma after the Fontan procedure. N Engl J Med 2013;368(18):1756–7.

28. Elder RW, Parekh S, Book WM. More on hepatocellular carcinoma after the Fontan procedure. N Engl J Med 2013;369(5):490.

29. Ghaferi AA, Hutchins GM. Progression of liver pathology in patients undergoing the Fontan procedure: chronic passive congestion, cardiac cirrhosis, hepatic adenoma, and hepatocellular carcinoma. J Thorac Cardiovasc Surg 2005;129(6): 1348–52.

30. Goldschlager N, Epstein AE, Naccarelli G, et al. Practical guidelines for clinicians who treat patients with amiodarone. Practice Guidelines Subcommittee, North American Society of Pacing and Electrophysiology. Arch Intern Med 2000; 160(12):1741–8.

31. Lewis JH, Ranard RC, Caruso A, et al. Amiodarone hepatotoxicity: prevalence and clinicopathologic correlations among 104 patients. Hepatology 1989;9(5): 679–85.

32. Richer M, Robert S. Fatal hepatotoxicity following oral administration of amiodarone. Ann Pharmacother 1995;29(6):582–6.

33. Felker GM, Adams KF Jr, Gattis WA, et al. Anemia as a risk factor and therapeutic target in heart failure. J Am Coll Cardiol 2004;44(5):959–66.

34. Kansagara D, Dyer E, Englander H, et al. Treatment of anemia in patients with heart disease: a systematic review. Ann Intern Med 2013;159(11):746–57.

35. Wilkinson KL, Brunskill SJ, Doree C, et al. Red cell transfusion management for patients undergoing cardiac surgery for congenital heart disease. Cochrane Database Syst Rev 2014;(2):CD009752.

36. Wang A, Book WM, McConnell M, et al. Prevalence of hepatitis C infection in adult patients who underwent congenital heart surgery prior to screening in 1992. Am J Cardiol 2007;100(8):1307–9.

37. Cox DA, Ginde S, Tweddell JS, et al. Outcomes of a hepatitis C screening protocol in at-risk adults with prior cardiac surgery. World J Pediatr Congenit Heart Surg 2014;5(4):503–6.

38. Alter MJ, Kruszon-Moran D, Nainan OV, et al. The prevalence of hepatitis C virus infection in the United States, 1988 through 1994. N Engl J Med 1999;341(8): 556–62.

39. Vogt M, Mühlbauer F, Braun SL, et al. Prevalence and risk factors of hepatitis C infection after cardiac surgery in childhood before and after blood donor screening. Infection 2004;32(3):134–7.
40. Zardi EM, Abbate A, Zardi DM, et al. Cirrhotic cardiomyopathy. J Am Coll Cardiol 2010;56(7):539–49.
41. Rodriguez-Roisin R, Krowka MJ. Hepatopulmonary syndrome: a liver-induced lung vascular disorder. N Engl J Med 2008;358(22):2378–87.
42. Cremona G, Higenbottam TW, Mayoral V, et al. Elevated exhaled nitric oxide in patients with hepatopulmonary syndrome. Eur Respir J 1995;8(11):1883–5.
43. Schenk P, Fuhrmann V, Madl C, et al. Hepatopulmonary syndrome: prevalence and predictive value of various cut offs for arterial oxygenation and their clinical consequences. Gut 2002;51(6):853–9.
44. Rodriguez-Roisin R, Krowka MJ, Hervé P, et al, ERS Task Force Pulmonary-Hepatic Vascular Disorders (PHD) Scientific Committee. Pulmonary-hepatic vascular disorders (PHD). Eur Respir J 2004;24(5):861–80.
45. Rodriguez-Roisin R, Krowka MJ. Is severe arterial hypoxaemia due to hepatic disease an indication for liver transplantation? A new therapeutic approach. Eur Respir J 1994;7(5):839–42.
46. Swanson KL, Wiesner RH, Krowka MJ. Natural history of hepatopulmonary syndrome: impact of liver transplantation. Hepatology 2005;41(5):1122–9.
47. Arguedas MR, Abrams GA, Krowka MJ, et al. Prospective evaluation of outcomes and predictors of mortality in patients with hepatopulmonary syndrome undergoing liver transplantation. Hepatology 2003;37(1):192–7.
48. Krowka MJ, Mandell MS, Ramsay MA, et al. Hepatopulmonary syndrome and portopulmonary hypertension: a report of the multicenter liver transplant database. Liver Transpl 2004;10(2):174–82.
49. Gupta S, Castel H, Rao RV, et al. Improved survival after liver transplantation in patients with hepatopulmonary syndrome. Am J Transplant 2010;10(2):354–63.
50. Collisson EA, Nourmand H, Fraiman MH, et al. Retrospective analysis of the results of liver transplantation for adults with severe hepatopulmonary syndrome. Liver Transpl 2002;8(10):925–31.
51. Badesch DB, Champion HC, Sanchez MA, et al. Diagnosis and assessment of pulmonary arterial hypertension. J Am Coll Cardiol 2009;54(1 Suppl):S55–66.
52. Krowka MJ, Swanson KL, Frantz RP, et al. Portopulmonary hypertension: results from a 10-year screening algorithm. Hepatology 2006;44(6):1502–10.
53. Castro M, Krowka MJ, Schroeder DR, et al. Frequency and clinical implications of increased pulmonary artery pressures in liver transplant patients. Mayo Clin Proc 1996;71(6):543–51.
54. Yang YY, Lin HC, Lee WC, et al. Portopulmonary hypertension: distinctive hemodynamic and clinical manifestations. J Gastroenterol 2001;36(3):181–6.
55. Humbert M, Lau EM, Montani D, et al. Advances in therapeutic interventions for patients with pulmonary arterial hypertension. Circulation 2014;130(24):2189–208.
56. Krowka MJ, Fallon MB, Kawut SM, et al. International liver transplant society practice guidelines: diagnosis and management of hepatopulmonary syndrome and portopulmonary hypertension. Transplantation 2016;100(7):1440–52.
57. Kaplowitz N. Liver and biliary diseases. Baltimore (MD): Williams & Wilkins; 1992.
58. Acierno LJ. Cardiac complications in acquired immunodeficiency syndrome (AIDS): a review. J Am Coll Cardiol 1989;13(5):1144–54.
59. Jones AL, Prescott LF. Unusual complications of paracetamol poisoning. QJM 1997;90(3):161–8.

60. Singal AK, Bataller R, Ahn J, et al. ACG clinical guideline: alcoholic liver disease. Am J Gastroenterol 2018;113(2):175–94.
61. Piano MR. Alcoholic cardiomyopathy: incidence, clinical characteristics, and pathophysiology. Chest 2002;121(5):1638–50.
62. Milani A, Zaccaria R, Bombardieri G, et al. Cirrhotic cardiomyopathy. Dig Liver Dis 2007;39(6):507–15.
63. Gertz MA, Kyle RA. Hepatic amyloidosis (primary [AL], immunoglobulin light chain): the natural history in 80 patients. Am J Med 1988;85(1):73–80.
64. Park MA, Mueller PS, Kyle RA, et al. Primary (AL) hepatic amyloidosis: clinical features and natural history in 98 patients. Medicine (Baltimore) 2003;82(5): 291–8.
65. Iwata T, Hoshii Y, Kawano H, et al. Hepatic amyloidosis in Japan: histological and morphometric analysis based on amyloid proteins. Hum Pathol 1995;26(10): 1148–53.
66. Kyle RA, Bayrd ED. Amyloidosis: review of 236 cases. Medicine (Baltimore) 1975; 54(4):271–99.
67. Dubrey SW, Cha K, Anderson J, et al. The clinical features of immunoglobulin light-chain (AL) amyloidosis with heart involvement. QJM 1998;91(2):141–57.
68. Gulati V, Harikrishnan P, Palaniswamy C, et al. Cardiac involvement in hemochromatosis. Cardiol Rev 2014;22(2):56–68.

Hepatobiliary Complications in Critically Ill Patients

Amanda Cheung, MD[a],*, Steven Flamm, MD[b]

KEYWORDS

- Critical illness • Hepatobiliary • Acute liver injury • Acute liver failure
- Hypoxic liver injury • Cholestatic liver injury

KEY POINTS

- The liver's response to the systemic inflammatory response syndrome may include acute liver injury, liver synthetic dysfunction, or acute liver failure.
- Underlying hepatic congestion is an important risk factor for liver injury in critically ill patients.
- Hypoxic liver injury occurs in the setting of decreased hepatic blood flow, arterial hypoxemia, and hepatic venous congestion.
- Intrahepatic cholestasis occurs commonly in critically ill patients due to altered bile acid synthesis, hepatobiliary transport, and feedback regulation.

INTRODUCTION

The systemic inflammatory response syndrome (SIRS) is a term used to describe the physiologic changes that occur in response to a wide range of insults and often leads to multiorgan dysfunction.[1] The liver plays a key role in the body's response to inflammation partly due to the abundance of resident macrophages, more specifically Kupffer cells, that are activated in response to bacteria and endotoxins released by damaged tissue.[2] The resulting production of proinflammatory cytokines, chemokines, and acute-phase proteins contributes to hepatotoxicity directly and indirectly.

ACUTE LIVER INJURY

Hepatic dysfunction varies in severity from mild liver chemistry abnormalities to acute liver failure (ALF). Acute liver injury (ALI) includes hepatocellular and cholestatic injury and may be accompanied by liver synthetic dysfunction or ALF in the most severe

Disclosure Statement: The authors have nothing to disclose.
[a] Division of Gastroenterology and Hepatology, Stanford University School of Medicine, 750 Welch Road, Suite 210, Palo Alto, CA 94304, USA; [b] Division of Gastroenterology and Hepatology, Northwestern Feinberg School of Medicine, 19-046 Arkes Building, 676 North Saint Clair, Chicago, IL 60611, USA
* Corresponding author.
E-mail address: cheungac@stanford.edu

Clin Liver Dis 23 (2019) 221–232
https://doi.org/10.1016/j.cld.2018.12.005
1089-3261/19/© 2018 Elsevier Inc. All rights reserved.

liver.theclinics.com

cases (**Fig. 1**). Hepatocellular injury is characterized by elevations in aspartate amino-transferase (AST) and alanine aminotransferase (ALT), with the latter more specific for liver injury. Common causes of hepatocellular injury in critical illness include hypoxic liver injury, congestive hepatopathy, and drug-induced liver injury (DILI). Cholestatic injury typically presents with increased alkaline phosphatase (ALP) and γ-glutamyl transpeptidase (GGT) and occurs in the setting of increased synthesis or decreased clearance of bile. Cholestasis may be a direct effect of the SIRS, DILI, or parenteral nutrition.

Markers of hepatic synthetic dysfunction include elevated bilirubin, decreased albumin, and prolonged prothrombin time. However, these parameters may be altered in critically ill patients even in the absence of hepatic dysfunction. Prothombin time is affected by dysfunctional pancreatic enzyme secretion, small bowel diseases, or vitamin K deficiency that may be related to prolonged fasting, altered gut flora in setting of antibiotic use, or fat malabsorption. In addition, critically ill patients may have increased factor consumption due to disseminated intravascular coagulation or massive bleeding. Although albumin synthesis only occurs in the liver, low albumin levels are not necessarily a sole reflection of liver dysfunction. Hepatocytes respond to critical illness by selectively decreasing production of negative acute phase proteins, including albumin.[2] Furthermore, increased capillary leakage with altered tissue distribution and changes in catabolism and degradation may contribute to low albumin levels.[3] Bilirubin elevation occurs with cholestatic injury or biliary tract obstruction, increased production in the setting of hemolysis, and decreased clearance in the setting of hepatic dysfunction.

The importance of hepatic dysfunction is clearly recognized as an important prognostic factor because bilirubin level has been included in the most utilized scoring algorithms to assess critically ill patients (**Table 1**).[4–6] Early hepatic dysfunction is a predictor of ICU and hospital mortality independent of severity of illness at presentation, even in critically ill patients with no underlying liver disease; furthermore, survival rates worsen incrementally with higher bilirubin levels.[7,8] Additionally, patients with preexisting liver disease, in particular those with cirrhosis or alcoholic liver disease, have an increased likelihood of developing ALI and death.[9]

ALF is defined by the presence of encephalopathy and impaired liver synthetic function in the setting of ALI.[10] The most common cause of ALF in the Western world is DILI, including acetaminophen overdose and idiosyncratic drug reactions. Viral hepatitis is the leading cause in the remainder of the world.[11] An additional important cause of ALF to consider in critically ill patients is hypoxic liver injury. Management of ALF depends on the underlying etiology, but all patients typically are managed in an ICU due to the high mortality risk.

HYPOXIC LIVER INJURY

Hypoxic hepatitis, shock liver, and ischemic hepatitis are terms used in the literature to describe the state in which the liver sustains injury due to decreased oxygen delivery

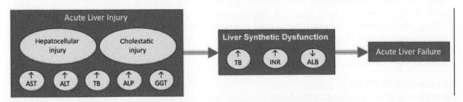

Fig. 1. Hepatic injury in critical illness. ALB, albumin; TB, total bilirubin.

Table 1
Scoring algorithms to assess prognosis in critically ill patients

	Components of Scoring Algorithm
SOFA score	Bilirubin, creatinine, FiO2, GCS, MAP or vasopressor use, PaO2, platelets
SAPS	Age, bilirubin, creatinine, GCS, HR, oxygenation (PaO2/FiO2 or PaO2), pH, platelet count, SBP, temperature, WBC, chronic health conditions, admission information, surgical status
APACHE III	Age, albumin, bilirubin, BUN, creatinine, FiO2, GCS, glucose, height, HR, RR, mechanical ventilation, MAP, PaCO2, PaO2, pH, sodium, temperature, urine output, WBC, chronic health conditions, admission information

Abbreviations: APACHE, acute physiology and chronic health evaluation; BUN, blood urea nitrogen; FiO2, fraction of inspired oxygen; GCS, Glasgow Coma Scale score; HR, heart rate; MAP, mean arterial pressure; PaO2, partial pressure arterial oxygen; RR, respiratory rate; SAPS, simplified acute physiology score; SBP, systolic blood pressure; SOFA, sequential organ failure assessment; WBC, white blood cell.

or utilization. All these terms, however, are technically misleading. Hepatitis implies the presence of inflammation in the liver, which typically is not present. Shock and ischemia also may not occur in a significant proportion of cases. Hemodynamic data (**Table 2**) provide an understanding of additional mechanisms that may contribute to hypoxic liver injury.[12,13]

Under normal physiological circumstances, the liver receives 30% of the total cardiac output with 25% coming from the oxygen-rich hepatic artery, and the other 75% from the nutrient-rich portal vein. The hepatic arterial buffer response ensures steady hepatic blood flow.[14] This regulatory mechanism is able to change the vascular tone of the hepatic artery to maintain constant total hepatic blood flow despite changes in the portal vein flow. Thus, the liver is able to accommodate to low flow states, highlighted by the fact that isolated hypovolemic shock rarely causes hypoxic liver injury.[12,13,15–17] Additional factors that contribute to hypoxic liver injury include hypoxemia, passive venous congestion, increased oxygen demand, impaired oxygen utilization, and reperfusion injury after a hypoxic event.

The group of cardiac failure patients in the critical care setting include decompensated congestive heart failure (CHF) and new-onset cardiac failure. Precipitating

Table 2
Pathophysiology of hypoxic liver injury

	Mechanism of Injury	Arterial Oxygen Pressure	Mean Arterial Pressure	Central Venous Pressure	Cardiac Index	Hepatic Blood Flow
Cardiac failure	Decreased oxygen delivery	⇔	⇓ ⇔	⇑	⇓	⇓
Respiratory failure	Decreased oxygen content in blood	⇓	⇔	⇔ ⇑	⇔ ⇑	⇔ ⇑
Septic shock	Decreased oxygen utilization	⇔	⇓	⇓	⇔ ⇑	⇔ ⇑
Hypovolemic shock	Decreased oxygen delivery	⇔	⇓	⇓	⇓	⇓

⇑ Increased
⇔ No change
⇓ Decreased

events leading to cardiac failure include myocardial infarction, acute pulmonary edema, arrhythmias, pulmonary embolism, pericardial tamponade, and trauma. The presence of shock is variable but more frequently seen in patients with acute cardiac failure, whereas patients with CHF often may not have significant hypotension.[12] In patients with cardiogenic shock, the severity of hypotension is not a predictor of developing hypoxic liver injury. Central venous pressure (CVP) is notably higher in those who do develop hypoxic damage, suggesting that passive congestion plays a key role in injury.[18]

The majority of patients who experience hypoxic liver injury in the setting of isolated respiratory failure, without additional cardiac or circulatory failure, have an underlying chronic respiratory disease such as pulmonary fibrosis, chronic obstructive pulmonary disease, or obstructive sleep apnea. In some cases of chronic respiratory failure, patients develop right-sided heart failure with a compensatory increase in cardiac index and hepatic blood flow; however, the hepatic venous congestion that occurs over time significantly predisposes to hepatic injury.[19,20]

Hepatic blood flow is preserved and often increased in the setting of sepsis due to the increased cardiac output in response to the drop in systemic vascular resistance. Oxygen content in blood is unchanged but unable to meet the increased demands in severe sepsis.[21] Utilization of oxygen by the hepatocytes is impaired by circulating endotoxins and inflammatory cytokines that are released by the disrupted gut mucosal barrier.[22]

The pooled incidence of hypoxic liver injury is estimated to be 2.5% of all admissions to the ICU, with up to 50% in-hospital mortality.[23] A significant proportion of identified cases is associated with cardiac failure (56%), followed in frequency by septic shock (23%) and respiratory failure (13%).[12,13,15–17] Hypotension is not a prerequisite for hypoxic liver injury; furthermore, some patients may develop significant liver injury after experiencing only 15 minutes of hypotension.[13,20] Patients at higher risk include those with baseline congestive hepatopathy or other underlying chronic liver disease. Portal hypertension in cirrhosis leads to portosystemic shunting, including intrahepatic shunting with decreased utilization.[24] Chronic alcohol use leads to increased mitochondrial oxygen consumption and release of cytokine mediators, particularly in zone 3.[25] These altered physiologic states may become problematic in the setting of compromised hepatic blood flow or oxygen delivery.

The most common laboratory finding is a rapid increase in aminotransferase levels within one to two days of the inciting event with AST typically peaking prior to ALT and normalization approximately one to two weeks after the injury.[26] Features that may distinguish hypoxic liver injury from viral hepatitis or DILI include a marked elevation of lactate dehydrogenase (LDH) and international normalized ratio (INR). An ALT-to-LDH ratio less than 1.5 has been suggested as a defining feature of hypoxic liver injury.[27] Although jaundice is not the predominant feature in hypoxic liver injury, elevations in bilirubin may occur, particularly in those with sepsis, vasopressor or mechanical ventilation requirements, and need for renal replacement therapy.[28] Additional evidence to support hypoxic liver injury includes injury to other organs, such as renal failure, in particular acute tubular necrosis, pancreatitis, rhabdomyolysis, and other end-organ dysfunction.

Although not required to make a diagnosis, a liver biopsy would demonstrate centrilobular necrosis with collapse of the hepatocyte architecture, particularly around zone 3, the most susceptible region to hypoxic injury due to its distance from the oxygen-rich blood.[29] Inflammatory cells are not a characteristic feature in hypoxic liver injury. Because hepatic venous congestion may be present in many of these cases, biopsy often has features of hepatic congestion, including dilated sinusoids with hepatocyte atrophy.[30]

The Sequential Organ Failure Assessment (SOFA) score is a widely recognized and validated predictor of outcomes in critically ill patients.[31] Moreover, it is also a predictor of mortality in the subset of patients with hypoxic liver injury.[15] Significantly elevated bilirubin reflects a greater severity of illness with increased complications and poor outcomes.[28] Although AST, ALT, and LDH levels are higher in nonsurvivors, these parameters are not independent risk factors for predicting death; on the other hand, significant coagulopathy, a marker reflective of liver synthetic dysfunction, is an independent risk factor for in-hospital mortality.[15,16]

Not only is septic shock a contributing cause of hypoxic liver injury, it is also an independent risk factor for in-hospital mortality.[15,16] The most common causes of death are septic shock and cardiac failure rather than liver-related causes.[15,17] Thus, management of patients with hypoxic liver injury is not focused on the liver itself but rather the underlying etiology and risk factors that led to the injury, including optimization of cardiac function and correction of hypoxemia, hypovolemia, and hypotension, if persistent.

CONGESTIVE HEPATOPATHY

Passive congestion of the liver occurs with any cause of longstanding right-sided heart failure, including left-sided heart failure, constrictive cardiomyopathy, and chronic respiratory failure with cor pulmonale. The increased central venous pressure is transmitted to the hepatic veins and sinusoids, leading to sinusoidal dilation with enlargement of the fenestrations, which may result in loss of protein-rich fluid to the lymphatic system.[32] Distinguishing features on physical examination include firm hepatomegaly, presence of hepatojugular reflux, and high protein ascites.

Histologic examination of the liver typically shows sinusoidal dilation and congestion, centrilobular hepatocyte atrophy, regenerative hyperplasia or nodules, and fibrosis starting in zone 3 and progressing to central-portal bridging fibrosis.[33] Unlike other causes of liver disease, the distribution of fibrosis is not homogenous. This may be explained by the proposed mechanism of injury that stasis leads to development of microthrombi with local hypoxia and resulting fibrosis.[34]

Patients with hepatic congestion may be asymptomatic due to the body's compensatory response until an inciting event occurs, including any cause for acute decompensated heart failure or hypoxic liver injury.[20] Mild liver chemistry abnormalities, typically in a cholestatic pattern, are common even in asymptomatic patients, and aminotransferase levels are mildly elevated unless there is concomitant hypoxic liver injury. Elevations in bilirubin, ALP, and GGT are correlated with right atrial pressure, disease severity classified by the New York Heart Association, and long-term prognosis.[35,36]

CHOLESTATIC LIVER DYSFUNCTION

Cholestasis in critical illness typically results in elevated direct bilirubin levels, up to a 3-fold increase in ALP and GGT levels, and minimal aminotransferase elevations.[37] Histologic examination is characterized by hepatocellular, canalicular, and ductular bilirubinostasis.[38] Additional findings may include hyperplasia of Kupffer cells, periportal mononuclear inflammatory infiltrate, ductular reaction, and sinusoidal dilation.[39] Risk factors include the presence of sepsis with gram-negative bacteria, shock requiring vasopressor support, preexisting chronic liver disease, and the need for mechanical ventilation, parenteral nutrition, or antibiotics.[7]

Under normal physiologic conditions (**Fig. 2**), unconjugated bile acids and bilirubin are transported into the hepatocyte via organic anion transporting polypeptides

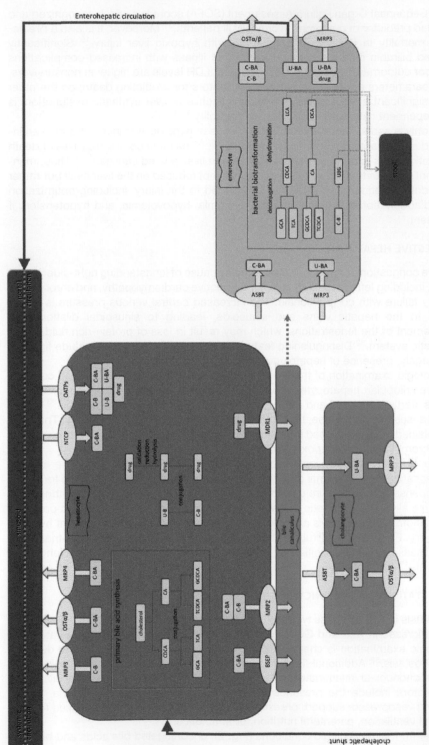

Fig. 2. Pathophysiology of bile synthesis and transport under normal physiologic conditions. CA, cholic acid; C-B, conjugated bilirubin; C-BA, conjugated bile acids; DCA, deoxycholic acid; GCA, glycocholic acid; GCDCA, glycochenodeoxycholic acid; GDCA, glycodeoxycholic acid; GLCA, glycolithocholic acid; TCA, taurocholic acid; TCDCA, taurochenodeoxycholic acid; TDCA, taurodeoxycholic acid; TLCA, taurolithocholic acid; U-B, ungonjugated bilirubin; U-BA, unconjugated bile acids; UBG, urobilinogen; UDCA, ursodeoxycholic acid.

(OATP) 1B1 on the sinusoidal membrane, whereas conjugated bile acids are transported via Na^+-dependent bile acid transporter (NTCP). Once in the hepatocyte, unconjugated bilirubin and bile acids undergo conjugation prior to transport out via multidrug resistance-associated protein (MRP) 2 and bile salt export pump (BSEP), respectively, into the bile canaliculus. Farnesoid X receptor (FXR) is the main regulator of bile acid homeostasis by modulating bile acid synthesis and transport.[40] Activation of hepatic FXR, primarily by chenodeoxycholic acid (CDCA), leads to up-regulation of BSEP and MRP2, the main canalicular efflux pumps, and suppresses cholesterol alpha-hydroxylase (CYP7A1), the rate-limiting step in bile acid synthesis, and bile acid uptake vita NTCP and OATP1B1. This feedback mechanism results in decreased bile acid synthesis and overall efflux of bile acid from the hepatocytes in response to elevated bile acids. Activation of enterocyte FXR increases intestinal organic solute transporter (OST) α/β and decreased apical sodium bile acid transporters (ASBTs), which similarly leads to efflux of bile salts from the enterocyte.[41]

Primary bile acids (CA and CDCA) are synthesized from cholesterol in the hepatocytes via cytochrome P450-mediated CYP7A1 whereas secondary bile acids (DCA and LCA) are present in the liver as a result of the enterohepatic circulation. Both primary and secondary bile acids are conjugated with glycine (GCA, GCDCA, GDCA, GLCA) or taurine (TCA, TCDCA, TDCA, TLCA) before export via BSEP or MRP2 into the bile canaliculus and delivered to the small intestine. Due to the pH of the proximal intestine, these conjugated forms are fully ionized and may be referred to as bile salts in this state.

The enterohepatic circulation returns about 95% of the bile acids to the liver in the portal venous circulation either in its original form or as secondary bile acids. Bile salts are transported into enterocytes in the terminal ileum via ASBT. The majority of the conjugated primary bile salts are reabsorbed in the small intestine. About 15% of the primary bile salts reach the distal ileum and are deconjugated by bacteria which may also be reabsorbed. In addition to deconjugation, CA and CDCA that reach the colon may be dehydroxylated to form secondary bile salts, DCA and LCA, respectively. A small proportion of CDCA also undergoes epimerization to UDCA. LCA is typically conjugated with sulfate which makes it poorly absorbable and the majority is lost in stool along with half the DCA, which totals about 5% of the entire bile salt pool. Bile salts enters the portal circulation via $OST\alpha/\beta$ or MRP3. Unconjugated bile acids are also able to enter circulation passively. Conjugated and unconjugated bile acids are then transported into hepatocytes from the portal circulation via NTCP and OATP-1B1, respectively.

Unconjugated bile acids may be passively absorbed by the cholangiocytes and subsequently returned to the sinusoids for hepatocyte uptake. A similar process occurs with conjugated bile acids via ASBT and $OST\alpha$-$OST\beta$ transporters. Overall this cholehepatic shunt pathway may be a mechanism to determine the bile acid composition and leads to downstream signaling.

Unconjugated bilirubin is a byproduct of heme degradation, primarily from senescent erythrocytes, and enters hepatocytes via OATP-1B1. Within the hepatocyte, bilirubin is conjugated with glucuronic acid prior to entering bile via MRP2 on the canalicular membrane. Though conjugated bilirubin may cross the sinusoidal membrane via MRP3, it typically re-enters the hepatocyte via OATP1B1 or OAT1B3, receptors that may also respond to excess conjugated bilirubin in the systemic circulation by increasing reuptake. Bilirubin in the bile is typically conjugated but undergoes bacterial deconjugation once it reaches the intestines leading to formation of urobilinogen. About 80% of urobilinogen is excreted in stool, and the remainder follows the enterohepatic circulation with some excretion in the urine.

Cholestatic liver dysfunction occurs in critically ill patients due to disturbance of bile acid synthesis, hepatobiliary transport, and feedback regulation.[42] An inflammatory state in the liver, whether from direct hepatotoxicity or as part of the systemic inflammatory response, leads to inhibition of hepatic FXR, which removes the negative feedback on CYP7A1 and allows novel bile acid synthesis. Bile acids in the hepatocytes typically activate BSEP and MRP2 in a positive feedback manner to promote efflux of bile acids and bilirubin out of the hepatocytes into bile. In the setting of cholestasis, however, there is accumulation of all the bile acids. Excess lithocholic acid (LCA) functions as a partial FXR antagonist and down-regulates BSEP.[40] Decreased transcription of efflux transporters, including BSEP and OSTα/β, on the canalicular membrane leads to accumulation of bile acids in the hepatocytes, and decreased expression of the enzymes needed for conjugation results in diminished bile acid detoxification.[41] Thus, the overall increase in bile acid levels, in particular those with potential toxicities, causes further inflammation and cholestasis.

In response to the accumulation of bilirubin and bile acids in the hepatocytes, MRP3, MRP4, and OSTα/β are up-regulated to transport conjugated bilirubin and bile acids across the basolateral membrane of the hepatocyte into the systemic circulation.[42] The inflammatory cytokine response in critical illness leads to suppression of important transcription factors for NCTP and OATP, disrupting the enterohepatic circulation and leading to elevated bilirubin and bile acid levels in the systemic circulation despite the concomitant sequestration of these compounds in the hepatocytes.[42]

Gut dysbiosis is often seen in critically ill patients due to lack of enteral nutrition, slowed gut motility, relative hypoxia, and use of antibiotics.[43] With this change in the intestinal microbiome, there is increased dehydroxylation of bile acids, leading to an altered bile acid pool with an increased proportion of secondary bile acids, which are cytotoxic when present at concentrations that exceed normal physiologic levels.[44] Additionally, in acute cholestatic liver injury, down-regulation of the intestinal tight junction proteins and increased intestinal permeability allow for translocation of bacteria and endotoxins independent of the changes in the microbiome.[45] Endotoxemia leads to hepatocellular injury with release of numerous cytokines that contribute to the physiologic changes in bile transport and handling, including decreased intestinal OSTα/β receptors and increased ASBT receptors, leading to influx of bile acids to the enterocytes.[46] The overall response in the gut is further production of endotoxins with translocation across the compromised gut barrier and entry into the enterohepatic circulation.[47]

ISCHEMIC/SCLEROSING CHOLANGIOPATHY

Ischemic cholangiopathy occurs when hepatic arterial blood flow is severely compromised because the bile ducts receive their blood supply exclusively from arteries. A majority of cases are iatrogenic, in which there was surgical manipulation of the artery, such as liver transplantation or accidental injury, embolization, or directed chemotherapy. Severe cases of shock or trauma with prolonged ischemia and hypoxia, however, may lead to ischemic cholangiopathy. This clinical entity is rare and has also been referred to as sclerosing cholangiopathy in critically ill patients.[48] The initial inciting event causes ischemic necrosis of the biliary duct mucosa, formation of biliary casts, and bile stasis, ultimately leading to fibrous changes during the healing process, leading to stricture formation.[49] The initial presentation is similar to the majority of the other critically ill patients with SIRS and cholestatic jaundice. Patients with sclerosing cholangiopathy, however, have persistent cholestasis.

Suspicion should be raised in patients with persistently elevated bilirubin, ALP, or γ-glutamyl transferase beyond two weeks that is expected in cholestasis related to critical illness alone.[48] The clinical course of sclerosing cholangiopathy includes increased risk for developing cholangitis and rapid progression to cirrhosis or liver failure with low likelihood of transplant-free survival.[50]

GALLBLADDER AND BILIARY DISEASE

Biliary obstruction from gallstones, biliary sludge, or malignancy causes a cholestatic pattern of liver chemistry abnormalities with characteristic dilation of the biliary tree. Depending on the level of obstruction, cholecystitis or cholangitis may occur from bacterial infection in the setting of obstruction and resulting biliary stasis. Acalculous cholecystitis is more commonly seen in critically ill patients as a result of gallbladder stasis, ischemia, inflammation, and secondary bacterial infection.[51] Although elevated bilirubin levels are more frequently due to cholestasis in SIRS, underlying disease of the gallbladder or biliary tree must be considered and can be evaluated easily with noninvasive imaging techniques.[52]

DRUG-INDUCED LIVER INJURY

The liver is particularly vulnerable to DILI because it is the primary site of drug processing. Hepatic metabolism includes a phase 1 reaction with drug transformation to reactive metabolites and a phase 2 reaction that conjugates these metabolites to detoxify them and allow for export and elimination. Limited export across the canalicular membrane and decreased hepatic biotransformation lead to the accumulation of drugs and its metabolites in the hepatocytes.[53] Accumulation of reactive metabolites is one of the underlying mechanisms of drug-induced hepatotoxicity.[54] Part of the inflammatory response in critical illness includes decreased expression of conjugating enzymes that may cause increased susceptibility to DILI in this patient population.[41] In addition to direct hepatotoxicity, drugs may also inhibit or damage the bile salt efflux pumps, contributing further to the toxic accumulation of bile salt, bilirubin, and other toxins.[40] These alterations in the normal processing of xenobiotics and the frequent need to use numerous pharmacologic agents in the critically ill patients make these patients uniquely vulnerable to DILI.

REFERENCES

1. Bone RC, Balk RA, Cerra FB, et al. Definitions for sepsis and organ failure and guidelines for the use of innovative therapies in sepsis. The ACCP/SCCM Consensus Conference Committee. American College of Chest Physicians/Society of Critical Care Medicine. Chest 1992;101:1644–55.

2. Dhainaut JF, Marin N, Mignon A, et al. Hepatic response to sepsis: interaction between coagulation and inflammatory processes. Crit Care Med 2001;29:S42–7.

3. Nicholson JP, Wolmarans MR, Park GR. The role of albumin in critical illness. Br J Anaesth 2000;85:599–610.

4. Vincent JL, Moreno R, Takala J, et al. The SOFA (Sepsis-related Organ Failure Assessment) score to describe organ dysfunction/failure. On behalf of the Working Group on Sepsis-Related Problems of the European Society of Intensive Care Medicine. Intensive Care Med 1996;22:707–10.

5. Moreno RP, Metnitz PG, Almeida E, et al. SAPS 3–From evaluation of the patient to evaluation of the intensive care unit. Part 2: development of a prognostic

model for hospital mortality at ICU admission. Intensive Care Med 2005;31: 1345–55.

6. Zimmerman JE, Kramer AA, McNair DS, et al. Acute Physiology and Chronic Health Evaluation (APACHE) IV: hospital mortality assessment for today's critically ill patients. Crit Care Med 2006;34:1297–310.

7. Brienza N, Dalfino L, Cinnella G, et al. Jaundice in critical illness: promoting factors of a concealed reality. Intensive Care Med 2006;32:267–74.

8. Kramer L, Jordan B, Druml W, et al. Incidence and prognosis of early hepatic dysfunction in critically ill patients–a prospective multicenter study. Crit Care Med 2007;35:1099–104.

9. Waseem N, Limketkai BN, Kim B, et al. Risk and prognosis of acute liver injury among hospitalized patients with hemodynamic instability: a nationwide analysis. Ann Hepatol 2018;17:119–24.

10. Lee WM, Stravitz RT, Larson AM. Introduction to the revised American Association for the Study of Liver Diseases Position Paper on acute liver failure 2011. Hepatology 2012;55:965–7.

11. Bernal W, Wendon J. Acute liver failure. N Engl J Med 2013;369:2525–34.

12. Henrion J, Schapira M, Luwaert R, et al. Hypoxic hepatitis: clinical and hemodynamic study in 142 consecutive cases. Medicine (Baltimore) 2003;82:392–406.

13. Birrer R, Takuda Y, Takara T. Hypoxic hepatopathy: pathophysiology and prognosis. Intern Med 2007;46:1063–70.

14. Shah V, Kamath P. Portal hypertension and variceal bleeding. In: Feldman MFL, Brandt L, editors. Sleisenger & Fordtran's gastrointestinal and liver disease : pathophysiology, diagnosis, management, vol. 1, 10th edition. Philadelphia: Elsevier/Saunders; 2016. p. 1524–52.

15. Fuhrmann V, Kneidinger N, Herkner H, et al. Hypoxic hepatitis: underlying conditions and risk factors for mortality in critically ill patients. Intensive Care Med 2009;35:1397–405.

16. Raurich JM, Llompart-Pou JA, Ferreruela M, et al. Hypoxic hepatitis in critically ill patients: incidence, etiology and risk factors for mortality. J Anesth 2011;25:50–6.

17. Chang PE, Goh BG, Ekstrom V, et al. Low serum albumin predicts early mortality in patients with severe hypoxic hepatitis. World J Hepatol 2017;9:959–66.

18. Henrion J, Descamps O, Luwaert R, et al. Hypoxic hepatitis in patients with cardiac failure: incidence in a coronary care unit and measurement of hepatic blood flow. J Hepatol 1994;21:696–703.

19. Ucgun I, Ozakyol A, Metintas M, et al. Relationship between hypoxic hepatitis and cor pulmonale in patients treated in the respiratory ICU. Int J Clin Pract 2005;59:1295–300.

20. Seeto RK, Fenn B, Rockey DC. Ischemic hepatitis: clinical presentation and pathogenesis. Am J Med 2000;109:109–13.

21. Ackland G, Grocott MP, Mythen MG. Understanding gastrointestinal perfusion in critical care: so near, and yet so far. Crit Care 2000;4:269–81.

22. Yoseph BP, Klingensmith NJ, Liang Z, et al. Mechanisms of intestinal barrier dysfunction in sepsis. Shock 2016;46:52–9.

23. Tapper EB, Sengupta N, Bonder A. The incidence and outcomes of ischemic hepatitis: a systematic review with meta-analysis. Am J Med 2015;128:1314–21.

24. Pan Z, Wu XJ, Li JS, et al. Functional hepatic flow in patients with liver cirrhosis. World J Gastroenterol 2004;10:915–8.

25. Cederbaum AI. Alcohol metabolism. Clin Liver Dis 2012;16:667–85.

26. Henrion J. Hypoxic hepatitis. Liver Int 2012;32:1039–52.

27. Cassidy WM, Reynolds TB. Serum lactic dehydrogenase in the differential diagnosis of acute hepatocellular injury. J Clin Gastroenterol 1994;19:118–21.
28. Jäger B, Drolz A, Michl B, et al. Jaundice increases the rate of complications and one-year mortality in patients with hypoxic hepatitis. Hepatology 2012;56:2297–304.
29. Wallach HF, Popper H. Central necrosis of the liver. AMA Arch Pathol 1950;49:33–42, illust.
30. Kotin P, Hall EM. "Cardiac" or congestive cirrhosis of liver. Am J Pathol 1951;27:561–71.
31. Ferreira FL, Bota DP, Bross A, et al. Serial evaluation of the SOFA score to predict outcome in critically ill patients. JAMA 2001;286:1754–8.
32. Giallourakis CC, Rosenberg PM, Friedman LS. The liver in heart failure. Clin Liver Dis 2002;6:947–67, viii-ix.
33. Louie CY, Pham MX, Daugherty TJ, et al. The liver in heart failure: a biopsy and explant series of the histopathologic and laboratory findings with a particular focus on pre-cardiac transplant evaluation. Mod Pathol 2015;28:932–43.
34. Wanless IR, Liu JJ, Butany J. Role of thrombosis in the pathogenesis of congestive hepatic fibrosis (cardiac cirrhosis). Hepatology 1995;21:1232–7.
35. Poelzl G, Ess M, Mussner-Seeber C, et al. Liver dysfunction in chronic heart failure: prevalence, characteristics and prognostic significance. Eur J Clin Invest 2012;42:153–63.
36. Allen LA, Felker GM, Pocock S, et al. Liver function abnormalities and outcome in patients with chronic heart failure: data from the Candesartan in Heart Failure: assessment of Reduction in Mortality and Morbidity (CHARM) program. Eur J Heart Fail 2009;11:170–7.
37. Thomson SJ, Cowan ML, Johnston I, et al. 'Liver function tests' on the intensive care unit: a prospective, observational study. Intensive Care Med 2009;35:1406–11.
38. Vanwijngaerden YM, Wauters J, Langouche L, et al. Critical illness evokes elevated circulating bile acids related to altered hepatic transporter and nuclear receptor expression. Hepatology 2011;54:1741–52.
39. Hirata K, Ikeda S, Honma T, et al. Sepsis and cholestasis: basic findings in the sinusoid and bile canaliculus. J Hepatobiliary Pancreat Surg 2001;8:20–6.
40. Kullak-Ublick GA, Stieger B, Meier PJ. Enterohepatic bile salt transporters in normal physiology and liver disease. Gastroenterology 2004;126:322–42.
41. Jia W, Xie G. Bile acid-microbiota crosstalk in gastrointestinal inflammation and carcinogenesis. Nat Rev Gastroenterol Hepatol 2018;15:111–28.
42. Jenniskens M, Langouche L, Vanwijngaerden YM, et al. Cholestatic liver (dys) function during sepsis and other critical illnesses. Intensive Care Med 2016;42:16–27.
43. Wolff NS, Hugenholtz F, Wiersinga WJ. The emerging role of the microbiota in the ICU. Crit Care 2018;22:78.
44. Hofmann AF. The continuing importance of bile acids in liver and intestinal disease. Arch Intern Med 1999;159:2647–58.
45. Fouts DE, Torralba M, Nelson KE, et al. Bacterial translocation and changes in the intestinal microbiome in mouse models of liver disease. J Hepatol 2012;56:1283–92.
46. Chand N, Sanyal AJ. Sepsis-induced cholestasis. Hepatology 2007;45:230–41.
47. Nolan JP. The role of intestinal endotoxin in liver injury: a long and evolving history. Hepatology 2010;52:1829–35.

48. Gelbmann CM, Rümmele P, Wimmer M, et al. Ischemic-like cholangiopathy with secondary sclerosing cholangitis in critically ill patients. Am J Gastroenterol 2007; 102:1221–9.

49. Engler S, Elsing C, Flechtenmacher C, et al. Progressive sclerosing cholangitis after septic shock: a new variant of vanishing bile duct disorders. Gut 2003;52: 688–93.

50. Leonhardt S, Veltzke-Schlieker W, Adler A, et al. Trigger mechanisms of secondary sclerosing cholangitis in critically ill patients. Crit Care 2015;19:131.

51. Ryu JK, Ryu KH, Kim KH. Clinical features of acute acalculous cholecystitis. J Clin Gastroenterol 2003;36:166–9.

52. Frankel HL, Kirkpatrick AW, Elbarbary M, et al. Guidelines for the appropriate use of bedside general and cardiac ultrasonography in the evaluation of critically ill patients-part I: general ultrasonography. Crit Care Med 2015;43:2479–502.

53. Gonnert FA, Recknagel P, Hilger I, et al. Hepatic excretory function in sepsis: implications from biophotonic analysis of transcellular xenobiotic transport in a rodent model. Crit Care 2013;17:R67.

54. Au JS, Navarro VJ, Rossi S. Review article: drug-induced liver injury–its pathophysiology and evolving diagnostic tools. Aliment Pharmacol Ther 2011;34: 11–20.

Endocrine Diseases and the Liver: An Update

Miguel Malespin, MD*, Ammar Nassri, MD

KEYWORDS

- Endocrine system • Liver disease • Hypothalamic-pituitary axis • Thyroid hormone
- Estrogen • Adrenal gland

KEY POINTS

- Endocrine diseases can lead to changes in hepatic function and metabolism.
- Alterations in lipid and carbohydrate metabolism can occur in the presence of endocrine dysfunction and can contribute to the development of nonalcoholic fatty liver disease.
- Impaired hepatic function can affect endocrine processes. There is a potential for recovery with resolution of liver disease or transplantation.

INTRODUCTION

The endocrine system is composed of a network of organs (hypothalamus, pituitary, pineal gland, thyroid, parathyroid, pancreas, adrenal glands, and ovaries or testes), whose primary function include hormonal production and secretion. The hypothalamus-pituitary axis (HPA) maintains control of this intricate system through the processing of intracorporeal and extracorporeal signals, resulting in the release of mediator hormones to target organs. These primary endocrine organs signal changes that can then lead to alterations in autocrine or paracrine function. Secondary endocrine organs (eg, liver) also contribute to hormonal signaling while carrying out other primary nonendocrine processes. Because of this interconnection, dysfunctions occurring within the endocrine network can manifest in primary and secondary organs. This article focuses on the symbiosis that exists between the endocrine system and the liver.

HYPOTHALAMUS-PITUITARY AXIS

The HPA is considered the central endocrine processing center. Autonomic, neural, and endocrine feedback signals influence hypothalamic processes, leading to the

Disclosures: M. Malespin receives research funding from Abbvie, Gilead, Intercept, and Novo Nordisk. A. Nassri has no relevant disclosures.
Department of Medicine, University of Florida Health, 4555 Emerson Street, Suite 300, Jacksonville, FL 32207, USA
* Corresponding author.
E-mail address: malespinm@gmail.com

production of inhibitory hormones (somatostatin, dopamine) or stimulatory hormones (corticotropin-releasing hormone, growth hormone-releasing hormone, gonadotropin-releasing hormone, prolactin-releasing factors, thyrotropin-releasing hormone [TRH]). Hormonal transport occurs at the primary capillary plexus to the anterior pituitary gland or through neuronal signaling to the posterior pituitary.[1] Pituitary hormones (corticotropin, growth hormone, luteinizing hormone [LH] or follicle-stimulating hormone [FSH], thyroid-stimulating hormone [TSH], prolactin) are subsequently secreted to the liver through systemic circulation.

Hepatic afferent nerves provide sensory feedback to the HPA for regulation of a variety of functions, including glucose, glycogen, lipid, and protein metabolism. Directly and indirectly, corticotropin and growth hormone contribute to hepatic glycogen and glucose metabolism.[2] Glucocorticoid production through corticotropin-mediated induction results in the release of amino acids and glycerol, forming the substrates for hepatic gluconeogenesis.[3] In cases of secondary adrenal insufficiency, inadequate corticotropin production occurring as a consequence of pituitary disease can result in ineffective hepatic gluconeogenesis, resulting in episodes of hypoglycemia.[4]

PINEAL GLAND

The pineal gland is located in the region of the brain known as the epithalamus and is involved in the synthesis of melatonin from tryptophan.[5] Hepatic clearance of melatonin occurs through cytochrome P450–induced oxidation before urinary or fecal excretion.[6] Melatonin's primary function is regulation of sleep–wake cycles with increased blood concentrations resulting in sleep initiation and maintenance.[7] There are also a variety of secondary functions, including regulation of hemodynamics, immune response, and bone metabolism.[8] Whether these changes occur in relation to the circadian rhythm or from the direct signaling effect of melatonin remains unclear. Melatonin also exhibits antioxidant properties and plays a further role in hepatic glycogen metabolism.[9–11] These secondary functions provide insight to the potential hepatoprotective benefits described in animal models evaluating drug-induced liver injury, alcohol-related liver disease, nonalcoholic fatty liver disease (NAFLD), and hepatic fibrosis.[12] Further research is needed to evaluate these findings in human subjects and, specifically, the effects of pinealectomy on hepatic function and hormonal signaling.

THE THYROID GLAND AND THE LIVER

Through a variety of feedback signals, the liver and thyroid gland work in conjunction to maintain adequate corporal processes. Release of TRH in the hypothalamus leads to production of TSH in the anterior pituitary gland, which then promotes thyroidal production of thyroxine (T4) and its active form: 3,5,3′-triiodothyronine (T3)[13] (**Fig. 1**). T3 induces hepatic metabolic and functional processes by binding to nuclear receptors and regulating gene expression.[14] Thyroidal T4 release takes place at a higher rate than active T3 with most T3 production occurring through T4 conversion by iodothyronine deiodinase type 1 (D1) and deiodinase type 2 (D2).[15,16] D2 expression mostly occurs within the central nervous system and pituitary gland in response to increased T4 levels.[17] On the other hand, D1 is found in a variety of organs, including the liver, and also functions in the production of inactive reverse T3 (rT3).[18] Thus, although proper hepatic function depends on adequate thyroid hormone production, hepatic disease states can also adversely affect thyroid hormone production through inadequate T4 conversion.

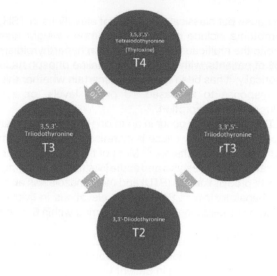

Fig. 1. Thyroid hormone metabolism.

Effects of Hypothyroidism on Liver Function

Primary hypothyroidism results from thyroidal dysfunction. Autoimmune thyroiditis or iodine deficiency are among the leading causes worldwide.[19] The prevalence of hypothyroidism within the United States ranges from approximately 3% to 4% of the population. Most individuals present with subclinical hypothyroidism (elevated TSH with normal T4) in comparison with a small subset with overt hypothyroidism (elevated TSH with low T4).[20,21] Secondary or tertiary (central) hypothyroidism occurs less commonly and in the presence of hypothalamic or pituitary disease, resulting in inadequate production of both TRH and TSH. Patients with secondary hypothyroidism do not appropriately respond to a low serum T4 and thus present with both decreased T4 and TSH levels.[22] The clinical impacts of hypothyroidism are variable and can lead to an elevation in aspartate (AST) and alanine aminotransferase (ALT) levels, or changes in hepatic metabolism.

The link between hypothyroidism and musculoskeletal dysfunction has been widely established as a nonhepatic cause of elevated liver enzymes.[23] Myopathies leading to elevated creatinine kinase level and a subsequent increase in AST or ALT occur in up to 80% of patients with hypothyroidism and result in a constellation of symptoms, including myalgias, muscle cramps, and weakness.[24–27] Thyroid hormone also plays a role in regulation of lipid metabolism, body weight, and insulin resistance. Hypothyroidism is present in 15% to 36% of patients with NAFLD.[28] Decreased cholesterol excretion and increased triglyceride deposition can give way to increased hepatic cholesterol and triglyceride concentrations.[29,30] Therefore, the occurrence of nonalcoholic steatohepatitis (NASH) secondary to hypothyroidism is considered among the hepatic causes of elevated aminotransferase levels. Alterations in hepatic function can also occur in the form of cholestasis. Although rarely reported, an increase in enzymatic Uridine 5′-diphospho-glucuronosyltransferase activity in conjunction with a decrease in p-nitrophenol transferase activity can result in biliary stasis.[31–33]

Effects of Hyperthyroidism on Liver Function

Hyperthyroidism occurs in approximately 1.3% of the population with Graves' disease and toxic multinodular goiter being the leading causes.[21] Serologic findings are variable based on cause but classically consists of elevations in TSH, T3, and free T4 levels. Typical symptoms include palpitations, tremors, weight loss, hyperhidrosis, and diarrhea. Despite the multicausality that exists in hyperthyroidism, abnormal liver tests occur in 39% of patients, with elevation of alkaline phosphatase occurring most commonly.[34] Historically, it has been difficult to ascertain whether this phenomenon is a direct hepatic response to increased T3 or T4 levels, or a consequence of thyrotoxicosis-induced bone resorption.

Elevations in ALT and AST levels occur in up to one-third of individuals with hyperthyroidism.[34,35] The presumed primary cause is increased metabolic demand, resulting in hypoperfusion and mild hepatic ischemia.[36] Most of these episodes are subclinical and self-limited, with intrahepatic cholestasis and acute liver failure occurring infrequently.[37,38] Thiamine therapy with propylthiouracil (PTU) and methimazole has also been associated with rare cases of hepatotoxicity.[39] PTU-related elevations in liver enzymes are also largely self-limited with normalization generally occurring within 6 months.[40–42]

Effects of Liver Disease Effects on Thyroid Function

Eighty-percent of daily T3 production occurs through D1 and D2 conversion[43] (see **Fig. 1**). Hepatic dysfunction occurring in patient with cirrhosis can result in decreased D1 activity and, in turn, inadequate free T3 levels.[44–46] Although most of these patients remain euthyroid, progressive hepatic dysfunction can lead a further decrease in free T3 levels and clinical manifestations related to this.[44,47,48] Moreover, circulatory T3 and T4 transport depends on hepatocyte production of T4-binding globulin (TBG), transthyretin, and albumin. Thus, in patients with endstage liver disease or acute liver failure, decreased total T4 and T3 are reflective of both a decrease in D1 and TBG synthesis.[49,50] These changes are reversible in the event of spontaneous hepatic recovery or liver transplantation.[43]

Furthermore, extrahepatic autoimmune conditions are particularly common in patients with primary biliary cholangitis (PBC) and autoimmune hepatitis. Twenty-six percent of patients with PBC develop thyroidal antibodies, with the prevalence of hypothyroidism secondary to Hashimoto thyroiditis ranging from approximately 20% to 30%.[51,52] Given this increased risk, current recommendations include yearly screening for thyroid disease with serum TSH for all patients with PBC.[53]

PARATHYROID

Parathyroid hormone (PTH) plays a central in role in calcium hemostasis, absorption, and bone turnover. Autoimmune polyendocrinopathy-candidiasis-ectodermal dystrophy (APECED) is a rare inherited autoimmune syndrome characterized by hypoparathyroidism; Addison disease; and, among other manifestations, idiopathic chronic active hepatitis.[54] Although the relationship between PTH and liver disease is poorly defined, cirrhosis is a major risk factor for osteopenia and osteoporosis in patients with cirrhosis, independent of age. The pathophysiology is poorly understood but hormonal imbalances play an important role. Low estrogen and testosterone levels resulting from hypogonadism increase the life span of osteoclasts and decreases it in osteoblasts, leading to higher bone resorption. Similarly, the synthesis of insulin-like growth factor (IGF)-1, an endocrine hormone usually produced in the liver, is deficient in cirrhosis, impairing osteoblastic activity and bone mineralization.[55]

PANCREAS

Glycogen hepatopathy is a rare complication of poorly controlled type 1 diabetes mellitus (DM) and is characterized by hepatomegaly, elevated liver enzymes, and glycogen accumulation. It is often misdiagnosed as NAFLD, and correct diagnosis depends on liver biopsy with Periodic acid-Schiff staining before and after diastase digestion[56] (**Fig. 2**).

Type I DM is characterized by islet cell autoimmunity, loss of pancreatic β-cells, and subsequent insulin deficiency. Insulin decreases hepatic gluconeogenesis by inhibiting gluconeogenic enzymes, modulating fatty acid synthesis, and downregulating Glucose transporter 2 expression.[57] Although not as well characterized as in type II DM, NAFLD is prevalent in patients with type I DM.[57] The lower incidence in type 1 DM may be explained by a suppression of lipolysis with insulin therapy, thus reducing intrahepatic triglyceride synthesis and free hepatic fatty acid flux.[58]

SEX HORMONES

Ovarian-produced 17B estradiol (E2) is the predominant circulating estrogen in women. In men and postmenopausal women, testosterone is the primary source of estrogen and is converted to E2 by peripheral aromatization in adipose tissue. Estrogens mediate their effects on the liver through a variety of mechanisms and are

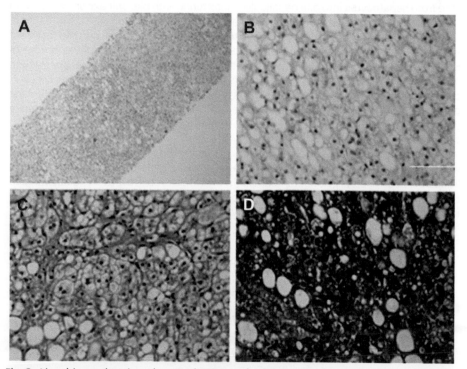

Fig. 2. Liver biopsy showing glycogen hepatopathy. HE staining (*A*, original magnification × 100; *B*, original magnification × 400) of liver biopsy demonstrating GH. It can be seen that the architecture is normal with diffuse hepatocellular change characterized by pale hepatocytes with cytoplasmic rarefaction and accentuation of the cell membranes. Few glycogenated nuclei are noted. No inflammation is seen. (*C*) Diastase and periodic acid-Schiff (PAS) staining (original magnification × 400), glycogen disappears after digestion with diastase. (*D*) PAS staining (original magnification × 400), demonstrating abundant cytoplasmic glycogen deposition. (*Reprinted from* Hepatobiliary & Pancreatic Diseases International Volume 17. Khoury K, Zohar Y, Shehadeh N, Saadi T. Glycogenic hepatopathy 113–18, © 2018; with permission from Elsevier.)

responsible for decreased de novo lipogenesis, reduced fatty acid delivery, increased Very-low-density lipoprotein-triglyceride export, and regulation of hepatic cholesterol uptake.[59] Estrogen deficiency occurring in menopause increases the risk of NAFLD with estrogen replacement, resulting in a reduction in transaminase levels.[60] Similarly, in younger patients with surgical or chemically induced menopause, the risk of NAFLD and steatohepatitis increases twofold.[59] Polycystic ovarian syndrome (PCOS) is a syndrome that comprises hyperandrogenism, anovulation, and polycystic ovarian morphology. Multiple studies have demonstrated an increased incidence of NAFLD, mainly resulting from obesity, central adiposity, and insulin resistance. However, some studies have shown associations of NAFLD with PCOS even when controlled for age, obesity, and central adiposity, likely secondary to hyperandrogenism.[61,62]

Estrogens can also cause intrahepatic cholestasis in premenopausal women using oral contraceptives, postmenopausal women on hormone replacement therapy, and in men receiving estrogen for prostate cancer. Similarly, increased levels of endogenous estrogen during pregnancy are associated with the development of intrahepatic cholestasis of pregnancy. Estrogens are thought to inhibit bile acid transport and uptake from hepatocytes into bile canaliculi by interfering with bile salt export pumps and inhibiting transporters on the basolateral membrane.[63]

A prothrombotic high estrogen state from oral contraceptives and, to a lesser extent, pregnancy has long been described as a risk factor for the development of Budd-Chiari syndrome.[64] On the other hand, extrahepatic portal vein obstruction has not been shown to have an association with estrogen use or pregnancy. Sinusoidal obstruction syndrome, also known as venocclusive disease, results from the drug-induced toxicity on liver sinusoidal endothelium (**Fig. 3**). One study suggests that patients receiving estrogen products are also at increased risk of sinusoidal obstruction syndrome.[64]

Hepatic adenomas are usually diagnosed in young women on oral contraceptives, with a dose-dependent association between estrogens and hepatic adenomas, and a 30 to 40 times increase in longstanding users of oral contraceptives.[63] The relationship between estrogens and other hepatic tumors, including hepatic hemangiomas and focal nodular hyperplasia, remains controversial and, to date, no strong association has been proven.[64]

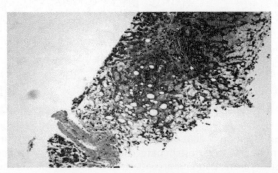

Fig. 3. Liver biopsy in sinusoidal obstruction syndrome. Microscopic finding of the liver biopsy. Venous dilatation and congestion in venoocclusive disease with fibrosis and subintimal edema (trichrome, original magnification × 200). (*From* Tavernier E, Chalayer E, Cornillon J, et al. Fulminant hepatitis due to very severe sinusoidal obstruction syndrome (SOS/VOD) after autologous peripheral stem cell transplantation: a case report. BMC Res Notes 2018;11:436; with permission.)

SEX HORMONES IN CIRRHOSIS

Low serum testosterone is found in up to 90% of patients with cirrhosis, and the degree of deficiency is related to the severity of liver disease.[65,66] Low testosterone is thought to contribute to many of the classic features of patients with liver disease, including testicular atrophy, gynecomastia, muscle wasting, and altered hair distribution.[65] There are multiple factors that are thought to contribute to primary hypogonadism, including ethanol-induced direct gonadal injury in patients with alcohol abuse. Central hypogonadism also occurs in patients with cirrhosis, resulting in decreased pituitary production of LH and increased prolactin levels. Estrogen levels are frequently elevated in men with cirrhosis as a result of increased peripheral aromatization of testosterone to estrogen and impaired hepatic metabolism.[65] For unclear reasons, LH and FSH levels fail to increase in response to a decrease in sex hormone production. Although this biochemical trend improves with liver transplantation, the clinical consequences of prior hormonal alterations, including sexual dysfunction and hypogonadism, may persist.[67–69] Furthermore, liver failure can downregulate GnRH secretion by the hypothalamus and lead to secondary testicular failure, thought to be from elevated cytokines such as interleukin (IL)-1, IL-6, and tumor necrosis factor (TNF)- α.[70] In a prospective study, low testosterone levels were found to be associated with increased mortality, infections, and the need for transplantation, independent of the Model for Endstage Liver Disease (MELD) score.[71]

ADRENAL GLANDS
Adrenal Insufficiency

Although not as widely recognized, there have been reports of mild elevation in transaminases in patients with Addison disease, as well as resolution with glucocorticoids.[72–74] Although the mechanisms are unclear, some investigators have postulated that infiltrating lymphocytes release cytokines, which then induce apoptosis and necrosis of hepatocytes, whereas others have implicated an immunologic reaction similar to that seen in autoimmune adrenalitis.[74]

Adrenal Excess

Increased glucocorticoid levels, such as that seen in Cushing syndrome, have been implicated in the pathogenies of insulin resistance, obesity, metabolic syndrome, and NAFLD. In animal models, chronically elevated glucocorticoid levels had a significant effect on the development of NAFLD, likely from increased hepatic cholesterol synthesis and reduced utilization.[75] Abnormalities in the peripheral metabolism of glucocorticoids, particularly relating to enzymes that inactivate or regenerate cortisol, such as 11-β-hydroxysteroid dehydrogenase 1, 11-β-hydroxysteroid dehydrogenase 2, and alpha-ring reductases, have also been implicated in the development of metabolic syndrome and NAFLD, and are increased in high cortisol states.[75] In a study comparing patients who received high cumulative doses of steroids compared with low doses, those who had received a high total dose had a significantly higher incidence of steatosis on liver biopsy.[76]

Hyperaldosteronism

The renin-angiotensin system is implicated in the pathogenesis of insulin resistance and NAFLD. In vitro studies have shown that aldosterone induces insulin resistance in hepatocytes by increasing messenger RNA (mRNA) expression of glyconeogenic enzymes, as well as degradation of the insulin receptor substrates via a reactive oxygen species-mediated pathway.[77,78] Patients with primary aldosteronism have an increased risk of metabolic syndrome, abnormal glucose metabolism, insulin resistance, and NAFLD compared with normotensive controls.[79,80] In a prospective study, subjects with primary aldosteronism who exhibited increased insulin resistance and impaired glucose metabolism showed improvement in insulin sensitivity after surgical or medical treatment.[81] Treatment with mineralocorticoid receptor antagonists can suppress local inflammation. In mouse models with DM and NAFLD or NASH, spironolactone and eplerenone treatment improved hepatic steatosis by reducing insulin resistance and hepatic inflammation, and decreased the progression of liver fibrosis.[82,83] In a metaanalysis comparing angiotensin receptor blockers (ARBs) and calcium channel blockers in nondiabetic patients, ARBs were found to be more effective in improving measures of insulin resistance.[84] Furthermore, when ARBs were used in NAFLD patients, they were found to improve liver steatosis, inflammation, and hepatic fibrosis.[85,86]

Adrenal Catecholamines

Pheochromocytomas are neuroendocrine tumors of chromaffin cells of the medulla or, more rarely, of extraadrenal chromaffin cells, and they result in excess catecholamine production. Patients with pheochromocytomas can present with markedly elevated liver transaminases, possibly due to repeated stimulation of adrenergic receptors, leading to increased resistance of hepatic arterioles and veins, with decreased blood flow to the liver.[87] In vitro and in vivo data suggest that catecholamines can exert fibrinogenic effects and be involved in the development of NAFLD because hepatic stellate cells express adrenergic receptors that produce norepinephrine and are inhibited by alpha and beta receptor antagonists.[88] These cells promote fibrogenesis in response to liver injury and were found to be markedly upregulated in NAFLD livers.[89]

ADRENAL GLANDS IN CIRRHOSIS

Numerous studies have demonstrated an association between cirrhosis and relative adrenal insufficiency (RAI), with some investigators referring to this clinical constellation as hepatoadrenal syndrome. RAI is the term given to inadequate production of cortisol relative to the severity of illness.[90] Initially reported in cirrhotic patients with septic shock or severe sepsis, more recent studies have demonstrated the presence of RAI in patients with noncritical chronic liver disease.[66,91–93] Two studies evaluating the incidence of RAI in nonseptic cirrhotic patients found an incidence of 26% to 47%.[92,94] Adrenal insufficiency in cirrhosis seems to predict early mortality, independent of Child-Pugh or MELD scores, as well as developing hepatorenal syndrome, infections, and sepsis.[94]

The precise cause of RAI in cirrhosis is unclear but one of the proposed mechanisms is the depletion or impaired synthesis of cholesterol, the main precursor for steroid biosynthesis, in the adrenal glands.[95] Several studies have demonstrated lower levels of cholesterol levels in cirrhotic subjects with RAI.[92,94] In addition, cytokines, such as IL-1, IL-6, and TNF-α, are increased in cirrhotic and septic states are thought to decrease the hepatic synthesis of apolipoprotein A-1, a major component of high-density lipoprotein (HDL), and increased levels of circulating endotoxins, such as lipopolysaccharide, impair normal metabolism and transport of cholesterol by downregulating HDL receptors.[96,97] TNF-α also inhibits the secretion of pituitary hormones and suppresses adrenal cortisol secretion.[98] Other causes include adrenal hemorrhage and infarction in the setting of coagulopathy, and hypotension, commonly seen in cirrhosis, leading to structural and functional damage of the adrenal gland.[99]

SUMMARY

The endocrine system is a complex network of organs interconnected through a bevy of signals aimed at maintaining the body's core processes and functions. Although classified as a secondary endocrine organ, the liver plays a crucial role in promoting homeostasis. Though gaps in knowledge remain in regard to fully understanding the hepato–endocrine interplay, it is well established that disease states of primary endocrine organs can lead to hepatic dysfunction and, inversely, hepatic disease can lead to alterations in endocrine function. In the past decades, there has occurred a rapid increase in the prevalence of NAFLD and complications related to disease progression. Hepatic lipid metabolism and cholesterol synthesis rely on proper endocrine function and feedback mechanisms. Therefore, there needs to be awareness to the potential of endocrine-related disease states in patients with NAFLD, and management of these conditions should be included within the context of conventional therapies. Furthermore, proper monitoring of endocrine function is essential in patients with advanced liver disease, particularly those with decompensated cirrhosis and acute liver failure.

REFERENCES

1. Chrousos GP. The hypothalamic-pituitary-adrenal axis and immune-mediated inflammation. N Engl J Med 1995;332(20):1351–62.
2. Ban T. The hypothalamus and liver metabolism. Acta Neuroveg (Wien) 1967; 30(1):137–44.
3. Uyama N, Geerts A, Reynaert H. Neural connections between the hypothalamus and the liver. Anat Rec A Discov Mol Cell Evol Biol 2004;280(1):808–20.
4. Nicolaides NC, Chrousos GP, Charmandari E. Adrenal insufficiency. In: De Groot LJ, Chrousos G, Dungan K, et al, editors. Endotext. South Dartmouth (MA): MDText.com, Inc.; 2000.
5. Zimmermann RC, McDougle CJ, Schumacher M, et al. Effects of acute tryptophan depletion on nocturnal melatonin secretion in humans. J Clin Endocrinol Metab 1993;76(5):1160–4.
6. Kopin IJ, Pare CM, Axelrod J, et al. 6-Hydroxylation, the major metabolic pathway for melatonin. Biochim Biophys Acta 1960;40:377–8.
7. Lynch HJ, Jimerson DC, Ozaki Y, et al. Entrainment of rhythmic melatonin secretion in man to a 12-hour phase shift in the light/dark cycle. Life Sci 1978;23(15): 1557–63.
8. Claustrat B, Leston J. Melatonin: physiological effects in humans. Neurochirurgie 2015;61(2–3):77–84.
9. Cardinali DP, Golombek DA, Rosenstein RE, et al. Melatonin site and mechanism of action: single or multiple? J Pineal Res 1997;23(1):32–9.
10. Manev H, Uz T, Kharlamov A, et al. In vivo protection against kainate-induced apoptosis by the pineal hormone melatonin: effect of exogenous melatonin and circadian rhythm. Restor Neurol Neurosci 1996;9(4):251–6.
11. Borges-Silva C, Takada J, Alonso-Vale MI, et al. Pinealectomy reduces hepatic and muscular glycogen content and attenuates aerobic power adaptability in trained rats. J Pineal Res 2007;43(1):96–103.
12. Zhang B, Wu ZY. Estrogen derivatives: novel therapeutic agents for liver cirrhosis and portal hypertension. Eur J Gastroenterol Hepatol 2013;25(3):263–70.
13. Peeters RP, Visser TJ. Metabolism of thyroid hormone. In: De Groot LJ, Chrousos G, Dungan K, et al, editors. Endotext. South Dartmouth (MA): MDText.com, Inc.; 2000.

14. Yen PM. Physiological and molecular basis of thyroid hormone action. Physiol Rev 2001;81(3):1097–142.
15. Bianco AC, Salvatore D, Gereben B, et al. Biochemistry, cellular and molecular biology, and physiological roles of the iodothyronine selenodeiodinases. Endocr Rev 2002;23(1):38–89.
16. Larsen PR, Zavacki AM. The role of the iodothyronine deiodinases in the physiology and pathophysiology of thyroid hormone action. Eur Thyroid J 2012;1(4): 232–42.
17. Riskind PN, Kolodny JM, Larsen PR. The regional hypothalamic distribution of type II 5'-monodeiodinase in euthyroid and hypothyroid rats. Brain Res 1987; 420(1):194–8.
18. Maia AL, Kim BW, Huang SA, et al. Type 2 iodothyronine deiodinase is the major source of plasma T3 in euthyroid humans. J Clin Invest 2005;115(9):2524–33.
19. Chakera AJ, Pearce SH, Vaidya B. Treatment for primary hypothyroidism: current approaches and future possibilities. Drug Des Devel Ther 2012;6:1–11.
20. Aoki Y, Belin RM, Clickner R, et al. Serum TSH and total T4 in the United States population and their association with participant characteristics: National Health and Nutrition Examination Survey (NHANES 1999-2002). Thyroid 2007;17(12): 1211–23.
21. Hollowell JG, Staehling NW, Flanders WD, et al. Serum TSH, T(4), and thyroid antibodies in the United States population (1988 to 1994): National Health and Nutrition Examination Survey (NHANES III). J Clin Endocrinol Metab 2002;87(2): 489–99.
22. Lania A, Persani L, Beck-Peccoz P. Central hypothyroidism. Pituitary 2008;11(2): 181–6.
23. Cakir M, Samanci N, Balci N, et al. Musculoskeletal manifestations in patients with thyroid disease. Clin Endocrinol 2003;59(2):162–7.
24. McKeran RO, Slavin G, Ward P, et al. Hypothyroid myopathy. A clinical and pathologaical study. J Pathol 1980;132(1):35–54.
25. Horak HA, Pourmand R. Endocrine myopathies. Neurol Clin 2000;18(1):203–13.
26. Madhu SV, Jain R, Kant S, et al. Myopathy presenting as a sole manifestation of hypothyroidism. J Assoc Physicians India 2010;58:569–70.
27. Monzani F, Caraccio N, Siciliano G, et al. Clinical and biochemical features of muscle dysfunction in subclinical hypothyroidism. J Clin Endocrinol Metab 1997;82(10):3315–8.
28. Eshraghian A, Hamidian Jahromi A. Non-alcoholic fatty liver disease and thyroid dysfunction: a systematic review. World J Gastroenterol 2014;20(25):8102–9.
29. Duntas LH. Thyroid disease and lipids. Thyroid 2002;12(4):287–93.
30. Adams AC, Astapova I, Fisher FM, et al. Thyroid hormone regulates hepatic expression of fibroblast growth factor 21 in a PPARalpha-dependent manner. J Biol Chem 2010;285(19):14078–82.
31. Huang MJ, Liaw YF. Clinical associations between thyroid and liver diseases. J Gastroenterol Hepatol 1995;10(3):344–50.
32. Ariza CR, Frati AC, Sierra I. Hypothyroidism-associated cholestasis. JAMA 1984; 252(17):2392.
33. Van Steenbergen W, Fevery J, De Vos R, et al. Thyroid hormones and the hepatic handling of bilirubin. I. Effects of hypothyroidism and hyperthyroidism on the hepatic transport of bilirubin mono- and diconjugates in the Wistar rat. Hepatology 1989;9(2):314–21.
34. Lin TY, Shekar AO, Li N, et al. Incidence of abnormal liver biochemical tests in hyperthyroidism. Clin Endocrinol 2017;86(5):755–9.

35. Thompson P Jr, Strum D, Boehm T, et al. Abnormalities of liver function tests in tyrotoxicosis. Mil Med 1978;143(8):548–51.

36. Myers JD, Brannon ES, Holland BC. A correlative study of the cardiac output and the hepatic circulation in hyperthyroidism. J Clin Invest 1950;29(8):1069–77.

37. Sola J, Pardo-Mindan FJ, Zozaya J, et al. Liver changes in patients with hyperthyroidism. Liver 1991;11(4):193–7.

38. Choudhary AM, Roberts I. Thyroid storm presenting with liver failure. J Clin Gastroenterol 1999;29(4):318–21.

39. Williams KV, Nayak S, Becker D, et al. Fifty years of experience with propylthiouracil-associated hepatotoxicity: what have we learned? J Clin Endocrinol Metab 1997;82(6):1727–33.

40. Cooper DS, Rivkees SA. Putting propylthiouracil in perspective. J Clin Endocrinol Metab 2009;94(6):1881–2.

41. Kim HJ, Kim BH, Han YS, et al. The incidence and clinical characteristics of symptomatic propylthiouracil-induced hepatic injury in patients with hyperthyroidism: a single-center retrospective study. Am J Gastroenterol 2001;96(1):165–9.

42. Gurlek A, Cobankara V, Bayraktar M. Liver tests in hyperthyroidism: effect of antithyroid therapy. J Clin Gastroenterol 1997;24(3):180–3.

43. Penteado KR, Coelho JC, Parolin MB, et al. The influence of end-stage liver disease and liver transplantation on thyroid hormones. Arq Gastroenterol 2015;52(2):124–8.

44. Borzio M, Caldara R, Borzio F, et al. Thyroid function tests in chronic liver disease: evidence for multiple abnormalities despite clinical euthyroidism. Gut 1983;24(7):631–6.

45. Green JR, Snitcher EJ, Mowat NA, et al. Thyroid function and thyroid regulation in euthyroid men with chronic liver disease: evidence of multiple abnormalities. Clin Endocrinol 1977;7(6):453–61.

46. L'Age M, Meinhold H, Wenzel KW, et al. Relations between serum levels of TSH, TBG, T4, T3, rT3 and various histologically classified chronic liver diseases. J Endocrinol Invest 1980;3(4):379–83.

47. Guven K, Kelestimur F, Yucesoy M. Thyroid function tests in non-alcoholic cirrhotic patients with hepatic encephalopathy. Eur J Med 1993;2(2):83–5.

48. Kayacetin E, Kisakol G, Kaya A. Low serum total thyroxine and free triiodothyronine in patients with hepatic encephalopathy due to non-alcoholic cirrhosis. Swiss Med Wkly 2003;133(13–14):210–3.

49. Kano T, Kojima T, Takahashi T, et al. Serum thyroid hormone levels in patients with fulminant hepatitis: usefulness of rT3 and the rT3/T3 ratio as prognostic indices. Gastroenterol Jpn 1987;22(3):344–53.

50. Kostopanagiotou G, Kalimeris K, Mourouzis I, et al. Thyroid hormones alterations during acute liver failure: possible underlying mechanisms and consequences. Endocrine 2009;36(2):198–204.

51. Crowe JP, Christensen E, Butler J, et al. Primary biliary cirrhosis: the prevalence of hypothyroidism and its relationship to thyroid autoantibodies and sicca syndrome. Gastroenterology 1980;78(6):1437–41.

52. Elta GH, Sepersky RA, Goldberg MJ, et al. Increased incidence of hypothyroidism in primary biliary cirrhosis. Dig Dis Sci 1983;28(11):971–5.

53. Lindor KD, Gershwin ME, Poupon R, et al. Primary biliary cirrhosis. Hepatology 2009;50(1):291–308.

54. Ahonen P, Myllarniemi S, Sipila I, et al. Clinical variation of autoimmune polyendocrinopathy-candidiasis-ectodermal dystrophy (APECED) in a series of 68 patients. N Engl J Med 1990;322(26):1829–36.
55. Santos LA, Romeiro FG. Diagnosis and management of cirrhosis-related osteoporosis. Biomed Res Int 2016;2016:1423462.
56. Asada S. Glycogenic hepatopathy in type 1 diabetes mellitus. Intern Med 2018; 57(8):1087–92.
57. Regnell SE, Lernmark A. Hepatic steatosis in type 1 diabetes. Rev Diabet Stud 2011;8(4):454–67.
58. Cusi K, Sanyal AJ, Zhang S, et al. Non-alcoholic fatty liver disease (NAFLD) prevalence and its metabolic associations in patients with type 1 diabetes and type 2 diabetes. Diabetes Obes Metab 2017;19(11):1630–4.
59. Palmisano BT, Zhu L, Stafford JM. Role of estrogens in the regulation of liver lipid metabolism. Adv Exp Med Biol 2017;1043:227–56.
60. McKenzie J, Fisher BM, Jaap AJ, et al. Effects of HRT on liver enzyme levels in women with type 2 diabetes: a randomized placebo-controlled trial. Clin Endocrinol 2006;65(1):40–4.
61. Vassilatou E. Nonalcoholic fatty liver disease and polycystic ovary syndrome. World J Gastroenterol 2014;20(26):8351–63.
62. Kim JJ, Kim D, Yim JY, et al. Polycystic ovary syndrome with hyperandrogenism as a risk factor for non-obese non-alcoholic fatty liver disease. Aliment Pharmacol Ther 2017;45(11):1403–12.
63. Chen J, Zhao KN, Liu GB. Estrogen-induced cholestasis: pathogenesis and therapeutic implications. Hepatogastroenterology 2013;60(126):1289–96.
64. Perarnau JM, Bacq Y. Hepatic vascular involvement related to pregnancy, oral contraceptives, and estrogen replacement therapy. Semin Liver Dis 2008;28(3): 315–27.
65. Sinclair M, Grossmann M, Gow PJ, et al. Testosterone in men with advanced liver disease: abnormalities and implications. J Gastroenterol Hepatol 2015;30(2): 244–51.
66. Zietz B, Lock G, Plach B, et al. Dysfunction of the hypothalamic-pituitary-glandular axes and relation to Child-Pugh classification in male patients with alcoholic and virus-related cirrhosis. Eur J Gastroenterol Hepatol 2003;15(5): 495–501.
67. Foresta C, Schipilliti M, Ciarleglio FA, et al. Male hypogonadism in cirrhosis and after liver transplantation. J Endocrinol Invest 2008;31(5):470–8.
68. Guechot J, Chazouilleres O, Loria A, et al. Effect of liver transplantation on sex-hormone disorders in male patients with alcohol-induced or post-viral hepatitis advanced liver disease. J Hepatol 1994;20(3):426–30.
69. Sorrell JH, Brown JR. Sexual functioning in patients with end-stage liver disease before and after transplantation. Liver Transplant 2006;12(10):1473–7.
70. Jones TH, Kennedy RL. Cytokines and hypothalamic-pituitary function. Cytokine 1993;5(6):531–8.
71. Sinclair M, Gow PJ, Grossmann M, et al. Low serum testosterone is associated with adverse outcome in men with cirrhosis independent of the model for end-stage liver disease score. Liver Transplant 2016;22(11):1482–90.
72. Boulton R, Hamilton MI, Dhillon AP, et al. Subclinical Addison's disease: a cause of persistent abnormalities in transaminase values. Gastroenterology 1995; 109(4):1324–7.
73. Olsson RG, Lindgren A, Zettergren L. Liver involvement in Addison's disease. Am J Gastroenterol 1990;85(4):435–8.

74. Ersan Ö, Demirezer B. Addison's disease: a rare cause of hypertransaminasaemia. Dig Dis Sci 2008;53(12):3269–71.
75. Papanastasiou L, Fountoulakis S, Vatalas IA. Adrenal disorders and non-alcoholic fatty liver disease. Minerva Endocrinol 2017;42(2):151–63.
76. Matsumoto T, Yamasaki S, Arakawa A, et al. Exposure to a high total dosage of glucocorticoids produces non-alcoholic steatohepatits. Pathol Int 2007;57(6): 388–9.
77. Wada T, Ohshima S, Fujisawa E, et al. Aldosterone inhibits insulin-induced glucose uptake by degradation of insulin receptor substrate (IRS) 1 and IRS2 via a reactive oxygen species-mediated pathway in 3T3-L1 adipocytes. Endocrinology 2009;150(4):1662–9.
78. Yamashita R, Kikuchi T, Mori Y, et al. Aldosterone stimulates gene expression of hepatic gluconeogenic enzymes through the glucocorticoid receptor in a manner independent of the protein kinase B cascade. Endocr J 2004;51(2):243–51.
79. Fallo F, Dalla Pozza A, Tecchio M, et al. Nonalcoholic fatty liver disease in primary aldosteronism: a pilot study. Am J Hypertens 2010;23(1):2–5.
80. Chen W, Li F, He C, et al. Elevated prevalence of abnormal glucose metabolism in patients with primary aldosteronism: a meta-analysis. Ir J Med Sci 2014;183(2): 283–91.
81. Catena C, Lapenna R, Baroselli S, et al. Insulin sensitivity in patients with primary aldosteronism: a follow-up study. J Clin Endocrinol Metab 2006;91(9):3457–63.
82. Wada T, Kenmochi H, Miyashita Y, et al. Spironolactone improves glucose and lipid metabolism by ameliorating hepatic steatosis and inflammation and suppressing enhanced gluconeogenesis induced by high-fat and high-fructose diet. Endocrinology 2010;151(5):2040–9.
83. Noguchi R, Yoshiji H, Ikenaka Y, et al. Selective aldosterone blocker ameliorates the progression of non-alcoholic steatohepatitis in rats. Int J Mol Med 2010;26(3): 407–13.
84. Yang Y, Wei RB, Xing Y, et al. A meta-analysis of the effect of angiotensin receptor blockers and calcium channel blockers on blood pressure, glycemia and the HOMA-IR index in non-diabetic patients. Metabolism 2013;62(12):1858–66.
85. Georgescu EF, Ionescu R, Niculescu M, et al. Angiotensin-receptor blockers as therapy for mild-to-moderate hypertension-associated non-alcoholic steatohepatitis. World J Gastroenterol 2009;15(8):942–54.
86. Goh GB, Pagadala MR, Dasarathy J, et al. Renin-angiotensin system and fibrosis in non-alcoholic fatty liver disease. Liver Int 2015;35(3):979–85.
87. Eun CR, Ahn JH, Seo JA, et al. Pheochromocytoma with markedly abnormal liver function tests and severe leukocytosis. Endocrinol Metab (Seoul) 2014;29(1): 83–90.
88. Oben JA, Roskams T, Yang S, et al. Hepatic fibrogenesis requires sympathetic neurotransmitters. Gut 2004;53(3):438–45.
89. Sigala B, McKee C, Soeda J, et al. Sympathetic nervous system catecholamines and neuropeptide Y neurotransmitters are upregulated in human NAFLD and modulate the fibrogenic function of hepatic stellate cells. PLoS One 2013;8(9): e72928.
90. Trifan A, Chiriac S, Stanciu C. Update on adrenal insufficiency in patients with liver cirrhosis. World J Gastroenterol 2013;19(4):445–56.
91. Fede G, Spadaro L, Privitera G, et al. Hypothalamus-pituitary dysfunction is common in patients with stable cirrhosis and abnormal low dose synacthen test. Dig Liver Dis 2015;47(12):1047–51.

92. Singh RR, Walia R, Sachdeva N, et al. Relative adrenal insufficiency in cirrhotic patients with ascites (hepatoadrenal syndrome). Dig Liver Dis 2018;50(11): 1232-7.
93. Park SH, Joo MS, Kim BH, et al. Clinical characteristics and prevalence of adrenal insufficiency in hemodynamically stable patients with cirrhosis. Medicine (Baltimore) 2018;97(26):e11046.
94. Acevedo J, Fernandez J, Prado V, et al. Relative adrenal insufficiency in decompensated cirrhosis: relationship to short-term risk of severe sepsis, hepatorenal syndrome, and death. Hepatology 2013;58(5):1757-65.
95. Yaguchi H, Tsutsumi K, Shimono K, et al. Involvement of high density lipoprotein as substrate cholesterol for steroidogenesis by bovine adrenal fasciculoreticularis cells. Life Sci 1998;62(16):1387-95.
96. Ettinger WH, Varma VK, Sorci-Thomas M, et al. Cytokines decrease apolipoprotein accumulation in medium from Hep G2 cells. Arterioscler Thromb 1994;14(1): 8-13.
97. Baranova I, Vishnyakova T, Bocharov A, et al. Lipopolysaccharide down regulates both scavenger receptor B1 and ATP binding cassette transporter A1 in RAW cells. Infect Immun 2002;70(6):2995-3003.
98. Gaillard RC, Turnill D, Sappino P, et al. Tumor necrosis factor alpha inhibits the hormonal response of the pituitary gland to hypothalamic releasing factors. Endocrinology 1990;127(1):101-6.
99. Cooper MS, Stewart PM. Corticosteroid insufficiency in acutely ill patients. N Engl J Med 2003;348(8):727-34.

Rheumatologic Diseases and the Liver

Agazi Gebreselassie, MD, MSc[a], Farshad Aduli, MD[b], Charles D. Howell, MD[c,]*

KEYWORDS

- Rheumatologic diseases • Liver injury • Elevated liver enzymes • Hepatotoxicity
- Autoimmune liver disease

KEY POINTS

- There is significant epidemiologic, genetic, and immunologic overlap between immune-mediated rheumatologic diseases and autoimmune liver diseases.
- Many rheumatologic diseases are associated with abnormal liver enzymes without significant parenchymal disease.
- Medications used to treat rheumatologic diseases may cause drug-induced liver injury.
- Primary liver diseases often have rheumatologic manifestations.

INTRODUCTION

Rheumatologic diseases encompass connective tissue disorders, vasculitides, arthritides, and immune-mediated diseases. Although the liver is a lymphoid organ exhibiting immune tolerance, it can be a target of autoimmune diseases.[1] The relationship between rheumatologic diseases and the liver is complex and not fully understood. There is a significant epidemiologic, genetic, and immunologic overlap between immune-mediated rheumatologic diseases and autoimmune liver diseases. Non-immune-mediated rheumatologic diseases may also affect the liver. Most rheumatologic diseases manifest with abnormal liver enzymes without significant parenchymal disease, and the associated liver lesions rarely progress to cirrhosis. A variety of medications used to treat rheumatologic diseases also affect the liver. Conversely, primary liver diseases can have rheumatologic manifestations related to viral hepatitis, autoimmune, and metabolic liver diseases. This article provides an overview on how rheumatologic

Disclosure Statement: The authors have nothing to disclose.
[a] Division of Gastroenterology and Hepatology, Department of Internal Medicine, Howard University Hospital, 2041 Georgia Avenue Northwest, Suite 4J19, Washington, DC 20060, USA;
[b] Division of Gastroenterology and Hepatology, Department of Internal Medicine, Howard University Hospital and College of Medicine, 2041 Georgia Avenue Northwest, Suite 5C22, Washington, DC 20060, USA; [c] Division of Gastroenterology and Hepatology, Department of Internal Medicine, Howard University Hospital and College of Medicine, 2041 Georgia Avenue Northwest, Suite 5C02, Washington, DC 20060, USA
* Corresponding author.
E-mail address: charles.howell@howard.edu

diseases and the medications used to treat them can affect the liver. A comprehensive list of rheumatologic diseases and medications that affect the liver disease is provided in **Tables 1** and **2**.

JOINT PAIN AND THE LIVER

Arthralgia (joint pain) with or without arthritis (joint inflammation), is a common reason for rheumatologic evaluation. There are a variety of liver diseases that manifest with arthralgia and arthritis. Acute viral hepatitis may present with diffuse joint pain that may mimic rheumatologic diseases. Up to 50% of individuals with hepatitis B virus (HBV) or hepatitis C virus (HCV) infection may have joint pain associated with cryoglobulinemia.[2] Some autoimmune liver diseases manifest with arthritis.[3] Metabolic liver diseases such as hemochromatosis and Wilson disease can affect the joints, mimicking osteoarthritis (OA).[4,5]

Table 1
Rheumatologic disorders associated with liver diseases

Rheumatologic Disorder	Associated Liver Disease
Polyarthritis	Acute viral hepatitis, HBV, HCV, autoimmune liver diseases
Mono/oligo arthritis	Hemochromatosis, Wilson disease
SLE	ELE, PBC, AIH, PSC, OS, NRH, BCS
Rheumatoid arthritis	ELE, PBC, AIH, PSC, OS, NAFLD, amyloidosis, EBV
Felty syndrome	ELE, hepatomegaly, NRH
Adult-onset Still disease	Fulminant liver failure
Primary systemic sclerosis	ELE, PBC, AIH, PSC,NRH, cirrhosis, HBV, HCV
Sjögren syndrome	ELE, PBC, AIH, PSC, NRH, pHTN
Fibromyalgia	HCV, cirrhosis
Psoriatic arthritis	NAFLD
MCTD	AIH
Gouty arthritis	NAFLD
Inflammatory myopathies	ELE, hepatitis C, HCC
Systemic vasculitis	
Takayasu arteritis and giant cell arthritis	Hepatic artery vasculitis
PAN	HBV. hepatic artery vasculitis, ELE
Polyangiitis, eosinophilic granulomatosis with polyangiitis, and microscopic polyangiitis	PBC, AIH
Cryoglobulinemic vasculitis	HCV, HBV
Lupus vasculitis, antiphospholipid syndrome	Hepatomegaly, steatosis, ELE, chronic active hepatitis, granulomatous disease and cirrhosis, BCS
IgG4 disease	Sclerosing cholangitis, obstructive jaundice (from external compression), ELE
Osteoporosis	Cholestasis, cirrhosis, glucocorticoids

Abbreviations: AIH, autoimmune hepatitis; BSC, Budd-Chiari syndrome; EBV, Epstein-Barr virus; ELE, elevated liver enzymes; HBV, hepatitis B virus; HCV, hepatitis C virus; IgG4, immunoglobulin G4; NAFLD, non-alcoholic fatty liver disease; NRH, nodular regenerative hyperplasia; OS, overlap syndrome; PBC, primary biliary cholangitis; pHTN, portal hypertension; PSC, primary sclerosing cholangitis.

Table 2	
Medications used in rheumatologic diseases and associated liver disorders	
Medication	**Associated Liver Disease**
Acetaminophen	ELE, liver failure
NSAIDs	ELE, acute hepatitis, cholestatic disease, acute liver failure and ductopenia
Colchicine	ELE
Allopurinol	ELE, DRESS, acute liver failure
Glucocorticoids	ELE, NAFLD, HBV reactivation, acute liver failure
Non-biologic DMARDs	
Methotrexate	ELE, NAFLD, fibrosis, acute necrosis
Thiopurines (azathioprine, mercaptopurine)	ELE, hypersensitivity, cholestasis, NRH, veno-occlusive disease
Hydroxychloroquine	Acute hepatitis
Penicillamine	ELE, cholestasis
Sulfasalazine	ELE, hypersensitivity (DRESS)
Leflunomide	ELE, DILI
Cyclophosphamide	ELE, DILI, veno-occlusive disease
Mycophenolate mofetil	ELE, DILI
Cyclosporine	ELE, biliary sludge, cholelithiasis
Apremilast	No reported hepatotoxicity so far (limited experience)
Biologic DMARDs and small molecules	
Anti-TNFs	ELE, hepatitis B reactivation, AIH cholestasis, fulminant hepatitis
Abatacept	ELE, AIH, possible HBV reactivation
Rituximab	ELE, HBV reactivation
Tocilizumab	ELE, DILI
Tofacitinib	ELE
Ustekinumab	ELE, HBV reactivation
Belimumab	Possible HBV reactivation
Interleukin 1b inhibitors	
Anakinra	ELE, DILI
Canakinumab	ELE
Rilonacept	ELE

Abbreviations: AIH, autoimmune hepatitis; DILI, drug-induced liver injury; DMARDs, disease-modifying anti-rheumatic drugs; DRESS, drug reaction with eosinophilia and systemic symptoms; ELE, elevated liver enzymes; HBV, hepatitis B virus; NAFLD, non-alcoholic fatty liver disease; NRH, nodular regenerative hyperplasia; NSAIDs, non-steroidal anti-inflammatory drugs; TNF, tumor necrosis factor.

Obesity and metabolic syndrome, which are risk factors for non-alcoholic fatty liver disease (NAFLD), are also associated with OA, rheumatoid arthritis (RA), and gouty arthritis.[6–9] Patients with cirrhosis are at risk for osteoporosis. Glucocorticoid therapy is associated with osteoporosis and bone fracture.[10]

SYSTEMIC LUPUS ERYTHEMATOSUS

Systemic lupus erythematosus (SLE) is a systemic autoimmune disease that affects multiple organs including the liver. The liver may be involved in 19.4% to 60% of patients with SLE at some point in their illness.[11,12] The most common finding is an elevation in liver enzymes. The leading cause of liver dysfunction in patients with SLE is drug-induced liver injury (31%), followed by SLE-associated hepatitis (29%). Other possible causes for liver disease in SLE are fatty liver disease (18%), autoimmune hepatitis (AIH) (5%), primary biliary cholangitis (PBC) (2%), cholangitis (1.6%), alcohol (1.6%), or viral hepatitis (0.8%).[11] Antiphospholipid syndrome, an autoimmune disorder that is commonly found with SLE, and manifests with arterial and venous thrombosis, is associated with Budd-Chiari syndrome.[13] Liver infarction and very rarely liver rupture from vasculitis have also been reported in patients with SLE.[14]

It is important to differentiate between SLE-associated hepatitis and AIH because of therapeutic and prognostic implications. SLE-associated hepatitis is associated with kidney disease and does not lead to significant liver disease. AIH, however, may lead to significant liver disease including liver failure. Both SLE-associated hepatitis and AIH manifest with polyarthralgia, elevated gamma globulins, and a positive antinuclear antibody creating a diagnostic dilemma. Serum antibodies, complement levels, and liver histology can help to differentiate between SLE-associated hepatitis and AIH. A summary of distinguishing characteristics between the 2 disease entities is given in **Table 3**. The liver histologic abnormalities in SLE include portal, periportal, or lobular hepatitis with or without necrosis, cholestasis, steatosis, small artery vasculitis, granulomatous hepatitis, nodular regenerative hyperplasia (NRH), and peliosis hepatitis.[15] The characteristic histologic features of AIH are portal mononuclear infiltrates that can invade the limiting plate, and infiltrate into the surrounding lobule causing periportal piecemeal necrosis. An AIH-SLE overlap syndrome may also occur.[16]

RA

RA is a systemic autoimmune disorder, which typically presents with symmetric inflammation of multiple joints. Liver enzyme elevation can occur in up to 50% of patients with RA. More than 60% of patients with RA may have abnormal liver histology.[17] The most common liver histologic findings in RA include mild chronic inflammatory infiltration of the portal tract, small foci of hepatocyte necrosis, and fatty liver. Fibrotic liver disease is rare thus limiting the need for routine liver biopsy before starting methotrexate therapy.[18]

Medications used to treat RA such as non-steroidal anti-inflammatory drugs (NSAIDs) and disease-modifying anti-rheumatic drugs (DMARDs) may also cause

Table 3		
Distinguishing characteristics between SLE-associated hepatitis and autoimmune hepatitis		
	SLE-Associated Hepatitis	AIH
C3/C4	Low	Normal
Anti-SMA antibodies	Negative	Positive
Anti-LKM and anti-LPA	Negative	Positive
Anti-ribosomal P antibodies	Elevated	Normal
Liver histology	Portal, periportal, or lobular hepatitis with or without hepatocyte necrosis	Mononuclear infiltrates that invade the limiting plate
Prognosis	Associated with kidney failure	May lead to liver failure

Abbreviations: AIH, autoimmune hepatitis; anti-LKM, anti-liver kidney microsomal; anti-LPA, anti-liver pancreas antigen; anti-SMA, anti-smooth muscle antibody.

elevation in liver enzymes. Liver dysfunction related to RA usually does not progress to cirrhosis. There are few reports of spontaneous liver rupture associated with RA, which is most likely related to rheumatoid vasculitis.[19] NRH with portal hypertension can also occur in the presence or absence of Felty syndrome (discussed later).[20,21]

There is an increased prevalence of autoimmune liver diseases such as PBC, AIH, and PSC (primary sclerosing cholangitis) in patients with RA.[22] PBC occurs in up to 10% of patients.[23] Up to 27% of patients with autoimmune liver disease have elevated levels of rheumatoid factor (RF). Anti-cyclic citrullinated peptide antibody positivity seems to be more specific than RF to diagnose RA in patients with autoimmune and HCV-related liver disease.[24]

Patients with RA are also at risk to develop NAFLD. Possible risk factors for NAFLD in RA are chronic inflammation, methotrexate, and steroid use.[25] Amyloidosis presenting with hepatomegaly can also be seen in patients with RA.[23]

Felty syndrome, a triad of RA, neutropenia, and splenomegaly, is associated with hepatomegaly, abnormal liver tests, NRH, and portal hypertension. Patients with Felty syndrome should be screened for the presence of liver disease, portal hypertension, and esophageal varices.[21]

SJÖGREN SYNDROME

Sjögren syndrome (SS) is an autoimmune disease primarily affecting the exocrine glands (salivary, lacrimal, pancreas, and other exocrine glands). The diagnosis is primarily based on typical sicca symptoms (dry mouth and eyes), as well as glandular and extra-glandular manifestations. Forty-nine percent of patients with SS have abnormal serum liver tests, and clinical evidence of liver disease is found in 27% of the patients.[26,27] Liver diseases associated with SS include, PBC, AIH, viral hepatitis (B and C), sclerosing cholangitis, NRH, and cirrhosis.[27–30] Up to 13% of patients with SS have HCV infection and there is a significant overlap between the two in terms of symptoms, histologic findings, and serum antibodies. There is predominance of cryoglobulins and low complement levels in viral hepatitis, whereas there is high frequency of autoantibodies (anti-Ro/SS-A and anti-La/SS-B antibodies) in SS.[27] SS also shares features of immunoglobulin G4 (IgG4)-related disease, which involves the pancreaticobiliary system.[31]

SYSTEMIC SCLEROSIS

Systemic sclerosis (SSc) is a systemic disease characterized by fibrosis, vasculopathy, and immune dysfunction.[32] The gastrointestinal tract is affected in up to 95% of patients with SSc. The liver is rarely affected in SSc (1.1%).[33] The most common associated liver disease is PBC occurring in up to 22%.[34] AIH, idiopathic portal hypertension, NRH, and PSC have been also reported in association with SSc.[32] PBC is more associated with the limited cutaneous type of SSc, which has positivity for anti-centromere antibodies and anti-topoisomerase antibodies.[34] PBC/SSc overlap liver disease has a slower progression when compared with PBC alone.[35]

SPONDYLOARTHRITIS

Spondyloarthritis (SpA) refers to a group of rheumatologic conditions that primarily affect the axial skeleton, tendons, and entheses (insertion of tendon to bone).[36] These include ankylosing spondylitis (AS), reactive arthritis, psoriatic arthritis, undifferentiated arthritis, and enteropathy-associated arthritis (inflammatory bowel disease-associated arthritis). Psoriatic arthritis has been shown to be associated with

NAFLD.[37] Generalized pustular psoriasis, an uncommon type of psoriasis has been associated with neutrophilic cholangitis with magnetic resonance cholangiopancreatography features similar to PSC.[38] Elevated alkaline phosphatase and gamma-glutamyl transpeptidase are reported with AS.[39] HLA-B27-positive enthesopathy has also been reported in PBC.[40]

CRYSTAL ARTHROPATHIES

Crystal arthropathies are characterized by deposition of crystals in the synovium with inflammation. These include entities such as gouty arthritis, calcium pyrophosphate deposition, and basic calcium phosphate deposition. Gout is the most common inflammatory arthritis and results from crystallization of excessive levels of uric acid. Hyperuricemia is closely associated with metabolic syndrome. There is a global rise in the prevalence of gouty arthritis, which parallels the increase in hypertension, cardiovascular disease, insulin resistance, and obesity.[8] Increased consumption of fructose also predisposes to hyperuricemia, which leads to NAFLD and liver inflammation.[41] There is some evidence that controlling hyperuricemia with medications might improve metabolic syndrome.[42] Medications used for gout treatment such as colchicine, allopurinol, and febuxostat can occasionally cause hepatotoxicity.[43-45]

SYSTEMIC VASCULITIS

Vasculitis refers to the inflammation of the vascular system including arteries, veins, or capillaries. Large-, medium-, or small-sized vessels can be affected. It can be idiopathic, secondary to antigen trigger, or an autoimmune condition. The liver is not usually a primary target of vasculitis diseases.[46] However, large-vessel vasculitis, such as Takayasu arteritis and giant cell arthritis, may involve the hepatic artery.[47,48] Polyarteritis nodosa (PAN) is a medium-vessel vasculitis that may also cause hepatomegaly and elevated liver enzymes as a result of hepatic vascular involvement.[49] HBV infections are also associated with PAN.[50] There are reports that small-vessel vasculitis, such as granulomatosis with polyangiitis, eosinophilic granulomatosis with polyangiitis, and microscopic polyangiitis, can be associated with autoimmune liver diseases such as PBC and AIH.[51-53] HBV and HCV infections are associated with cryoglobulinemic vasculitis, which is characterized by palpable purpura, joint pain, peripheral neuropathy, glomerulonephritis, and involvement of other organs.[54,55] Lupus cytoclastic vasculitis is associated with hepatomegaly, steatosis, abnormal liver enzymes, chronic active hepatitis, granulomatous disease, and cirrhosis.[46] Antiphospholipid syndrome may result in Budd-Chiarl syndrome due to thrombosis of the hepatic vein.[13]

INFLAMMATORY AND VIRAL MYOPATHIES

Inflammatory myopathies are a group of disorders characterized by immune-mediated muscle inflammation, which results in muscle weakness. The group includes polymyositis, dermatomyositis, inclusion body myositis, immune-medicated necrotizing myopathy, and overlap syndromes (with another systemic rheumatic disease). There is usually an elevation of aspartate aminotransferase (AST) and alanine aminotransferase (ALT) in inflammatory myopathies. The origin of the enzyme elevation is from muscle and not the liver, and AST is usually more elevated than ALT.[56] Muscle-specific enzymes such as creatinine phosphokinase and myoglobin are usually concomitantly elevated.[57] A cholestatic pattern of enzyme elevation should alert the possibility of underlying liver disease.

Dermatomyositis can occur with a PBC-AIH overlap syndrome or as a paraneoplastic manifestation of hepatocellular carcinoma.[58–60] Hepatitis C and E are occasionally associated with myositis.[61,62]

OTHER RHEUMATOLOGIC DISORDERS AND THE LIVER

Mixed connective tissue disease (MCTD) is an overlap syndrome of SLE, SSc, and polymyositis along with high levels of anti-U1RNP antibodies. There are few case reports of AIH associated with MCTD.[63,64]

Adult-onset Still disease is characterized by polyarthralgia, rash, fever, and leukocytosis. Elevated liver enzymes and hepatomegaly have been reported in up to 62% and 11% of patients, respectively. There are also reports fulminant liver failure in adult-onset Still disease.[65,66]

Fibromyalgia (FM) is a clinical condition characterized by widespread chronic pain, tenderness of skin and muscle to pressure, fatigue, sleep disturbance, and exercise intolerance.[67] The prevalence of FM among patients with HCV infection was found to be 19%.[68] Up to 27% of patients with cirrhosis have FM. HCV and non-alcoholic steatohepatitis-related cirrhosis are significantly associated with FM.[69]

IgG4 disease is an immune-mediated fibroinflammatory disease that is characterized by infiltration of plasma cells in tissues. Almost any organ can be affected by the disease. It predominantly affects middle-aged to elderly patients.[70] It causes sclerosing cholangitis in 4% to 10% of affected individuals.[71,72] Among patients with auto-immune pancreatitis, up to 24% have associated liver involvement.[73,74] When the liver is affected, patients usually present with obstructive jaundice and abnormal liver tests.[31,75] Diagnosis is made by tissue biopsy and demonstration of characteristic histology. Treatment involves immunosuppressive therapy with rapid improvement but relapse is common.[72]

VIRAL HEPATITIS AND RHEUMATOLOGIC DISEASES

Acute and chronic viral hepatitis can cause diffuse joint and muscle pain mimicking a variety of rheumatologic disorders. HBV infection is associated with PAN, mixed cryoglobulinemia, and arthritis.[54] HCV infection is associated with mixed cryoglobulinemia, cryoglobulinemic vasculitis, arthralgia, arthritis, fibromyalgia, PAN, Behcet disease, vasculitis, Raynaud syndrome, Sjögren syndrome, and SLE.[27,55,76] Antiviral therapy for HBV and HCV infection has an important role in the treatment of cryoglobulinemia.[77] It is important to screen patients with rheumatologic diseases for HBV and HCV infections to provide early treatment and prevent viral reactivation or worsening of preexisting disease after starting immunosuppressive therapy.

MEDICATION-RELATED LIVER TOXICITY

A variety of medications are used to treat rheumatologic diseases (see **Table 2**). Most of these medications cause a transient elevation in liver enzymes, but the liver damage can sometimes progress to chronic liver disease, fibrosis, cirrhosis, or fulminant liver failure. Some medications have a direct hepatotoxic effect, whereas others affect the liver indirectly by reactivating latent infections or inducing an autoimmune disease.

Acetaminophen

Acetaminophen is commonly used as a pain reliever in patients with arthritis. It is usually the first-line medication recommended for mild to moderate OA because of its analgesic efficacy and presumed tolerability. Acetaminophen can cause dose-dependent liver failure specially when associated with alcohol abuse. Acetaminophen doses should be limited to 4 g daily in patients who do not have preexisting liver disease. In patients with underlying liver disease and the elderly, doses should be limited to 2 g daily or less.[78]

NSAIDs

Non-steroidal anti-inflammatory drugs are the most frequently used medications, both as prescription and as over-the-counter drugs. They can cause mild elevation of liver enzymes in up to 15% of patients, which normalizes after discontinuation.[79,80] Acute hepatitis, cholestatic disease, acute liver failure, and ductopenia have been reported with NSAID use.[81,82] Salicylates cause dose-dependent liver damage. Although almost all types of NSAIDs are reported to cause elevation in liver enzymes, diclofenac and sulindac are more likely to be associated with hepatotoxicity.[79] Ibuprofen and naproxen are the least hepatotoxic.[81] Cyclooxygenase-2 inhibitors, such as celecoxib, seem to be less hepatotoxic than non-selective NSAIDs.[83] Concomitant use of other anti-rheumatic medications with NSAIDs increases the risk of hepatotoxicity.[79]

Glucocorticoids

Glucocorticoids are extensively prescribed for a variety of rheumatologic diseases. Chronic corticosteroid use is associated with fatty liver disease.[84] A short course of high-dose intravenous corticosteroids, such as methylprednisolone, may also cause acute liver failure.[85] There is a risk of HBV infection reactivation depending on the dose and duration of use of the glucocorticoid and the hepatitis B surface antigen (HBsAg)/hepatitis B core antibody (HBc) status of the patient. Patients on prednisone (or equivalent) doses of ≥10 mg daily for ≥ 4 weeks and who are HBsAg-positive/anti-HBc-positive are considered to be high risk (>10%) for HBV reactivation. Patients on prednisone doses ≥10 mg daily for ≥4 weeks, but who are HBsAg-negative/HBc-positive are considered moderate risk (1%–10%). Those who are on a low dose of prednisone (<10 mg) for ≥4 weeks and HBsAg-positive/HBc-positive are also considered moderate risk. Anti-viral prophylaxis is recommended for both the- high and moderate-risk groups.[86]

Non-biologic (synthetic) DMARDs

Sulfasalazine can cause acute liver injury in 0.1% of patients with arthritis. The liver injury can be part of hypersensitivity or DRESS (drug rash, eosinophilia, systemic symptoms) syndrome. It usually occurs in the first month of treatment and has hepatocellular or cholestatic pattern.[87] Liver enzyme elevations can occur in 5% of patients on leflunomide, which usually occurs in the first 6 months of treatment. Cases of acute liver failure have been reported and close monitoring is suggested in the first few months after starting treatment.[87]

Methotrexate is a commonly used DMARD to treat various rheumatologic diseases, particularly RA. It can cause asymptomatic elevation of liver enzymes, steatosis, liver fibrosis, and, rarely, acute necrosis.[88] A recent meta-analysis showed that liver-related adverse effects occurred in 11.2% of patients on methotrexate-treated patients compared with 6.3% in the control group. The prevalence of minor liver enzyme elevation (≤3 upper limit of normal) was 7.9% in the methotrexate group and 5.2% in the control group. Major enzyme elevations (>3 upper limit of normal) were found to be 3.3% and 1%, respectively. The occurrence of liver failure, fibrosis, cirrhosis, or death was very rare.[89] Other confounding factors, such as alcohol use, fatty liver disease, and concomitant NSAIDs, may also contribute to elevation in liver enzymes.[90] Serious liver complications are not common with methotrexate use.[89] As methotrexate is a corner stone in the therapy of many rheumatologic disorders, other potential causes of mild liver enzyme elevation should be ruled out before stopping treatment.[91] If methotrexate-related hepatotoxicity is suspected, doses can be reduced and patients should be monitored closely. Methotrexate is usually stopped when liver enzymes increase to more than 3 times the upper limit after it is initiated.[92] When there is mild liver enzyme elevation, treatment can be continued with close monitoring.[91] Cumulative doses of 1 to 10 g are associated with liver histologic abnormalities and some degree of fibrosis. The risk of liver fibrosis with prolonged use of low-dose methotrexate (10 mg/wk) is very low. Liver biopsy is rarely needed. It is only indicated to rule out other potential causes of liver enzyme elevation and persistence of elevated liver enzymes despite stopping the medication.[87,92] Folate administration with methotrexate may reduce the frequency of liver enzyme elevations.

Thiopurine analogues (azathioprine and mercaptopurine) are used in a variety of inflammatory disorders. Liver injury is reported in 0.1% to 2% of patients on azathioprine.[87] Asymptomatic elevation of liver enzymes usually improves with or without dosage modifications.[93] Thiopurine-induced hepatotoxicity may be a hypersensitivity reaction, an idiosyncratic cholestatic reaction, or vascular endothelial cell injury.[94] Endothelial injury may lead to NRH and hepatic veno-occlusive disease.[87]

Biologic DMARDs

Biologic DMARDs are molecules, usually monoclonal antibodies, that are directed to inhibit a specific activity in the cascade of immune response. They are being increasingly used for a variety of inflammatory disorders including rheumatologic diseases.

Anti-tumor necrosis factor (anti-TNF) drugs (infliximab, etanercept, adalimumab, golimumab, certolizumab) are commonly used after failure of non-biologic DMARDs. Asymptomatic liver enzyme elevation of 2 to 3 times the upper normal limit can occur in 37% to 42% of patients at some point during treatment. It is usually possible to continue anti-TNF drugs with close monitoring in patients with mildly elevated liver enzymes.[95] Other potential causes of liver enzyme elevation should also be ruled out. Immune-mediated hepatitis (including AIH-like entities), cholestatic liver disease, and fulminant hepatitis secondary to hepatitis B reactivation, have been reported with anti-TNF drugs.[95] HBsAg-positive individuals should be started on prophylactic anti-viral treatment before anti-TNF drugs are started, whereas those who have positive HBc require close monitoring.[96] Anti-TNF medications seem to be safe to use in patients with hepatitis C infection, although further studies are needed to assess this.[87,97]

Rituximab is an anti-CD 20 antibody that is used in the treatment of moderate to severe RA in combination to methotrexate when anti-TNF medications fail. It is associated with reactivation of hepatitis B in HBsAg-positive and HBsAg-negative/HBc-positive patients.[98] Thus, anti-viral prophylaxis should be offered to these patients. Elevation in liver enzymes has been observed in patients with hepatitis C infection when started on rituximab. Careful monitoring is suggested if anti-viral therapy is not provided.[99]

SUMMARY

Rheumatologic diseases are common and can coexist with immune-mediated and non-immune-mediated liver disorders. Patients with SLE, RA, SS, and SSc can develop autoimmune liver diseases such as PBC, AIH, PSC, or overlap syndrome. NRH can occur with SLE, RA, SS, and azathioprine use. Gout, a non-immunologic rheumatic disease is associated with NAFLD. It is important for the health care providers to consider rheumatologic diseases and their treatment as part of the differential diagnoses of abnormal liver enzymes and liver dysfunction. The armamentarium for the treatment of rheumatologic diseases is ever increasing, thus mandating an awareness of the potential side effects of these medications and a close working relationship and collaboration with rheumatologists.

REFERENCES

1. Gao B. Basic liver immunology. Cell Mol Immunol 2016;13(3):265–6.
2. Aydeniz A, Namiduru M, Karaoglan I, et al. Rheumatic manifestations of hepatitis B and C and their association with viral load and fibrosis of the liver. Rheumatol Int 2010;30(4):515–7.
3. Selmi C, Generali E, Gershwin ME. Rheumatic manifestations in autoimmune liver disease. Rheum Dis Clin North Am 2018;44(1):65–87.
4. Yu H, Xie JJ, Chen YC, et al. Clinical features and outcome in patients with osseomuscular type of Wilson's disease. BMC Neurol 2017;17(1):34.
5. Dallos T, Sahinbegovic E, Stamm T, et al. Idiopathic hand osteoarthritis vs haemochromatosis arthropathy–a clinical, functional and radiographic study. Rheumatology (Oxford) 2013;52(5):910–5.
6. Lementowski PW, Zelicof SB. Obesity and osteoarthritis. Am J Orthop (Belle Mead NJ) 2008;37(3):148–51.
7. Bellentani S, Marino M. Epidemiology and natural history of non-alcoholic fatty liver disease (NAFLD). Ann Hepatol 2009;8(Suppl 1):S4–8.
8. Thottam GE, Krasnokutsky S, Pillinger MH. Gout and metabolic syndrome: a tangled web. Curr Rheumatol Rep 2017;19(10):60.
9. Qin B, Yang M, Fu H, et al. Body mass index and the risk of rheumatoid arthritis: a systematic review and dose-response meta-analysis. Arthritis Res Ther 2015; 17:86.
10. Santos LA, Romeiro FG. Diagnosis and management of cirrhosis-related osteoporosis. Biomed Res Int 2016;2016:1423462.
11. Takahashi A, Abe K, Saito R, et al. Liver dysfunction in patients with systemic lupus erythematosus. Intern Med 2013;52(13):1461–5.
12. Efe C, Purnak T, Ozaslan E, et al. Autoimmune liver disease in patients with systemic lupus erythematosus: a retrospective analysis of 147 cases. Scand J Gastroenterol 2011;46(6):732–7.
13. Uthman I, Khamashta M. The abdominal manifestations of the antiphospholipid syndrome. Rheumatology (Oxford) 2007;46(11):1641–7.
14. Mor F, Beigel Y, Inbal A, et al. Hepatic infarction in a patient with the lupus anticoagulant. Arthritis Rheum 1989;32(4):491–5.
15. Matsumoto T, Yoshimine T, Shimouchi K, et al. The liver in systemic lupus erythematosus: pathologic analysis of 52 cases and review of Japanese Autopsy Registry Data. Hum Pathol 1992;23(10):1151–8.
16. Adiga A, Nugent K. Lupus hepatitis and autoimmune hepatitis (lupoid hepatitis). Am J Med Sci 2017;353(4):329–35.
17. Selmi C, De Santis M, Gershwin ME. Liver involvement in subjects with rheumatic disease. Arthritis Res Ther 2011;13(3):226.
18. Ruderman EM, Crawford JM, Maier A, et al. Histologic liver abnormalities in an autopsy series of patients with rheumatoid arthritis. Br J Rheumatol 1997;36(2): 210–3.

19. Lee JE, Kim IJ, Cho MS, et al. A case of rheumatoid vasculitis involving hepatic artery in early rheumatoid arthritis. J Korean Med Sci 2017;32(7):1207–10.

20. Goritsas C, Roussos A, Ferti A, et al. Nodular regenerative hyperplasia in a rheumatoid arthritis patient without Felty's syndrome. J Clin Gastroenterol 2002;35(4): 363–4.

21. Thorne C, Urowitz MB, Wanless I, et al. Liver disease in Felty's syndrome. Am J Med 1982;73(1):35–40.

22. Liaskos C, Bogdanos DP, Rigopoulou EI, et al. Development of antimitochondrial antibodies in patients with autoimmune hepatitis: art of facts or an artifact? J Gastroenterol Hepatol 2007;22(3):454–5.

23. Radovanovic-Dinic B, Tesic-Rajkovic S, Zivkovic V, et al. Clinical connection between rheumatoid arthritis and liver damage. Rheumatol Int 2018;38(5):715–24.

24. Koga T, Migita K, Miyashita T, et al. Determination of anti-cyclic citrullinated peptide antibodies in the sera of patients with liver diseases. Clin Exp Rheumatol 2008;26(1):121–4.

25. Chalasani N, Younossi Z, Lavine JE, et al. The diagnosis and management of non-alcoholic fatty liver disease: practice guideline by the American Association for the Study of Liver Diseases, American College of Gastroenterology, and the American Gastroenterological Association. Am J Gastroenterol 2012;107(6): 811–26.

26. Kaplan MJ, Ike RW. The liver is a common non-exocrine target in primary Sjogren's syndrome: a retrospective review. BMC Gastroenterol 2002;2:21.

27. Ramos-Casals M, Sanchez-Tapias JM, Pares A, et al. Characterization and differentiation of autoimmune versus viral liver involvement in patients with Sjogren's syndrome. J Rheumatol 2006;33(8):1593–9.

28. Montefusco PP, Geiss AC, Bronzo RL, et al. Sclerosing cholangitis, chronic pancreatitis, and Sjogren's syndrome: a syndrome complex. Am J Surg 1984; 147(6):822–6.

29. Lindgren S, Manthorpe R, Eriksson S. Autoimmune liver disease in patients with primary Sjogren's syndrome. J Hepatol 1994;20(3):354–8.

30. Scott CA, Avellini C, Desinan L, et al. Chronic lymphocytic sialoadenitis in HCV-related chronic liver disease: comparison of Sjogren's syndrome. Histopathology 1997;30(1):41–8.

31. Ghazale A, Chari ST, Zhang L, et al. Immunoglobulin G4-associated cholangitis: clinical profile and response to therapy. Gastroenterology 2008;134(3):706–15.

32. Frech TM, Mar D. Gastrointestinal and hepatic disease in systemic sclerosis. Rheum Dis Clin North Am 2018;44(1):15–28.

33. Forbes A, Marie I. Gastrointestinal complications: the most frequent internal complications of systemic sclerosis. Rheumatology (Oxford) 2009;48(Suppl 3):iii36–9.

34. Assassi S, Fritzler MJ, Arnett FC, et al. Primary biliary cirrhosis (PBC), PBC autoantibodies, and hepatic parameter abnormalities in a large population of systemic sclerosis patients. J Rheumatol 2009;36(10):2250–6.

35. Liberal R, Grant CR, Sakkas L, et al. Diagnostic and clinical significance of anti-centromere antibodies in primary biliary cirrhosis. Clin Res Hepatol Gastroenterol 2013;37(6):572–85.

36. Caplan L, Kuhn KA. Gastrointestinal and hepatic disease in spondyloarthritis. Rheum Dis Clin North Am 2018;44(1):153–64.

37. van der Voort EA, Koehler EM, Dowlatshahi EA, et al. Psoriasis is independently associated with nonalcoholic fatty liver disease in patients 55 years old or older: results from a population-based study. J Am Acad Dermatol 2014;70(3):517–24.

38. Viguier M, Allez M, Zagdanski AM, et al. High frequency of cholestasis in generalized pustular psoriasis: evidence for neutrophilic involvement of the biliary tract. Hepatology 2004;40(2):452–8.
39. Robinson AC, Teeling M, Casey EB. Hepatic function in ankylosing spondylitis. Ann Rheum Dis 1983;42(5):550–2.
40. Kung YY, Tsai CY, Tsai YY, et al. Enthesopathy in a case of primary biliary cirrhosis with positive HLA-B27. Clin Exp Rheumatol 1997;15(6):708–9.
41. Johnson RJ, Perez-Pozo SE, Sautin YY, et al. Hypothesis: could excessive fructose intake and uric acid cause type 2 diabetes? Endocr Rev 2009;30(1):96–116.
42. Lanaspa MA, Sanchez-Lozada LG, Cicerchi C, et al. Uric acid stimulates fructokinase and accelerates fructose metabolism in the development of fatty liver. PLoS One 2012;7(10):e47948.
43. Bohm M, Vuppalanchi R, Chalasani N. Drug-Induced Liver Injury Network. Febuxostat-induced acute liver injury. Hepatology 2016;63(3):1047–9.
44. Abbott CE, Xu R, Sigal SH. Colchicine-induced hepatotoxicity. ACG Case Rep J 2017;4:e120.
45. Iqbal U, Siddiqui HU, Anwar H, et al. Allopurinol-induced granulomatous hepatitis: a case report and review of literature. J Investig Med High Impact Case Rep 2017;5(3). 2324709617728302.
46. Bailey M, Chapin W, Licht H, et al. The effects of vasculitis on the gastrointestinal tract and liver. Gastroenterol Clin North Am 1998;27(4):747–82, v-vi.
47. Nakao K, Ikeda M, Kimata S, et al. Takayasu's arteritis. Clinical report of eighty-four cases and immunological studies of seven cases. Circulation 1967;35(6): 1141–55.
48. Lee S, Childerhouse A, Moss K. Gastrointestinal symptoms and granulomatous vasculitis involving the liver in giant cell arteritis: a case report and review of the literature. Rheumatology (Oxford) 2011;50(12):2316–7.
49. Bassel K, Harford W. Gastrointestinal manifestations of collagen-vascular diseases. Semin Gastrointest Dis 1995;6(4):228–40.
50. Guillevin L, Le Thi Huong D, Godeau P, et al. Clinical findings and prognosis of polyarteritis nodosa and Churg-Strauss angiitis: a study in 165 patients. Br J Rheumatol 1988;27(4):258–64.
51. Ruiz-Ferreras E, Martin-Arribas A, Tabernero-Fernandez G, et al. Microscopic polyangiitis in a patient with primary biliary cirrhosis: treatment complications. Nefrologia 2016;36(1):78–80.
52. Tovoli F, Vannini A, Fusconi M, et al. Autoimmune liver disorders and small-vessel vasculitis: four case reports and review of the literature. Ann Hepatol 2013;13(1): 136–41.
53. Lohani S, Nazir S, Tachamo N, et al. Autoimmune hepatitis and eosinophilic granulomatosis with polyangiitis: a rare association. BMJ Case Rep 2017;2017.
54. Han SH. Extrahepatic manifestations of chronic hepatitis B. Clin Liver Dis 2004; 8(2):403–18.
55. Cacoub P, Comarmond C, Domont F, et al. Extrahepatic manifestations of chronic hepatitis C virus infection. Ther Adv Infect Dis 2016;3(1):3–14.
56. Schneeberger EE, Arriola MS, Fainboim H, et al. Idiophatic inflammatory myophaties: its asociation with liver disorders. Rev Fac Cien Med Univ Nac Cordoba 2012;69(3):139–43 [in Spanish].
57. Volochayev R, Csako G, Wesley R, et al. Laboratory test abnormalities are common in polymyositis and dermatomyositis and differ among clinical and demographic groups. Open Rheumatol J 2012;6:54–63.

58. Pamfil C, Candrea E, Berki E, et al. Primary biliary cirrhosis–autoimmune hepatitis overlap syndrome associated with dermatomyositis, autoimmune thyroiditis and antiphospholipid syndrome. J Gastrointestin Liver Dis 2015;24(1):101–4.

59. Shimizu J. Clinical and histopathological features of myositis associated with anti-mitochondrial antibodies. Rinsho Shinkeigaku 2013;53(11):1114–6 [in Japanese].

60. Shiba H, Takeuchi T, Isoda K, et al. Dermatomyositis as a complication of interferon-alpha therapy: a case report and review of the literature. Rheumatol Int 2014;34(9):1319–22.

61. Mengel AM, Stenzel W, Meisel A, et al. Hepatitis E-induced severe myositis. Muscle Nerve 2016;53(2):317–20.

62. Del Bello A, Arne-Bes MC, Lavayssiere L, et al. Hepatitis E virus-induced severe myositis. J Hepatol 2012;57(5):1152–3.

63. Marshall JB, Ravendhran N, Sharp GC. Liver disease in mixed connective tissue disease. Arch Intern Med 1983;143(9):1817–8.

64. Zold E, Bodolay E, Dezso B, et al. Mixed connective tissue disease associated with autoimmune hepatitis and pulmonary fibrosis. Isr Med Assoc J 2014; 16(11):733–4.

65. Taccone FS, Lucidi V, Donckier V, et al. Fulminant hepatitis requiring MARS and liver transplantation in a patient with Still's disease. Eur J Intern Med 2008; 19(6):e26–8.

66. Zhu G, Liu G, Liu Y, et al. Liver abnormalities in adult onset Still's disease: a retrospective study of 77 Chinese patients. J Clin Rheumatol 2009;15(6):284–8.

67. Wolfe F, Clauw DJ, Fitzcharles MA, et al. Fibromyalgia criteria and severity scales for clinical and epidemiological studies: a modification of the ACR preliminary diagnostic criteria for fibromyalgia. J Rheumatol 2011;38(6):1113–22.

68. Kozanoglu E, Canataroglu A, Abayli B, et al. Fibromyalgia syndrome in patients with hepatitis C infection. Rheumatol Int 2003;23(5):248–51.

69. Rogal SS, Bielefeldt K, Wasan AD, et al. Fibromyalgia symptoms and cirrhosis. Dig Dis Sci 2015;60(5):1482–9.

70. Chen JH, Deshpande V. IgG4-related disease and the liver. Gastroenterol Clin North Am 2017;46(2):195–216.

71. Wallace ZS, Deshpande V, Mattoo H, et al. IgG4-related disease: clinical and laboratory features in one hundred twenty-five patients. Arthritis Rheumatol 2015; 67(9):2466–75.

72. Inoue D, Yoshida K, Yoneda N, et al. IgG4-related disease: dataset of 235 consecutive patients. Medicine (Baltimore) 2015;94(15):e680.

73. Kanno A, Masamune A, Okazaki K, et al. Nationwide epidemiological survey of autoimmune pancreatitis in Japan in 2011. Pancreas 2015;44(4):535–9.

74. Kanno A, Nishimori I, Masamune A, et al. Nationwide epidemiological survey of autoimmune pancreatitis in Japan. Pancreas 2012;41(6):835–9.

75. Huggett MT, Culver EL, Kumar M, et al. Type 1 autoimmune pancreatitis and IgG4-related sclerosing cholangitis is associated with extrapancreatic organ failure, malignancy, and mortality in a prospective UK cohort. Am J Gastroenterol 2014;109(10):1675–83.

76. Samuel DG, Rees IW. Extrahepatic manifestations of hepatitis C virus (HCV). Frontline Gastroenterol 2013;4(4):249–54.

77. Bonacci M, Lens S, Londono MC, et al. Virologic, clinical, and immune response outcomes of patients with hepatitis C virus-associated cryoglobulinemia treated with direct-acting antivirals. Clin Gastroenterol Hepatol 2017;15(4):575–83.e571.

78. Lewis JH, Stine JG. Review article: prescribing medications in patients with cirrhosis - a practical guide. Aliment Pharmacol Ther 2013;37(12):1132–56.

79. Crofford LJ. Use of NSAIDs in treating patients with arthritis. Arthritis Res Ther 2013;15(Suppl 3):S2.

80. Rostom A, Goldkind L, Laine L. Nonsteroidal anti-inflammatory drugs and hepatic toxicity: a systematic review of randomized controlled trials in arthritis patients. Clin Gastroenterol Hepatol 2005;3(5):489–98.

81. Teoh NC, Farrell GC. Hepatotoxicity associated with non-steroidal anti-inflammatory drugs. Clin Liver Dis 2003;7(2):401–13.

82. Paulose-Ram R, Hirsch R, Dillon C, et al. Prescription and non-prescription analgesic use among the US adult population: results from the third National Health and Nutrition Examination Survey (NHANES III). Pharmacoepidemiol Drug Saf 2003;12(4):315–26.

83. Soni P, Shell B, Cawkwell G, et al. The hepatic safety and tolerability of the cyclooxygenase-2 selective NSAID celecoxib: pooled analysis of 41 randomized controlled trials. Curr Med Res Opin 2009;25(8):1841–51.

84. Woods CP, Hazlehurst JM, Tomlinson JW. Glucocorticoids and non-alcoholic fatty liver disease. J Steroid Biochem Mol Biol 2015;154:94–103.

85. Ferraro D, Mirante VG, Losi L, et al. Methylprednisolone-induced toxic hepatitis after intravenous pulsed therapy for multiple sclerosis relapses. Neurologist 2015;19(6):153–4.

86. Perrillo RP, Gish R, Falck-Ytter YT. American Gastroenterological Association Institute technical review on prevention and treatment of hepatitis B virus reactivation during immunosuppressive drug therapy. Gastroenterology 2015;148(1): 221–44.e3.

87. Anelli MG, Scioscia C, Grattagliano I, et al. Old and new antirheumatic drugs and the risk of hepatotoxicity. Ther Drug Monit 2012;34(6):622–8.

88. Huang D, Aghdassi E, Su J, et al. Prevalence and risk factors for liver biochemical abnormalities in Canadian patients with systemic lupus erythematosus. J Rheumatol 2012;39(2):254–61.

89. Conway R, Low C, Coughlan RJ, et al. Risk of liver injury among methotrexate users: a meta-analysis of randomised controlled trials. Semin Arthritis Rheum 2015;45(2):156–62.

90. Schmajuk G, Miao Y, Yazdany J, et al. Identification of risk factors for elevated transaminases in methotrexate users through an electronic health record. Arthritis Care Res (Hoboken) 2014;66(8):1159–66.

91. Conway R, Carey JJ. Risk of liver disease in methotrexate treated patients. World J Hepatol 2017;9(26):1092–100.

92. Visser K, Katchamart W, Loza E, et al. Multinational evidence-based recommendations for the use of methotrexate in rheumatic disorders with a focus on rheumatoid arthritis: integrating systematic literature research and expert opinion of a broad international panel of rheumatologists in the 3E Initiative. Ann Rheum Dis 2009;68(7):1086–93.

93. Bastida G, Nos P, Aguas M, et al. Incidence, risk factors and clinical course of thiopurine-induced liver injury in patients with inflammatory bowel disease. Aliment Pharmacol Ther 2005;22(9):775–82.

94. Gisbert JP, Gonzalez-Lama Y, Mate J. Thiopurine-induced liver injury in patients with inflammatory bowel disease: a systematic review. Am J Gastroenterol 2007; 102(7):1518–27.

95. Rossi RE, Parisi I, Despott EJ, et al. Anti-tumour necrosis factor agent and liver injury: literature review, recommendations for management. World J Gastroenterol 2014;20(46):17352–9.

96. Pauly MP, Tucker LY, Szpakowski JL, et al. Incidence of hepatitis B virus reactivation and hepatotoxicity in patients receiving long-term treatment with tumor necrosis factor antagonists. Clin Gastroenterol Hepatol 2018;16(12):1964–73.e1.

97. Vigano M, Degasperi E, Aghemo A, et al. Anti-TNF drugs in patients with hepatitis B or C virus infection: safety and clinical management. Expert Opin Biol Ther 2012;12(2):193–207.

98. Mozessohn L, Chan KK, Feld JJ, et al. Hepatitis B reactivation in HBsAg-negative/HBcAb-positive patients receiving rituximab for lymphoma: a meta-analysis. J Viral Hepat 2015;22(10):842–9.

99. Chen YM, Chen HH, Chen YH, et al. A comparison of safety profiles of tumour necrosis factor alpha inhibitors and rituximab therapy in patients with rheumatoid arthritis and chronic hepatitis C. Ann Rheum Dis 2015;74(3):626–7.

Hepatic Manifestations of Cystic Fibrosis

Sasan Sakiani, MD[a],*, David E. Kleiner, MD, PhD[b], Theo Heller, MD[c], Christopher Koh, MD, MHSc[c],*

KEYWORDS

- Cystic fibrosis liver disease • CFLD • Liver disease in cystic fibrosis
- Focal biliary cirrhosis • Non-cirrhotic portal hypertension

KEY POINTS

- Cystic fibrosis liver disease is the third leading cause of death in patients with cystic fibrosis.
- There are no clear guidelines for diagnosing cystic fibrosis liver disease and several diagnostic criteria have been proposed in the past.
- Most patients with cystic fibrosis liver disease are diagnosed before puberty, although, as life expectancies improve, adult-onset cystic fibrosis liver disease is becoming increasingly recognized.
- There are no proven therapies for cystic fibrosis liver disease, although ursodeoxycholic acid is commonly used.
- Liver transplant is a viable option, either alone or in combination with lung transplantation for patients with advanced liver disease from cystic fibrosis.

INTRODUCTION

Cystic fibrosis (CF) is the most common autosomal recessive genetic disorder in white people,[1,2] and is also one of the most lethal.[3,4] It is caused by a mutation in the gene coding for the CF transmembrane conductance regulator (CFTR) protein on chromosome 7.[2] With advances in medical care, the life expectancy of patients with CF has increased from 16 years in 1970 to 47.7 years in 2016.[5] Given this improved longevity,

Disclosure Statement: The authors have nothing to disclose.
[a] Division of Gastroenterology and Hepatology, University of Maryland School of Medicine, University of Maryland Medical Center, 22 South Greene Street, N3W50, Baltimore, MD 21201, USA; [b] Laboratory of Pathology, National Cancer Institute, National Institutes of Health, 10 Center Drive, Building 10, Room 2S235, MSC 1500, Bethesda, MD 20892, USA; [c] Liver Diseases Branch, National Institute of Diabetes and Digestive and Kidney Diseases, National Institutes of Health, 10 Center Drive, Building 10, Room 9B-16, MSC 1800, Bethesda, MD 20892, USA
* Corresponding author.
E-mail addresses: ssakiani@som.umaryland.edu (S.S.); christopher.koh@nih.gov (C.K.)

the extrapulmonary manifestations related to CF are identified more often. Although the leading cause of death in CF patients continues to be from complications of pulmonary disease, followed by complications of lung transplantation, liver disease has been identified as the third most common and the most important non-pulmonary cause of death in these patients.[5] In the current era of CF management, the prevalence of cystic fibrosis liver disease (CFLD) has been described to approach 40% in patients with CF,[6,7] and accounts for 2% to 5% of overall CF mortality.[8–10]

Cystic fibrosis liver disease is well described in pediatric patients, and studies have demonstrated that most patients present with evidence of CFLD before puberty.[7,11] A large retrospective study by Boelle and colleagues[12] evaluating 3328 CF patients born after 1985 demonstrated that the incidence of CFLD increased by approximately 1% each year after the age of 5 and reached 10% by the age of 30. Risk factors identified for CFLD in this study included male sex, CFTR F508del homozygosity, and history of meconium ileus.[12] With improved life expectancy, a larger proportion of patients with CF now consist of adults over the age of 18 (52% in 2016 compared with just 29% in 1986).[5] A recent study involving a longitudinal cohort of adult patients followed over a median of 24.5 years at the NIH Clinical Center in the United States demonstrated that adult-onset CFLD occurred at a median age of 37 in patients who did not have evidence of CFLD during childhood.[3]

PATHOPHYSIOLOGY

The CFTR gene encodes for a protein that is found on the apical surface of cholangiocytes and gallbladder epithelia (**Fig. 1**).[1,13] This CFTR protein is responsible for regulating the fluid and electrolyte content of bile by increasing apical biliary chloride secretion to create a transmembrane gradient of Cl, which can then be used to increase bile acid independent bile flow via the Cl^-/HCO_3^- exchanger along with passive movement of water.[1,14] This leads to increased fluidity of bile as well as alkalinization of the bile. Thus, mutations in the CFTR protein can lead to impaired secretion of Cl^- and thus lead to the development of viscous bile with reduced flow and alkalinity.[14,15] Whereas the mechanism of the development of cirrhosis in CF is still unclear, it seems that these changes can lead to stagnation of the bile, which leads to accumulation of toxic bile acids and increased infections. As such, liver biopsies early in pediatric patients have demonstrated mucus plugging in cholangiocytes.[16] These changes can lead to periductal inflammation, damage to cholangiocytes, bile duct proliferation, and periportal fibrosis (**Fig. 2A**).[14] For this reason, CFLD typically presents as a cholestatic liver disease with the typical, well-described hepatic lesion of focal biliary cirrhosis, particularly in the pediatric population and in patients with more severe mutations (**Fig. 2B**).[1,17] In addition to these changes, a recent study demonstrated that CFTR regulates Toll-like receptor 4-dependent inflammatory responses by inhibiting Rous sarcoma oncogene cellular homologue (Src) activity, and mutations in CFTR lead to self-activation of Src leading to increased inflammatory cytokines and disruption of the epithelial barrier.[9,18] This, in turn, can lead to translocation of bacteria into the portal circulation, hepatic inflammation, and fibrosis.[19]

In addition to focal biliary cirrhosis, many patients with CF can present with hepatic steatosis (**Fig. 2C**). Traditionally, hepatic steatosis in the CF population has been associated with nutritional deficiencies, particularly essential fatty acids.[20] More recently it has been described that steatosis in patients with CF is multifactorial and includes etiologies similar to those in the general population, such as nonalcoholic fatty liver disease (NAFLD) and alcoholic liver disease. A questionnaire-based study performed in the United Kingdom found that 83% of patients with

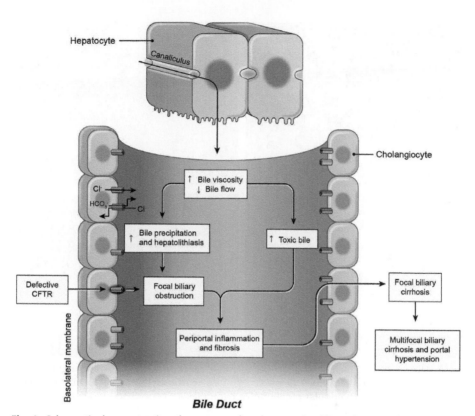

Bile Duct

Fig. 1. Schematic demonstrating the proposed pathogenesis of liver disease related to cystic fibrosis. Defective functioning of cystic fibrosis transmembrane conductance regulators (CFTR) expressed in the intra- and extra-hepatic cholangiocytes results in impaired Cl⁻ secretion across the apical membrane, leading to decreased bile flow and increased bile precipitation. This results in ductular obstruction with subsequent periportal inflammation and fibrosis and focal biliary cirrhosis. Progressive disease may manifest as multifocal biliary cirrhosis and portal hypertension.

CF drink alcohol, with 13% falling in the excessive or at-risk category, although this was less than the general population, in which this was found to be 23%.[21] Also, patients with CF are not immune to the obesity epidemic. With improvements in nutritional support, according to the 2016 Cystic Fibrosis Foundation annual report, the median BMI for adult patients with CF has increased by 3 points over the past 20 years. Of adult patients, 18.3% are obese with BMI greater than 30, with most having CF mutations other than F508del.[5] In addition, a study characterizing adult patients with CF demonstrated that these patients also develop other metabolic risk factors typically associated with NAFLD, including diabetes mellitus or impaired glucose tolerance and hypertriglyceridemia, particularly with increasing age.[22] It remains unclear whether or not these metabolic risk factors also predispose CF patients to the development of non-alcoholic steatohepatitis similar to the general population.

Whereas hepatic steatosis and focal biliary cirrhosis are more common findings in pediatric patients with CF, focal biliary cirrhosis is not believed to be as common in adult patients with CF. Several studies have recently demonstrated that the liver

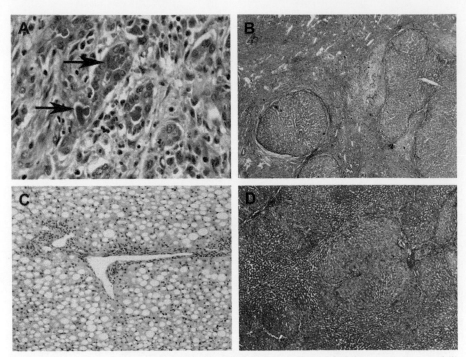

Fig. 2. Liver histology demonstrating: (A) ductular reaction with bile stasis, neutrophilic infiltration, and granular debris (*arrows*); (B) focal cirrhosis changes; (C) marked, pan-acinar steatosis; and (D) nodular regenerative hyperplasia.

disease and portal hypertension associated with CFLD is not entirely due to the development of fibrosis or cirrhosis, but that non-cirrhotic portal hypertension (NCPH) also plays a role. Studies have shown that only 20% to 27% of patients with CF presenting with signs of portal hypertension actually have underlying cirrhosis.[9,23] Portal hypertension in these patients seems to be due to NCPH, and explants have demonstrated evidence of presinusoidal-type portal hypertension because of obliterative venopathy with fibrosis within portal vein branches, which is consistent with this diagnosis.[24] Biopsies from patients with CFLD have also shown evidence of nodular regenerative hyperplasia, which is a type of NCPH and may be related to recurrent vascular and infectious complications and possibly drug-induced liver injury (**Fig. 2**D).[3]

Finally, another notable condition that leads to chronic liver injury in patients with CF is the development of hepatolithiasis owing to changes in the composition and stagnation of bile. This can lead to stricturing biliary diseases and sclerosing cholangitis, which can itself lead to a secondary biliary cirrhosis. A prospective study evaluating 27 patients with CF via magnetic resonance cholangiopancreatography (MRCP) demonstrated that, of 9 patients who met clinical, biochemical, or ultrasonographic (US) criteria of liver disease, all had abnormal MRCP results, with features resembling primary sclerosing cholangitis (PSC) in 5, and simple biliary lesions in the remaining 4; 9 patients who did not meet criteria for liver disease also had abnormal findings (5 PSC-like and 4 simple biliary lesions).[25] In addition, a recent study demonstrated that 19% of patients with PSC carry mutations in CFTR and that 50% had CFTR polymorphisms.[26]

CLINICAL PRESENTATION AND DIAGNOSIS

Patients with CFLD may have a wide array of presentations, from asymptomatic and mild elevations in hepatic and biliary enzymes, to steatosis and hepatosplenomegaly, to findings of decompensated cirrhosis with portal hypertension, ascites, and variceal bleeding. Whereas hepatomegaly and splenomegaly are common in patients with CFLD, traditional physical examinations are typically inaccurate in identifying subtle changes in organomegaly. Also, although elevated hepatic enzymes are common in patients with CF, these alone have been not shown to be accurate in diagnosing CFLD. Studies have demonstrated that 53% to 93% of patients with CF have at least one abnormal value of aspartate aminotransferase (AST) or alanine aminotransferase (ALT), although more than one-third have abnormal levels of gamma glutamyl-transferase (GGT) by the age of 21.[9,20,27] These frequently abnormal liver tests may be due to the multiple infections and medications that patients with CF experience. In addition, while not specifically studied in CF patients, a large study evaluating the sensitivity and specificity of ALT thresholds currently used by children's hospitals in detecting NAFLD, hepatitis B virus, and hepatitis C virus, demonstrated sensitivity of only 32% to 48% and specificity of 92% and 96% in boys and girls, respectively.[28] However, Woodruff and colleagues[27] demonstrated that AST greater than 1.5× upper limit of normal (ULN) or GGT greater than 1.5× ULN were strong predictors of under-lying liver disease in patients with CF and Bodewes and colleagues[29] demonstrated a strong correlation between persistently elevated GGT and the development of cirrhosis within 2 years. Therefore, patients presenting with significant or persistently elevated liver biochemistries warrant further investigation for evidence of CFLD. A proposed algorithm for the evaluation of CFLD patients with abnormal liver tests is presented in **Fig. 3**.

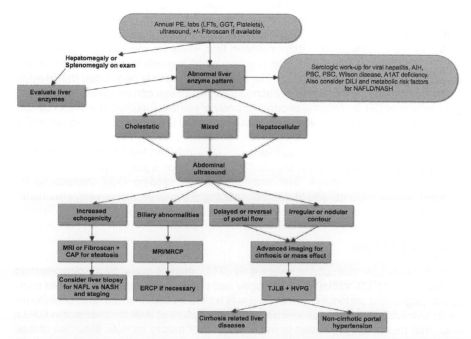

Fig. 3. Algorithmic evaluation for cystic fibrosis liver disease in patients with cystic fibrosis and abnormal liver tests.

With the evolution and advancements in hepatic imaging, subtle changes that occur early in the course of CFLD have become more easily identifiable. A recent study proposing a classification system based on a short unenhanced MRI protocol demonstrated a sensitivity of 94.1% and specificity of 84.6% when discriminating CFLD from controls, and that disease severity significantly corresponded to these findings.[30] This study also demonstrated that the albumin-bilirubin score was better than Child-Pugh score in assessing the severity of liver disease in these patients. Interestingly, this study did not find any significant difference in hepatic fat fraction in CF patients compared with controls, suggesting that these findings were more related to other patient characteristics such as history of diabetes or medication exposure. Statistically significant differences between CF patients and controls were noted in amount of periportal fat deposition, periportal tracking on diffusion-weighted images, bile duct abnormalities, heterogeneous liver parenchyma, gallbladder alterations, periportal fibrosis, and widening of fissures and hilum.[30]

In addition to simple laboratory values and imaging, other non-invasive measures of liver disease have been used in staging and diagnosing CFLD. Two lab-based markers, AST-to-platelet ratio index (APRI) and the fibrosis-4 score (FIB-4) have been described to correlate with the presence of CFLD as diagnosed by dual-pass liver biopsies, with area under the receiver operating characteristics (AUROC) of 0.75 for APRI and 0.60 for FIB-4.[31] Another non-invasive measure of liver disease that has been studied in CFLD includes vibration-controlled transient elastography (VCTE). VCTE, particularly FibroScan (Echosens, Paris), has been approved by the US Food and Drug Administration for use in staging of other liver diseases such as hepatitis C, and as such it is becoming increasingly available. Whereas official cutoffs have yet to be established in CFLD, a study by Kitson and colleagues[32] demonstrated that liver stiffness measurements (LSM) by FibroScan greater than 6.8 kPa had a 76% sensitivity and 92% specificity for detecting CFLD. In addition, liver stiffness has been shown to directly correlate with the severity of CFLD and was believed to be better than APRI with AUROC of 0.91 versus 0.78, respectively.[33] A recent study by Gominon and colleagues[34] demonstrated that, while the median LSM progressed by 0.23 kPa/y in patients with CF, it progressed at a much faster rate (0.94 kPa/y, $P = .02$) in those who develop CFLD. The authors of this study concluded that in addition to the baseline LSM, the rate of change in liver stiffness can be used to predict the development of CFLD. With the expanding body of literature exploring VCTE in CF patients, there may be clinical utility in performing annual LSM as a screening tool in CF patients.

Owing to the challenges in diagnosing CFLD, which can lead to delayed medical management, patients with CF should be screened for signs of liver disease with yearly physical examinations, liver enzyme testing including GGT, monitoring for declining platelets counts, and abdominal imaging. If available, non-invasive measurements of fibrosis including VCTE and APRI should be performed in at-risk patients.

DIAGNOSTIC CRITERIA

Given the wide spectrum of diseases within CFLD, there is currently no clear method for diagnosing CFLD. Although liver biopsy has been described to be the gold standard of diagnosing underlying CFLD, its use is limited by the inherited risks of performing an invasive liver biopsy, as well as the patchy nature of liver involvement in CFLD, which may be underrepresented or missed by a liver biopsy sample. Because of this, several diagnostic criteria have been proposed for the diagnosis of CFLD. The most commonly used is one that was proposed by Debray and colleagues[17] in 2011, which involved at least 2 of following after ruling out other causes of liver disease: hepato-megaly or splenomegaly, abnormal LFTs above the ULN in at least 3 consecutive de-terminations over 12 months, or ultrasound evidence of liver involvement, with liver biopsies being performed if there was any doubt. Another commonly used definition was one that was proposed by the Cystic Fibrosis Foundation after a meeting was convened in 2007, which proposed classifying CFLD as (1) CF-related liver disease with clinical examination, imaging, histologic, or laparoscopic findings of cirrhosis or portal hypertension, (2) liver involvement without cirrhosis consisting of at least one of: persistent or intermittent elevations of AST, ALT, GGT at least 2× ULN, steatosis or fibrosis on histology, cholangiopathy based on imaging, or US findings other than those consistent with cirrhosis, or (3) pre-clinical with no examination, radiologic, or biochemical evidence of liver disease.[35] More recently, a new diagnostic criteria was proposed based on the findings of a longitudinal study at the NIH that incorpo-rated the use of non-invasive fibrosis markers of liver disease such as transient elas-tography, APRI, and FIB-4 with previously proposed criteria.[3] These latter criteria were shown to be able to detect more cases of CFLD compared with previously proposed criteria by Debray and colleagues (47% vs 22%, respectively), suggesting that prior studies may be underestimating the prevalence of actual disease. A recent longitudi-nal study by Alexopoulou and colleagues (unpublished data) evaluating a cohort of 62 patients with CF compared the old criteria (Debray) and new criteria (NIH) and found similar findings, with 25.8% and 43.5% of patients meeting criteria for CFLD, respec-tively. However, the clinical significance of this higher rate of diagnosis still needs to be determined. **Table 1** describes the features of each of these diagnostic criteria.

DIFFERENTIAL DIAGNOSIS

Aside from the more common presentations of CFLD, patients with CF are at risk for other causes of chronic liver injury. Therefore, patients with CF presenting with abnormal liver enzymes or abnormal hepatic imaging should be screened for other causes of chronic liver disease. Because CFLD is primarily a cholestatic liver disease, diseases such as PSC and primary biliary cholangitis (PBC) need to be ruled out. Also, patients need to be screened for biliary diseases such as choledocholithiasis and dis-ease related to an obstructive process; MRCP/MRI may be indicated in these patients. Drug-induced liver injury is another important etiology of liver disease in these patients and often leads to intermittent or persistently elevated liver function tests. This in-cludes antibiotics that are well established as causes of drug-induced liver injury, as well as newly developed medications that are used to directly modulate the CFTR pro-tein, such as ivacaftor and lumacaftor. These newer medications have demonstrated an ability to cause elevations in serum aminotransferases up to 3× ULN in up to 25% of patients.[36] Finally, all patients need to be screened for concomitant alcohol abuse (screening questionnaires such as CAGE), viral hepatitis such as hepatitis A, B, and C (serum serologies and/or PCR), and autoimmune hepatitis (ANA, ASMA, anti-LKM, and total immunoglobulins), Wilson disease (ceruloplasmin), celiac disease (anti-transglutaminase antibody and/or duodenal biopsies), alpha-1-antitrypsin deficiency (A1AT level and phenotype), as well as metabolic risk factors for NAFLD (diabetes or glucose intolerance, central adiposity, hypertension, hypertriglyceridemia, low lhigh-density lipoprotein).

MANAGEMENT

Once CFLD has been diagnosed, the goals of treatment consist of managing the sequelae associated with each specific disease, particularly those associated with

Table 1
Features of each of the diagnostic criteria

	Debray Criteria	NIH Criteria	CF Foundation Classification
Any of:		Radiologic evidence of diffuse liver disease, cirrhosis, or portal hypertension	Evidence of cirrhosis or portal hypertension based on any of: Clinical examination
	Liver biopsy consistent with CFLD (performed if any doubt)	Liver biopsy consistent with CFLD (performed for any reason)	Imaging Histology Laparoscopy
At least 2 of:	Hepatomegaly or splenomegaly on examination and confirmed by ultrasound	Hepatomegaly or splenomegaly on imaging	Liver involvement without cirrhosis with at least 1 of: Persistent/intermittent elevations of AST, ALT, GGT >2× ULN
	Abnormal ALT, AST, or GGT above the ULN at least 3 consecutive determinations over 12 mo	At least 2 persistently abnormal ALT, AST, GGT, or ALP over 2 y	Steatosis/fibrosis on histology Cholangiopathy on imaging
	US evidence of liver involvement or portal hypertension		US findings other than cirrhotic features
		Persistently abnormal APRI, FIB-4, or AAR Abnormal FibroScan at any time	
			Pre-clinical with no examination, radiologic, or biochemical evidence of liver disease

portal hypertension, and treatment to delay the progression of disease. All patients with CFLD should have monitoring of liver enzymes and markers associated with hepatic synthetic function including coagulation (prothrombin time/international normalized ratio [INR]) and albumin every 3 to 6 months.

Portal Hypertension

The diagnosis and management of portal hypertension is crucial given the potential severe consequences associated with esophageal or gastric variceal bleeding. However, there are no clear guidelines as to when and how to initiate screening or how often to perform this. A retrospective study evaluating episodes of gastrointestinal bleeding at a tertiary referral center in London, England, which is also a referral center for cystic fibrosis patients, described 18 patients with CFLD who presented with gastrointestinal bleeding, with the median age of first bleed at 20 years (range 9.7–30.9).[37] This wide age range suggests that screening for portal hypertension should occur once the diagnosis of CFLD has been made, and that screening should occur annually.[17]

With respect to how the screening should be performed, although transjugular measurements of hepatic portal pressures is the current gold standard in detecting and quantifying portal hypertension, this diagnostic modality is invasive and not uniformly available. In addition, hepatic venous pressure gradient measurements are poor at detecting pre-sinusoidal portal hypertension, which is often a component of different diseases within the NCPH spectrum. Whereas additional studies are still required for validation, several non-invasive measures of portal hypertension have been shown to predict the presence of portal hypertension and esophageal varices in patients with CFLD. For example, progressively lower levels of platelets on longitudinal follow up have previously been shown to correlate with presence and severity of liver disease and may possibly be associated with increased risks of mortality.[3] A Cochrane review evaluating the presence of esophageal varices in patients with liver diseases and portal hypertension from diseases other than CFLD demonstrated that the platelet count-to-spleen length ratio is a more accurate predictor than either alone in adult patients, whereas other studies have suggested that platelet counts alone may be better in pediatric populations.[38,39] As such, the British Society of Pediatric Gastroenterology, Hepatology and Nutrition recommends screening endoscopies in patients with platelet counts less than $120 \times 10^9/L$.[38] As these recommendations were based on studies involving liver diseases other than CFLD, studies are necessary to validate these findings in CFLD. Finally, CT, MRI, and US findings suggestive of portal hypertension, such as recanalization of the umbilical vein and visualization of varices, are also very helpful in determining those patients with portal hypertension.

Once the diagnosis of portal hypertension has been made, upper endoscopic evaluation is the method of choice for determining the presence of esophageal and gastric varices, and screening allows for detection of varices before bleeding. In patients with high risk varices (ie, grade 2 or 3), band ligation is preferred to non-selective beta-blockers given the increased risk of pulmonary complications in these patients. Patients with esophageal varices can then be placed in a banding protocol that consists of endoscopies at regular intervals until the varices are successfully eradicated.[9,38] However, given their concomitant underlying pulmonary disease, patients with CF are at increased risk for endoscopic procedures and anesthesia, and the risks of general anesthesia should be weighed against the risks of bleeding. Indeed, one survey demonstrated that pediatric patients with CF are typically screened at lower rates than those with other forms of liver disease.[40] Unfortunately there is currently no non-invasive measure that has been validated to help predict who would benefit from endoscopic procedures in patients with CFLD, as is the case of the Baveno VI recommendations in cirrhotic patients of other etiologies.[41] However, the non-invasive measures that are used in other causes of portal hypertension may still be helpful in determining which patients would benefit from endoscopic screening.

Patients who fail medical management of portal hypertension and have variceal bleeding or other complications, such as ascites, hypersplenism, and severe thrombocytopenia, may benefit from transhepatic porto-systemic shunts (TIPS), creation of surgical shunts, or splenectomy or partial splenic embolization.[42,43] There is no clear consensus as to which modality is best, and this typically depends on the patient's symptoms, underlying anatomy, center experience, and transplant candidacy. In the study by Gooding and colleagues,[37] of the 38 episodes of variceal bleeding in patients with CFLD, 30 were controlled endoscopically (band ligation and/or sclerotherapy, with 1 patient requiring glue injection for gastric varices), whereas 2 patients required TIPS after failed endoscopic treatment and 1 patient requiring surgical splenorenal shunt after failed endoscopic treatment. It should be noted that this study was performed in 2005, and a large proportion of patients underwent sclerotherapy rather than band ligation, which is currently the preferred treatment option for esophageal varices. Although decompressive shunts are not recommended as primary prophylaxis, they are typically the best option for long-term prevention of recurrent esophageal and gastric variceal rebleeding.[42]

Medical Management of CFLD

Unfortunately, medical treatments to delay progression or improve CFLD are still lacking.

Traditionally, once diagnosed with CFLD, patients have been started on ursodeoxycholic acid (UDCA). Although its exact mechanism of action is controversial, UDCA is a hydrophilic secondary bile acid that is believed to increase the fluidity and change the hydrophobicity of bile while also providing cytoprotective and anti-apoptotic effects.[44,45] Most of the data for the use of UDCA comes from its use in other cholestatic liver diseases such as PSC and PBC, and, although its utility in PBC is well established its benefit in PSC is more debatable. Similarly, a recent Cochrane review performed on CFLD patients found that data to support the use of UDCA is limited, with mostly low-quality studies and an absence of data regarding long-term outcomes such as death or need for liver transplantation.[46] Furthermore, in the study by Boelle and colleagues,[12] UDCA did not prevent the development of severe CFLD. On the other hand, a study by van der Feen and colleagues[47] demonstrated a decrease in liver stiffness as measured by transient elastography by 0.70 kPa/y in those with mild liver disease but not in those with CF-related cirrhosis. Whether or not UDCA is beneficial in CFLD has yet to be proven, although at this time, given the lack of alternative therapies and overall good tolerance, particularly at low and medium doses less than 20 mg/kg/d, most patients who are diagnosed with CFLD are still started on this medication.[7]

Recently, new therapies have been approved for patients with CF that directly target the CFTR protein and show promising results in pulmonary function.[48] These include Ivacaftor, a CFTR modulator that improves chloride transport through CFTR channels, which has been available since 2012, and Lumacaftor, which is used in conjunction with Ivacaftor and increases membrane expression of the CFTR protein. Although these medications show promise in other gastrointestinal complications associated with CF, their effects on the development and treatment of CFLD have not been directly evaluated in any trials.[49] Unfortunately, specific therapies for the treatment of CFLD are still lacking and further research is certainly needed in this area. Currently, there is a single ongoing phase II clinical trial evaluating different formulations of ursodiol in patients with CFLD (NCT00004315). In addition, in vitro studies looking at inhibiting Src using a kinase inhibitor have shown that, when used in combination with ivacaftor and lumacaftor, cholangiocyte fluid secretion is restored to normal.[50] However, human studies have not yet been performed.

Nutrition

Nutrition is a key part of the management of patients with CF and is associated with better lung function and survival in children with CF.[43] Malnutrition is multifactorial, including pancreatic insufficiency, as well as CFLD, which can lead to malabsorption of fats and fat-soluble vitamins. Severe malnutrition itself can also lead to hepatic steatosis, which is in the spectrum of CFLD. Screening for and repleting fat-soluble vitamins is thus important in these patients. Patients also often require higher calorie intakes (110%–200% of the general population) along with high fat diets to achieve their nutritional goals.[43] Patients with pancreatic insufficiency will benefit from pancreatic enzyme replacement therapy.[43] Unfortunately, medical treatment of CFLD has not yet been shown to improve nutritional outcomes in patients with CFLD. However, liver transplantation in patients with CFLD has been shown to preserve nutritional status with one study showing mild improvement in median BMI 5 years post-transplantation compared with pre-transplantation (19.6 vs 18.0 kg/m^2), though the difference was not statistically significant.[51]

Cancer Screening

Finally, whereas there is no clear data on the risk of development of hepatocellular carcinoma in patients with CFLD, once patients are found to have advanced fibrosis or cirrhosis, they should also be placed on a screening protocol for hepatocellular carcinoma with ultrasounds every 6 months based on guidelines for cirrhosis of other etiologies.[52]

Transplantation

According to the Cystic Fibrosis Patient Registry, 1642 patients with CF were reported to have had a solid organ transplant by 2016.[5] Lung transplantation is the most common organ transplanted in these patients. However, patients with planned lung transplantations that demonstrate severe portal hypertension from CFLD have been described to benefit from simultaneous liver and lung transplantations.[53] Unfortunately, most recent studies evaluating combined liver and lung transplantations within the past decade only consist of single-center experiences. Alternatively, liver transplantation alone has been performed in CF patients with hepatic decompensation and manifestations of portal hypertension such as variceal bleeding who have preserved lung function.[53,54] A study evaluating the effects of liver transplantation on lung function demonstrated that liver transplantation was neither beneficial nor detrimental to pulmonary function, with no difference in the rate of forced expiratory volume in the first second of expiration (FEV$_1$) decline after transplantation.[55] However, a different study performed in the United Kingdom demonstrated that the rate of decline in FEV$_1$ was lower (-0.74%, $P = .04$) compared with a predicted 3% annual decline in patients with CF up to 4 years after transplantation.[51] Finally, a single-center retrospective analysis evaluating the long-term outcomes of 9 patients with CF who underwent liver transplantation demonstrated that 3 required subsequent lung transplantation and one required combined liver and lung transplant within 10 years of the initial liver transplant procedure. In addition, 4 other patients were undergoing evaluation for lung transplantation.[56] Taken together, while liver transplantation may slow decline in pulmonary function, it appears not to halt the disease process and patients may ultimately require lung transplantation as well.

There are currently no clear guidelines to aid in determining which CFLD patients should be evaluated for liver transplantation. In general, patients with CFLD are considered for liver transplant if there is evidence of hepatic decompensation, such as coagulopathy (INR >1.5), ascites, jaundice, or extensive variceal bleeding that cannot be controlled by a portosystemic shunt.[8] In addition, there remains controversy regarding the timing of transplantation. Most liver transplants performed for CFLD are in children, with 79% (182 out of 230) of liver transplants in CF patients being performed in children between 1987 and 2008.[35,54] Contraindications to isolated liver transplant include active pulmonary infections or poor pulmonary function as expressed by FEV$_1$ less than 50%, extensive pulmonary fibrosis on imaging, or pulmonary hypertension (>35 mm Hg).[35] In these patients, combined liver and lung transplantations should be considered. However, the rates of combined liver and lung transplantation remains low, consisting of only 6% of transplants between 1987 and 2008 and only 50 cases recorded in the Scientific Registry of Transplant Recipients, for all causes, between 2005 and 2015.[54,57] Cystic fibrosis patients requiring combined liver-lung transplants must show signs of decreased pulmonary function with

FEV_1 lower than 40%, and their diagnosis must have been confirmed by genetic analysis. Exception points can be requested for these patients. Patients who are over the age of 18 are assigned a score that is 3 points below the median allocation model for end-stage liver disease (MELD) at transplant for liver recipients in the same donation service area (DSA). Patients under the age of 12 who meet the requirements for standardized pediatric end-stage liver disease scores, as well as patients between the ages of 12 to 17, are assigned a score equal to the median MELD at transplant for all liver recipients in the same DSA.[57]

A retrospective study reviewing the United Network for Organ Sharing database evaluated long-term outcomes for patients with CF undergoing liver transplantation. Although somewhat lower than that of other etiologies of liver disease, the 5-year survival rate of CFLD-related transplants was described to be respectable at 85.5% in children and 72.7% in adults. More importantly, this was significantly better than the 5-year survival rates in patients who remained on the transplant list, with hazard ratios of 0.33 and 0.25 in pediatric and adult patients respectively.[58] In another study evaluating isolated liver transplantation as well as combined liver-lung transplantation, 1- and 5-year survivals were not significant different between the 2 groups (80% and 80% vs 83.9% and 75.7%, respectively).[54] The major causes of death in these patients is pulmonary disease (22.7%) and hemorrhage (18.2%).[54] Thus, in patients with decompensated cirrhosis or uncontrollable bleeding due to portal hypertension that is not amenable to surgical shunts or TIPS, liver transplantation is a viable option, either alone or in combination with lung transplantation.

SUMMARY

Significant advancement in medical management has resulted in dramatically improved life expectancies in patients with CF compared with even just 10 years ago. Although prognosis has historically been intertwined with declining pulmonary status in CF patients, CFLD is now the third leading cause of death, the most common non-pulmonary cause of CF-related deaths, and accounts for up to 5% of deaths in patients with CF. Up until recently, most patients with CFLD presented in childhood; however, recent evidence seems to suggest a possible second wave of liver disease that becomes evident in adulthood.[3] It remains unclear if this liver disease is a result of underlying CF, or if it is the result of secondary complications such as chronic infections, therapeutics, or a yet to be understood process. There remains no consensus methodology for the diagnosis of CFLD, particularly given its patchy nature and variable presentations. However, different diagnostic algorithms have been described, some of which include newer imaging techniques and non-Invasive measures of liver disease. Further exploration in this area is needed given the importance of early diagnosis and intervention. Currently, medical treatment for CFLD remains limited, and is a burgeoning area for exploration. For patients with progressive disease, liver transplantation, either alone or in combination with lung transplantation, seems to be a feasible alternative, with improved outcomes and prolonged survival.

REFERENCES

1. Colombo C. Liver disease in cystic fibrosis. Curr Opin Pulm Med 2007;13:529–36.
2. Rowe SM, Miller S, Sorscher EJ. Mechanisms of disease: cystic fibrosis. N Engl J Med 2005;352:1992–2001.
3. Koh C, Sakiani S, Surana P, et al. Adult-onset cystic fibrosis liver disease: diagnosis and characterization of an underappreciated entity. Hepatology 2017;66: 591–601.

4. Strausbaugh SD, Davis PB. Cystic fibrosis: a review of epidemiology and patho-biology. Clin Chest Med 2007;28:279–88.
5. Cystic Fibrosis Foundation: Patient registry 2016 annual data report. Bethesda, Maryland, ©2017 Cystic Fibrosis Foundation.
6. Bhardwaj S, Canlas K, Kahi C, et al. Hepatobiliary abnormalities and disease in cystic fibrosis epidemiology and outcomes through adulthood. J Clin Gastroen-terol 2009;43:858–64.
7. Colombo C, Alicandro G. Liver disease in cystic fibrosis: illuminating the black box. Hepatology 2018. https://doi.org/10.1002/hep.30255.
8. Leung DH, Narkewicz MR. Cystic fibrosis-related cirrhosis. J Cyst Fibros 2017; 16(Suppl 2):S50–61.
9. Kamal N, Surana P, Koh C. Liver disease in patients with cystic fibrosis. Curr Opin Gastroenterol 2018;34:146–51.
10. Chatterjee K, Goyal A, Shah N, et al. Contemporary national trends of cystic fibrosis hospitalizations and co-morbidities in the United States. Adv Respir Med 2016;84:316–23.
11. Lamireau T, Monnereau S, Martin S, et al. Epidemiology of liver disease in cystic fibrosis: a longitudinal study. J Hepatol 2004;41:920–5.
12. Boelle PY, Debray D, Guillot L, et al. Cystic fibrosis liver disease: outcomes and risk factors in a large cohort of French patients. Hepatology 2018. https://doi.org/10.1002/hep.30148.
13. Cohn JA, Strong TV, Picciotto MR, et al. Localization of the cystic fibrosis trans-membrane conductance regulator in human bile duct epithelial cells. Gastroen-terology 1993;105:1857–64.
14. Kobelska-Dubiel N, Klincewicz B, Cichy W. Liver disease in cystic fibrosis. Prz Gastroenterol 2014;9:136–41.
15. Spirli C, Granato A, Zsembery K, et al. Functional polarity of Na^+/H^+ and Cl^-/HCO_3^- exchangers in a rat cholangiocyte cell line. Am J Physiol 1998;275: G1236–45.
16. Colombo C, Battezzati PM, Crosignani A, et al. Liver disease in cystic fibrosis: a prospective study on incidence, risk factors, and outcome. Hepatology 2002;36: 1374–82.
17. Debray D, Kelly D, Houwen R, et al. Best practice guidance for the diagnosis and management of cystic fibrosis-associated liver disease. J Cyst Fibros 2011;10: S29–36.
18. Fiorotto R, Villani A, Kourtidis A, et al. The cystic fibrosis transmembrane conduc-tance regulator controls biliary epithelial inflammation and permeability by regu-lating Src tyrosine kinase activity. Hepatology 2016;64:2118–34.
19. Flass T, Tong S, Frank DN, et al. Intestinal lesions are associated with altered in-testinal microbiome and are more frequent in children and young adults with cystic fibrosis and cirrhosis. PLoS One 2015;10:e0116967.
20. Lindblad A, Glaumann H, Strandvik B. Natural history of liver disease in cystic fibrosis. Hepatology 1999;30:1151–8.
21. Mc Ewan FA, Hodson ME, Simmonds NJ. The prevalence of "risky behaviour" in adults with cystic fibrosis. J Cyst Fibros 2012;11:56–8.
22. Georgiopoulou VV, Denker A, Bishop KL, et al. Metabolic abnormalities in adults with cystic fibrosis. Respirology 2010;15:823–9.
23. Hillaire S, Cazals-Hatem D, Bruno O, et al. Liver transplantation in adult cystic fibrosis: clinical, imaging, and pathological evidence of obliterative portal veno-pathy. Liver Transpl 2017;23:1342–7.

24. Witters P, Libbrecht L, Roskams T, et al. Liver disease in cystic fibrosis presents as non-cirrhotic portal hypertension. J Cyst Fibros 2017;16:e11–3.

25. Durieu I, Pellet O, Simonot L, et al. Sclerosing cholangitis in adults with cystic fibrosis: a magnetic resonance cholangiographic prospective study. J Hepatol 1999;30:1052–6.

26. Werlin S, Scotet V, Uguen K, et al. Primary sclerosing cholangitis is associated with abnormalities in CFTR. J Cyst Fibros 2018;17:666–71.

27. Woodruff SA, Sontag MK, Accurso FJ, et al. Prevalence of elevated liver enzymes in children with cystic fibrosis diagnosed by newborn screen. J Cyst Fibros 2017; 16:139–45.

28. Schwimmer JB, Dunn W, Norman GJ, et al. SAFETY study: alanine aminotransferase cutoff values are set too high for reliable detection of pediatric chronic liver disease. Gastroenterology 2010;138:1357–64, 1364.e1-2.

29. Bodewes FA, van der Doef HP, Houwen RH, et al. Increase of serum gamma-glutamyltransferase associated with development of cirrhotic cystic fibrosis liver disease. J Pediatr Gastroenterol Nutr 2015;61:113–8.

30. Poetter-Lang S, Staufer K, Baltzer P, et al. The efficacy of MRI in the diagnostic workup of cystic fibrosis-associated liver disease: a clinical observational cohort study. Eur Radiol 2019;29(2):1048–58.

31. Leung DH, Khan M, Minard CG, et al. Aspartate aminotransferase to platelet ratio and fibrosis-4 as biomarkers in biopsy-validated pediatric cystic fibrosis liver disease. Hepatology 2015;62:1576–83.

32. Kitson MT, Kemp WW, Iser DM, et al. Utility of transient elastography in the non-invasive evaluation of cystic fibrosis liver disease. Liver Int 2013;33:698–705.

33. Aqul A, Jonas MM, Harney S, et al. Correlation of transient elastography with severity of cystic fibrosis-related liver disease. J Pediatr Gastroenterol Nutr 2017;64:505–11.

34. Gominon AL, Frison E, Hiriart JB, et al. Assessment of liver disease progression in cystic fibrosis using transient elastography. J Pediatr Gastroenterol Nutr 2018;66: 455–60.

35. Flass T, Narkewicz MR. Cirrhosis and other liver disease in cystic fibrosis. J Cyst Fibros 2013;12:116–24.

36. LiverTox: Cystic fibrosis agents - ivacaftor and lumacaftor. https://livertox.nlm.nih.gov/IvacaftorLumacaftor.htm. Accessed September, 2018.

37. Gooding I, Dondos V, Gyi KM, et al. Variceal hemorrhage and cystic fibrosis: outcomes and implications for liver transplantation. Liver Transpl 2005;11:1522–6.

38. Davison S. Assessment of liver disease in cystic fibrosis. Paediatr Respir Rev 2018;27:24–7.

39. Colli A, Gana JC, Yap J, et al. Platelet count, spleen length, and platelet count-to-spleen length ratio for the diagnosis of oesophageal varices in people with chronic liver disease or portal vein thrombosis. Cochrane Database Syst Rev 2017;(4):CD008759.

40. Jeanniard-Malet O, Duche M, Fabre A. Survey on clinical practice of primary prophylaxis in portal hypertension in children. J Pediatr Gastroenterol Nutr 2017;64: 524–7.

41. Maurice JB, Brodkin E, Arnold F, et al. Validation of the Baveno VI criteria to identify low risk cirrhotic patients not requiring endoscopic surveillance for varices. J Hepatol 2016;65:899–905.

42. Marti J, Gunasekaran G, Iyer K, et al. Surgical management of noncirrhotic portal hypertension. Clin Liver Dis 2015;5:112–5.

43. Bolia R, Ooi CY, Lewindon P, et al. Practical approach to the gastrointestinal manifestations of cystic fibrosis. J Paediatr Child Health 2018;54:609–19.
44. Paumgartner G, Beuers U. Ursodeoxycholic acid in cholestatic liver disease: mechanisms of action and therapeutic use revisited. Hepatology 2002;36:525–31.
45. Kappler M, Espach C, Schweiger-Kabesch A, et al. Ursodeoxycholic acid therapy in cystic fibrosis liver disease–a retrospective long-term follow-up case-control study. Aliment Pharmacol Ther 2012;36:266–73.
46. Cheng K, Ashby D, Smyth RL. Ursodeoxycholic acid for cystic fibrosis-related liver disease. Cochrane Database Syst Rev 2017;(9):CD000222.
47. van der Feen C, van der Doef HP, van der Ent CK, et al. Ursodeoxycholic acid treatment is associated with improvement of liver stiffness in cystic fibrosis patients. J Cyst Fibros 2016;15:834–8.
48. Ramsey BW, Davies J, McElvaney NG, et al. A CFTR potentiator in patients with cystic fibrosis and the G551D mutation. N Engl J Med 2011;365:1663–72.
49. Houwen RHJ, van der Woerd WL, Slae M, et al. Effects of new and emerging therapies on gastrointestinal outcomes in cystic fibrosis. Curr Opin Pulm Med 2017;23:551–5.
50. Fiorotto R, Amenduni M, Mariotti V, et al. Src kinase inhibition reduces inflammatory and cytoskeletal changes in DeltaF508 human cholangiocytes and improves cystic fibrosis transmembrane conductance regulator correctors efficacy. Hepatology 2018;67:972–88.
51. Dowman JK, Watson D, Loganathan S, et al. Long-term impact of liver transplantation on respiratory function and nutritional status in children and adults with cystic fibrosis. Am J Transplant 2012;12:954–64.
52. Marrero JA, Kulik LM, Sirlin CB, et al. Diagnosis, staging, and management of hepatocellular carcinoma: 2018 practice guidance by the American Association for the Study of Liver Diseases. Hepatology 2018;68:723–50.
53. Halldorson J, AlQahtani K. Outcomes of combined liver/lung transplantation for cystic fibrosis using SRTR analysis. Am J Transplant 2017;17(Suppl 3). https://atcmeetingabstracts.com/abstract/outcomes-of-combined-liverlung-transplantation-for-cystic-fibrosis-using-srtr-analysis/.
54. Arnon R, Annunziato RA, Miloh T, et al. Liver and combined lung and liver transplantation for cystic fibrosis: analysis of the UNOS database. Pediatr Transplant 2011;15:254–64.
55. Miller MR, Sokol RJ, Narkewicz MR, et al. Pulmonary function in individuals who underwent liver transplantation: from the US cystic fibrosis foundation registry. Liver Transpl 2012;18:585–93.
56. Sivam S, Al-Hindawi Y, Di Michiel J, et al. Liver and lung transplantation in cystic fibrosis: an adult cystic fibrosis centre's experience. Intern Med J 2016;46:852–4.
57. OPTN/UNOS liver review board policy. 2017.
58. Mendizabal M, Reddy KR, Cassuto J, et al. Liver transplantation in patients with cystic fibrosis: analysis of United Network for Organ Sharing data. Liver Transpl 2011;17:243–50.

Intestinal Failure-Associated Liver Disease

Loris Pironi, MD*, Anna Simona Sasdelli, MD

KEYWORDS

- Liver disease • Steatosis • Cholestasis • Intestinal failure • Short bowel syndrome
- Parenteral nutrition • Lipid emulsion

KEY POINTS

- Intestinal failure-associated liver disease (IFALD) refers to a liver injury owing to one or more factors relating to intestinal failure including, but not limited to, parenteral nutrition and occurring in the absence of another primary parenchymal liver pathology (eg, viral or autoimmune hepatitis), other hepatotoxic factors (eg, alcohol/medication), or biliary obstruction.
- IFALD is more frequent in infants, who mainly develop cholestasis, than in older children and adults, who mainly develop steatosis.
- The diagnosis of IFALD is based on clinical, biochemical, radiological, and, when required, histologic information; no formally agreed criteria have been yet defined and the epidemiology is not clear.
- The pathogenesis of IFALD is multifactorial: intestinal failure-related, including total oral fasting, parenteral nutrition-related, and systemic-related factors play a role; alterations of the bile acids enterohepatic circulation, gut microbiome, and intestinal permeability, summarized in the concept of gut-liver axis, seem to be the main mechanisms.
- Prevention and treatment consist in avoiding and promptly treating all the risk factors in the individual patient.

INTRODUCTION

Intravenous supplementation (IVS) of parenteral nutrition (PN) admixtures and/or fluid and electrolyte solutions is the primary treatment of intestinal failure (IF), defined as "the reduction of gut function below the minimum necessary for the absorption of macronutrients and/or water and electrolytes, such that IVS is required to maintain health and/or growth".[1] The definition of IF precludes IVS as being considered

Disclosure Statement: Dr L. Pironi is a consultant for Baxter, Fresenius-Kabi, Shire. Dr A.S. Sasdelli has nothing to disclose.
Department of Medical and Surgical Science, Centre for Chronic Intestinal Failure, University of Bologna, St. Orsola-Malpighi Hospital, Via Massarenti, 9, 40138 Bologna, Italy
* Corresponding author.
E-mail address: loris.pironi@unibo.it

Clin Liver Dis 23 (2019) 279–291
https://doi.org/10.1016/j.cld.2018.12.009
1089-3261/19/© 2018 Elsevier Inc. All rights reserved.

synonymous with IF. Indeed, there may be patients receiving IVS notwithstanding normal intestinal absorptive function, because of refusal of an otherwise effective enteral nutrition. Intestinal failure is classified as acute (AIF), prolonged AIF or chronic IF (CIF).[1] Patients with AIF are metabolically unstable, require IVS for days, weeks, or months and are treated in a hospital setting.[1] Most cases of AIF are reversible within days with return to normal intestinal function. Around 50% of prolonged AIF evolves to CIF. Patients with CIF are metabolically stable, require IVS over months or years (reversible CIF) or life-long (irreversible CIF) and are treated at home (home parenteral nutrition [HPN]).[1,2] Parenteral nutrition is categorized as supplemental PN, when patients satisfy part of the energy requirement by oral/enteral feeding, or total PN when patients are on oral/enteral fasting and are totally dependent on IVS. In patients with AIF, elevation of liver function tests (LFTs) is mild, is mostly related to the underlying metabolic impairment, and often normalizes, despite continuing PN, when the metabolic state becomes stable and enteral or oral diet is reinstated.[1] In patients with CIF, alterations of liver function may evolve to liver failure, which is a criterion for combined liver and intestinal transplantation.[2]

DEFINITION

Alterations of liver function occurring in patients on PN were initially defined as PN-associated liver disease (PNALD).[3] However, a growing amount of evidence suggested that the deterioration of hepatic function in conjunction with long-term HPN was not the consequence of PN administration per se but because of IF and associated complications. Therefore, the term PNALD has been replaced with IF-associated liver disease (IFALD). The European Society for Clinical Nutrition and Metabolism (ESPEN) position paper on IFALD recommends that "the term IFALD refers to liver injury as a result of one or more factors relating to IF including, but not limited to, PN and occurring in the absence of another primary parenchymal liver pathology (eg, viral or autoimmune hepatitis), other hepatotoxic factors (eg, alcohol/medication) or biliary obstruction".[4]

DIAGNOSIS AND EPIDEMIOLOGY

The diagnosis of IFALD is based on clinical, biochemical, radiological and, when required, histologic information. A persistent elevation of liver enzymes, alkaline phosphatase and γ-glutamyl transferase $\geq$1.5 above the upper limit reference range that persists for $\geq$6 months in adults or $\geq$6 weeks in children are widely accepted criteria,[5,6] even though no formally agreed criteria have been defined so far. As a consequence, a wide range of prevalence and incidence (0%–50%) of IFALD, with higher percentages in children than in adults, have been reported.[1,2] The impact of the diagnostic criteria used in the literature[5,7–13] (Table 1) on the prevalence and incidence of IFALD in adults was analyzed in a recent cross-sectional and retrospective follow-up study on an individual cohort of patients on long-term HPN for CIF.[14]

At cross-sectional evaluation, depending on the used diagnostic criteria, the range of the frequency of IFALD was 5% to 15% for cholestasis, 19% to 43% for steatosis, 11% to 22% for fibrosis, and 7% to 40% for unclassified criteria. The retrospective follow-up showed that IFALD was present at HPN initiation, probably due to the liver derangement associated with the prolonged AIF that evolved in CIF, but resolved thereafter in a percentage of patients.[14] The ESPEN position paper recommends that the diagnosis of IFALD should be based on the presence of abnormal LFTs and/or evidence of radiological and/or histologic liver abnormalities.[4] Liver histology

Table 1
Diagnostic criteria for intestinal failure-associated liver disease categories

Category	Criteria
IFALD-cholestasis	• Cavicchi et al. criterion[7]: a value ≥1.5 the ULN on 2 of γ-GT, ALP, and serum conjugated bilirubin for ≥6 mo • ESPEN database (a) ConBil criterion[8]: conjugated bilirubin >0.3 mg/dL for ≥6 mo • ESPEN database (b) TotBil criterion[8]: total bilirubin >1 mg/dL and conjugated bilirubin >0.3 mg/dL for ≥6 mo
IFALD-steatosis	• AAR index, according to Sorbi et al.[9]: AST/ALT ratio <1 when AST and ALT > ULN • Ultrasound criterion, according to the European Association for the Study of the Liver (EASL) guidelines[10]: liver ultrasound echogenic appearance of steatosis
IFALD-fibrosis	• APRI index, according to Rath et al.[11]: AST to PLT ratio index = $[(AST/ULN\ AST) \times 100]/PLT\ (10^9/L) > 0.88$ • FIB-4 index, according to Sterling et al.[12]: Fibrosis-4 index = Age (y) × AST/[PLT $(10^9/L)$ × ALT$^{1/2}$]; advanced fibrosis: ≥2.67
IFALD-unclassified	• Luman and Shaffer criterion[13]: any deranged LFT ≥1.5 the ULN after >6 mo of HPN starting • Beath and Kelly criterion[5]: ALP and γ-GT ≥1.5 the ULN and US signs of liver steatosis

Abbreviations: ALP, alkaline phosphatase; ALT, alanine aminotransferase; AST, aspartate aminotransferase; ESPEN, European Society for Clinical Nutrition and Metabolism; γ-GT, gamma-glutamyl transferase; LFT, liver functional test; PTL, platelets; ULN, upper limit of normal; US, ultrasound.

is not considered mandatory for the diagnosis of IFALD and its need should be evaluated on a case-by-case basis.[1,4]

PATHOLOGY

A hallmark of IFALD is the concomitant presence of cholestasis and steatosis.[15,16] Cholestasis is more frequent in newborns and infants, whereas steatosis is more common in older children and adults.[7,15,16] IFALD-associated cholestasis shows feature of biliary obstruction with portal inflammation by neutrophils, portal edema, ductular proliferation, and ductopenia.[15,16] IFALD-associated steatosis consists of a combination of macro- and micro-vesicular periportal steatosis, mostly presenting with many small fat vacuoles (liposomes) into the hepatocyte cytoplasm with the nucleus centrally placed; this histologic feature implies active lipid turnover, metabolic instability, and mitochondrial injury and differs greatly from macrovesicular centrilobular steatosis observed in non-alcoholic fatty liver disease (NAFLD), which is associated with more a stable and equilibrated biochemical pattern. Steatohepatitis, a primary finding in NAFLD, is less frequently observed in IFALD.[15,16] IFALD-associated fibrosis presents with a "jigsaw" pattern with a portal, periportal, and portal-portal bridging development, different from the sinusoidal centrilobular fibrosis characteristic of NAFLD.[15,16] The finding of a combination of portal and perivenular fibrosis was considered a characteristic of PN injury.[15,16]

NATURAL HISTORY, ASSESSMENT, AND MONITORING

The progression of IFALD can ultimately end in liver failure, a mandatory indication for a life-saving combined liver and small bowel transplantation (ITx).[1] Infants are more susceptible to IF/PN-related hepatocellular injury and develop fibrosis, as well as progression to high-stage fibrosis more rapidly than older children and adults.[15] In 22 adult case series and 16 children cohorts, IFALD-related death represented 4% to 5% and 16% to 60% of total death on HPN, respectively, with a mortality rate greater in premature infants and babies.[17]

Monitoring the evolution of IFALD is therefore mandatory to prevent the evolution to end-stage liver disease as well as for the timing of patient referral for ITx. Routine assessment of LFTs every 3 to 4 months is recommended.[4] An international panel of experts proposed a severity categorization of IFALD, based on LFTs, abdominal ultrasound, liver histology features, and clinical features[18] (**Table 2**).

Determining when hepatic fibrosis is progressing to irreversible cirrhosis is a key issue for the timing for referral to ITx as well as for the type of transplantation. No association was found between the LFTs and the histologic degree or the rate of progression of hepatocellular injury or fibrosis.[15] The role of transient elastography (FibroScan), a non-invasive marker of liver fibrosis in various liver disease, in patients on HPN for CIF remains to be clarified. In adults, the FibroScan score was found to be significantly correlated with the histologic score of cholestasis but not of fibrosis.[19] On the contrary, the results of a study in children showed that it could be a promising non-invasive method for monitoring the development of IF-related liver histopathology.[20]

Ultimately, liver histology remains the gold standard for assessing IFALD, even though this also may be misleading owing to patchy hepatic injury.[1] The decision to perform a liver biopsy should be taken on an individual basis. A persistent abnormal conjugated bilirubin would be a "red flag" alerting for the need of liver histology.[1,4]

PATHOGENESIS

The pathogenesis of IFALD is multifactorial. Intestinal failure-related, PN-related, and systemic-related factors play a role.[3,5,6,21–23] The potential mechanisms are summarized in **Fig. 1**.

The IF-related factors are essentially represented by the interplay of 3 mechanisms that are synergistic in the pathogenesis of liver injury: (a) lack of enteral/oral feeding;

Table 2
Proposed classification of intestinal failure-associated liver disease severity

	Type 1 Early/ Mild	Type 2 Established/ Moderate	Type 3 Late/Severe
Enzymes (ALP, γ–GT) A: >6 mo C: >6 wk	>1.5 × ULN	>1.5 × ULN	>3 × ULN
Total bilirubin (with increased direct fraction)	<50 μmol/L (3 mg/dL)	50–100 μmol/L (3–6 mg/dL)	>100 μmol/L (6 mg/dL)
Hepatic ultrasound	Some echogenicity	Enlarged spleen, biliary sludge, marked echogenicity	Enlarged spleen, irregular liver, ascites, varices
Histology	Steatosis <25% Fibrosis <50% portal tracts	Steatosis >25% Fibrosis>50% portal tracts	Coagulopathy and thrombocytopaenia C/I for biopsy

Abbreviations: A, adults; ALP, alkaline phosphatase; C, children; C/I, contraindication; γ-GT, gamma-glutamyl transferase; ULN, upper limit of normal.

Parenteral nutrition-related factors

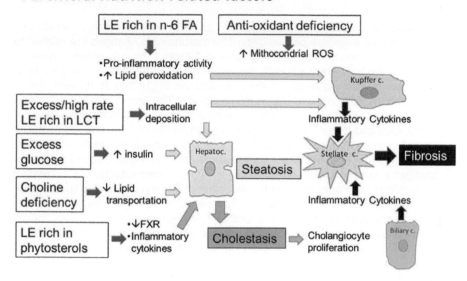

Gastrointestinal disease and systemic-related factors

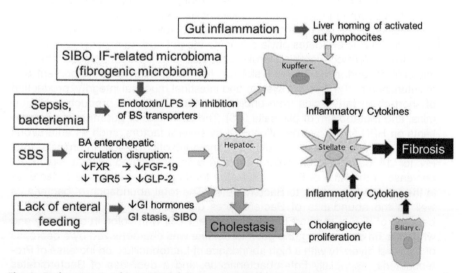

Fig. 1. Pathogenesis of intestinal failure-associated liver disease.

(b) alteration of the enterohepatic circulation of bile acids (BAs); and (c) changes in the gut microbiome. These factors have also been described under the term gut-liver axis, which indicates the gut-liver crosstalk through the portal vein blood flow, which provides the liver with gut-derived nutrients, signaling molecules, metabolic end products, as well as gut-derived toxins. The IF-related mechanisms of IFALD have been extensively discussed in recent reviews[5,6,21–23] and are summarized as follows:

- The absence of nutrients in the gut lumen can result in intestinal mucosal atrophy and increased intestinal permeability. The morphologic changes are related to the reduced secretion of intestinal growth factors. The gut growth hormone glucagon-like peptide-2 (GLP-2), secreted by the enteroendocrine L-cells of the ileum, plays a major role in the maintenance of gut health. Its secretion is stimulated by nutrients and BAs in the gut lumen. The secretion of GLP-2 mediated by BAs occurs through the BA activation of the G protein-coupled receptor TGR5, localized in gut mucosal crypts. The alteration of intestinal permeability, leading to the loss of epithelial barrier function, is probably due to the production of pro-inflammatory cytokines by intestinal immune cells, secondary to the changes in gut microbiota composition occurring during total fasting. Increased permeability facilitates massive translocation of intestinal bacterial lipopolysaccharide (LPS), a potent hepatotoxic inflammatory compound, into the portal circulation, mesenteric lymph nodes, and liver, with consequent liver injury, mainly characterized by cholestasis. Human and animal studies have shown that the severity of liver injury occurring during total PN associated with absence of enteral feeding, is typically reduced on introduction of enteral nutrition. Decreased hepatic injury was observed with concomitant supply of even a small amount of enteral nutrition.
- The human intestinal microbiota genome, or the gut microbiome, consists of 100 trillion commensal organisms and thousands of species, representing 200,000 to 300,000 genes. This is 10 times that of the aggregate human host genome. The composition of the gut microbiome varies among individuals, depending mainly on factors occurring during the first years of life. In individual healthy adults, the composition of the gut microbiome is relatively stable. Bacteria belonging to Firmicutes and Bacteroidetes phyla dominate the gut and, to a lesser extent, species from Verrucomicrobia, Proteobacteria, and Actinobacteria. The gut microbiome perform critical physiologic functions, such as development and maintenance of the immune system and intestinal mucosal integrity, production of short-chain fatty acids from undigested carbohydrates, production of vitamins, and metabolism of bile salts (BS). The variations of gut microbiota in patients on HPN for IF can be influenced by several factors, such as enteral/oral feeding, the gut anatomy and disease, and antibiotic therapy. In animals, total PN for 14 days without enteral feeding was associated with a significant decrease in the ratio of Firmicutes to the total bacteria, as well as a decrease in the ratio of Firmicutes to Bacteroidetes. The total abundance of bacteria as well as the abundance of Bacteroidetes did not differ. In patients on HPN because of IF due to short bowel syndrome (SBS) with colon in continuity and who were on oral feeding, the gut microbiome was characterized by a decrease of bacterial diversity with a high abundance of Lactobacillus, an increase of Proteobacteria, especially Enterobacteriaceae, and a decrease of Bacteroidetes and often Firmicutes. The changes did not differ between primary pathology and underlying disease or between children and adults. Increased abundance of Proteobacteria has been strongly associated with the pathogenesis of IFALD, especially liver steatosis and liver fibrosis. Possible mechanisms would be the Proteobacteria-induced pro-inflammatory status in the intestinal mucosa, with increased permeability and liver overload of gut-derived LPS, promoting inflammation and fibrogenesis. In patients with IF, a substantial increase in

Lactobacillus level, representing less than 1% of the gut microbiome in healthy subjects, has also been reported to be associated with diarrhea, D-lactic acidosis, and the development of IFALD, especially steatosis, via excessive BA deconjugation. In patients with impaired intestinal motility, as well as those with a small bowel closed loop, small intestinal bacterial overgrowth (SIBO) may develop, contributing to the pathogenesis of IFALD.

- The alteration of enterohepatic BAs circulation following BA malabsorption, such as in SBS, and/or changes in intestinal microbiota is a key mechanism implicated in the pathogenesis of IFALD-cholestasis due to the disruption of the gut-liver axis. In humans, primary BAs, chenodeoxycholic and cholic acids, are synthesized and conjugated to taurine or glycine in the liver and, as BSs, are secreted into bile. Approximately 95% of BAs are reabsorbed in the small intestine via enterohepatic circulation, whereas a minor fraction escapes before being further metabolized by the gut microbiota in the colon to the secondary BAs, deoxycholic, urodeoxycholic, and lithocholic acids. In addition to facilitating intestinal absorption of dietary fat and fat-soluble vitamins, BAs have direct antibacterial effects, regulate the host glucose and lipid metabolism, as well as energy homeostasis, and exert a trophic stimulation on the intestinal mucosa. Bile acid malabsorption causes a dysfunction of farnesoid-X receptor (FXR)/fibroblast growth factor-19 (FGF19) signaling. In healthy subjects, BAs activate the BA receptor FXR in the enterocyte of the distal ileum and in the liver, during the enterohepatic cycle. In the enterocyte, FXR stimulates the secretion of FGF19, which reaches the liver through the portal vein. In the hepatocyte, FGF19 downregulates cholesterol-7-alpha-hydroxylase-1, the rate-limiting key enzyme for the conversion of cholesterol into BAs, thus providing negative feedback control of BA synthesis. Hepatic FXR further acts as a safeguard against BA toxicity by controlling import and efflux of BS in the liver. The Farnesoid-X receptor seems to play a role also in maintaining intestinal permeability, thus protecting against bacterial and/or LPS translocation. Translocation of microbial products activates resident macrophages in the liver, with subsequent release of pro-inflammatory cytokines such as interleukin-6 and tumor necrosis factor alpha, which interferes with liver BA export. In IFALD, liver injury may arise from intrahepatic accumulation of BAs, and impaired FXR/FGF19-mediated liver repair. In patients with IF, serum FGF19 levels were found to be significantly lower than in healthy subjects and to correlate with portal inflammation or fibrosis, thus probably contributing to cellular apoptosis, fibrotic changes, and ultimately liver injury.
- Finally, linked to the gut-liver axis, the presence of inflammation in the gut, such as in exacerbations of Crohn's disease and necrotizing enterocolitis, would represent an increased risk of IFALD, possibly via the phenomenon of homing of activated gut lymphocytes to the liver.

The PN-related factors are mainly represented by excess of macronutrients in the PN admixture in comparison with the patient's requirements. Deficiency of micronutrients may also be involved. Excess of PN energy, delivered as either glucose or fat, promotes hepatic IFALD-steatosis. Glucose overfeeding can result in greater plasma insulin concentration, hepatic lipogenesis, and the build-up of triglycerides within hepatocytes. Fat supplied intravenously is carried by liposomes, rather than chylomicrons, which results in steatosis, characterized by fat deposition in Kupffer cells and hepatic lysosomes.[1] Hepatic steatosis may be induced by deficiency of choline,[16] essential fatty acids, and carnitine.[1,16] In comparison with 24-h continuous PN infusion, cyclic PN infusion (usually 10–14 h) is associated with a reduction in hyperinsulinemia, lower dextrose use, increased lipid oxidation, and lower fat deposition in the liver.[24,25] Excess amino acids may be associated with development of IFALD in children, and deficiency of taurine and cysteine may play a role in premature infants.[6] In adults, soybean-based (SO) intravenous fat emulsions (IVFEs) in excess of 1 g/kg/d have been shown to cause liver damage, especially IFALD-cholestasis.[7] Implicated mechanism would be the activation of the Kupffer cells because of the high content of pro-inflammatory ω-6 polyunsaturated fatty acid (PUFA), linoleic acid, the peroxidation of PUFAs, and the low content of α-tocopherol, a major lipophilic antioxidant agent, and fat overloading.[5,6,26] Furthermore, SO-IVFEs have a high content of plant sterols (especially sigmasterol), which have been shown to interrupt hepatocyte FXR signaling and the expression of downstream BA transporters, thus decreasing bile flow.[5,6,27,28]

Systemic-related risk factors for IFALD are mainly represented by recurrent catheter-related blood stream infection (CRBSI), which acts through the inhibition of BA transporters in the hepatocytes by endotoxin, leading to cholestasis.[1,5,6]

Overall, the consequence of chronic cholestasis is ductular proliferation. Proliferating cholangiocytes secrete pro-inflammatory and chemotactic cytokines.[6] Whatever the cause (microbiota or sepsis endotoxins, BA depletion, gut inflammation, excess SO-IVFE), activation of Kupffer cells within the liver stimulates the release of pro-inflammatory cytokines. Intrahepatic cytokines activate the liver stellate cells, which, in combination with immature or depleted intracellular antioxidant capacity (decreased α-tocopherol), seems to be the common pathway to hepatic fibrosis.[5]

Steatosis is favored by PN overfeeding of lipid emulsion (LE) and glucose and by choline deficiency. Fat deposition form LEs can occur also in Kupffer cells. Disruption of the enterohepatic BA circulation because of malabsorption (ie, SBS), or lack of oral or enteral feeding, increases intestinal absorption of bacterial LPS, circulating endotoxins associated with sepsis, and phytosterols contained in Les, cause cholestasis. The secondary effect of chronic cholestasis is ductular proliferation. Proliferating cholangiocytes secrete pro-inflammatory and chemotactic cytokines. Liver homing of activated lymphocytes from intestinal inflammation, excess of soybean-based LE rich in ω-6 PUFA, and depleted antioxidant capacity activates Kupffer cells to release pro-inflammatory cytokines.

PREVENTION AND TREATMENT

A schematic view of the pathophysiology, and the associated potential preventive and curative treatments of IFALD are summarized in **Table 3**.

For the prevention of IFALD, the ESPEN guideline recommendation can be summarized as follows:

- Preventing any infective/inflammatory foci (particularly CRBSI and SIBO)
- Preserving small intestinal length as long as possible and retaining the colon in continuity during surgical procedures
- Maintaining oral/enteral feeding
- Avoiding continuous PN infusion, instead, cycle PN infusion
- Avoiding PN overfeeding
- Limiting the dose of SO-IVFE to less than 1 g/kg/d in adults.[1]

Available data in adults do not support PN supplementation with taurine and carnitine,[1] whereas choline replacement has been reported to improve liver transaminases.[3,16] A few studies would support the efficacy of oral ursodeoxycholic acid,

Table 3
Proposed pathophysiology and associated preventive and curative measures for intestinal failure-associated liver disease

Pathogenic Factor	Intervention
Lack of oral feeding	Minimal oral/enteral feeding
Short bowel syndrome	Non-transplant surgery: restore intestinal continuity, intestinal lengthening procedures Ursodeoxycholic acid: 20–30 mg/kg/d
Small intestine bacterial overgrowth	Oral metronidazole, other antibiotics Prophylactic prokinetic drugs in dysmotility (ie, erythromycin)
Sepsis	Treat rapidly and optimize CVC management
Oxidative stress	α-Tocopherol (and other antioxidants ?) supplementation
Excess PN energy	Avoiding overfeeding Maintenance low-mid range BMI
Excess PN amino acids	Avoiding amount exceeding needs
Excess PN glucose	<7 mg/kg/min Cyclic PN (stop for 8 h)
Excess PN lipids Soybean LE (n-6 PUFA) Phytosterols phospholipids	Soybean-based LEs ≤1 g/kg/d ↓ ω-6 PUFA: LCT-MCT, olive oil, fish oil ↓ Phytosterols: FO, LCT-MCT, OO ↓ Phospholipids: LE concentration 30% <20% <10%
PN amino acid deficiency	Taurine-enriched AA solution (children)
Other PN deficiencies	Intravenous choline, 2 g/d Oral Lecithin, 20 g × 2/d Balanced IVFEs to avoid EFAD

Abbreviations: AA, amino acid; BMI, body mass index; CVC, central venous catheter; EFAD, essential fatty acids deficiency; FO, fish oil; IVFEs, intravenous fat emulsions; LCT-MCT, long-chain triglycerides-medium-chain triglycerides; OO, olive oil; PN, parenteral nutrition; PUFA, polyunsaturated fatty acid.

which displaces hepatotoxic BS and protects against hepatocellular injury.[1] Treatment of IFALD is based on the re-consideration of all the preventive measures, the revision of the LE type and dosage in the PN admixture, and the search for and treatment of potential inflammatory/infective foci.[1] In individual cases, antibiotics such as metronidazole and tetracycline may have beneficial effects.[29,30] According to the severity classification of IFALD, persistent hyperbilirubinemia from 3 to 6 mg/dL (50–100 μmol/L) would be a criterion for referral to an IF rehabilitation unit, and persistent concentration greater than 6 mg/dL a criterion for consultation or referral for transplantation assessment and listing.[1,18]

The most debated strategy is concerning the type and the amount of LEs.[1,6] To decrease the ω-6 PUFA load with PN admixtures, a new generation of LEs has been developed, containing lower amounts of PUFAs (medium chain triglycerides/soybean or olive/soybean-based IVFEs) and or enriched with ω-3 PUFAs (soybean/MCT/olive/fish or soybean/MCT/fish oil-based IVFEs), as well as pure fish oil-based IVFEs.[31] In addition to the lower content of the pro-inflammatory ω-6 PUFA, the potential advantages of fish oil containing IVFEs include the presence of the antiinflammatory ω-3 PUFAs, docosahexaenoic and eicosapentaenoic acid,[31] the higher content of the antioxidant α-tocopherol, and the lower or absent content of phytosterols.[32,33]

Most of the studies on the efficacy of the new generation of IVFEs in the prevention and treatment of IFALD have been carried out in newborns/infants and children. At

Table 4
Studies on treatment of IFALD with fish oil-based IVFE in adults, reporting the changes on liver histology

Author	Patient No.	IVFE Type and Dosage	Liver Histology Score			
			Baseline		End of Treatment	
Pironi et al.,[40] 2010	1	Omegaven 0.20 g/kg/d + Clinoleic for 8 mo	Cholestasis Steatosis Inflammation Fibrosis	0 2 2 3	Cholestasis Steatosis Inflammation Fibrosis	0 1 1 3
Jurewitsch et al.,[41] 2011	1	Omegaven 0.25 g/kg/d alone for 4 mo	• No steatosis • Heavy lobular and portal cholestasis • Fibrosis 2		• No steatosis • Portal hepatitis, cholangiopathy, no cholestasis • Fibrosis 2	
Xu et al.,[42] 2012	15	Omegaven 0.15–0.25 g/kg/d + Lipofundin for 1 mo	Cholestasis Steatosis Inflammation Fibrosis	Mean 1.5 2.2 2.8 1.9	Cholestasis Steatosis Inflammation Fibrosis	Mean 1.0 1.5 1.5 1.7

Abbreviations: IVFE, intravenous fat emulsion; Pironi and Xu, liver histology according to Brunt classification.

present, there is no evidence to strongly support the use of new-generation IVFEs to prevent IFALD, when the recommended standard dosage of lipids are <1 g/kg body weight/d in adults and 15% to 30% of non-protein calories as fat in children.[1,6,34–36] A debate is ongoing about the risk of essential fatty acids deficiency (EFAD) associated with the long-term use of low SO-IVFEs, especially in infants and children.[35,37]

Replacing SO-IVFEs with fish oil-based IVFEs has been suggested to play a role in the reversal of IFALD-cholestasis and steatosis in children on long-term HPN.[33,38,39] In the presence of IFALD-cholestasis, an alternative strategy would be reducing or temporally discontinuing IVS. This should be considered and balanced against the risks of giving insufficient energy, increased amount of glucose, and to generate an EFAD.[37] In children, a minimum 0.5 g/kg/d of soybean oil-based IVFE is recommended to prevent the development of EFAD.[6] Two case reports[40,41] and a case series[42] in which liver biopsy was performed before and at the end of the treatment, supported the role of pure fish oil-based IVFE for IFALD in adults (**Table 4**). Fish oil was added to the current IVFE in 2 studies[40,42] and replaced the IVFE in 1 case.[41] The dosage of fish oil ranged from 0.15 to 2.5 g/kg body weight/d of infusion. All the results showed a resolution or improvement of cholestasis, steatosis, and inflammation, but no changes were observed for liver fibrosis.[40–42]

SUMMARY

A liver injury, named IFALD, is a potential complication of patients on long-term HPN for CIF, characterized by either liver steatosis or cholestasis. Infants are more at risk of IFALD than older children and adults, even though the diagnostic criteria and, consequently, the epidemiology remain to be fully defined. Cholestasis is more frequent in infants, in whom the evolution to severe hepatic fibrosis, cirrhosis, and end-stage liver failure is more rapid. When liver failure occurs, IFALD is an indication for combined liver and intestinal transplantation.

The pathogenesis of IFALD is multifactorial. The main pathogenetic factors are related to the underlying gastrointestinal condition, now summarized by the concept of the gut-liver axis, including altered BA enterohepatic circulation, altered gut microbiome, increased intestinal permeability, and intraabdominal inflammation. Patients forced to total oral/enteral fasting are at increased risk of IFALD in comparison with those who are allowed to eat. Sepsis, most frequently CRBSI, is also a major pathogenetic factor. The PN-related factors are mainly represented by PN overfeeding of energy and/or of SO-IVFEs. Prevention and treatment are based on avoiding and promptly treating all the risk factors in the individual patient.

Future research should aim to further clarify the alteration of the so-called gut-liver axis, to find novel methods for diagnosis and monitoring, to generate evidence for current preventative strategies (eg, new IVFE and antibiotic therapy) and to develop novel therapeutic targets.[43]

REFERENCES

1. Pironi L, Arends J, Bozzetti F, et al, Home Artificial Nutrition & Chronic Intestinal Failure Special Interest Group of ESPEN. ESPEN guidelines on chronic intestinal failure in adults. Clin Nutr 2016;35(2):247–307.

2. Staun M, Pironi L, Bozzetti F, et al. ESPEN guidelines on parenteral nutrition: home parenteral nutrition (HPN) in adult patients. Clin Nutr 2009;28(4):467–79.

3. Buchman AL, Iyer K, Fryer J. Parenteral nutrition-associated liver disease and the role of isolated intestine and intestine/liver transplantation. Hepatology 2006;43: 9–19.

4. Lal S, Pironi L, Wanten G, et al, Home Artificial Nutrition & Chronic Intestinal Failure Special Interest Group of the European Society for Clinical Nutrition and Metabolism (ESPEN). Clinical approach to the management of intestinal failure associated liver disease (IFALD) in adults: a position paper from the home artificial nutrition and chronic intestinal failure special interest group of ESPEN. Clin Nutr 2018. https://doi.org/10.1016/j.clnu.2018.07.006.

5. Beath SV, Kelly DA. Total parenteral nutrition-induced cholestasis: prevention and management. Clin Liver Dis 2016;20(1):159–76.

6. Lacaille F, Gupte G, Colomb V, et al, ESPGHAN Working Group of Intestinal Failure and Intestinal Transplantation. Intestinal failure-associated liver disease: a position paper of the ESPGHAN Working Group of intestinal failure and intestinal transplantation. J Pediatr Gastroenterol Nutr 2015;60(2):272–83.

7. Cavicchi M, Beau P, Crenn P, et al. Prevalence of liver disease and contributing factors in patients receiving home parenteral nutrition for permanent intestinal failure. Ann Intern Med 2000;132:525–32.

8. Pironi L, Konrad D, Brandt C, et al. Clinical classification of adult patients with chronic intestinal failure due to benign disease: an international multicentre cross-sectional survey. Clin Nutr 2018;37(2):728–38.

9. Sorbi D, Boynton J, Lindor KD. The ratio of aspartate aminotransferase to alanine aminotransferase: potential value in differentiating non-alcoholic steatohepatitis from alcoholic liver disease. Am J Gastroenterol 1999;94(4):1018e22.

10. Byrne CD, Targher G. EASL-EASD-EASO Clinical Practice Guidelines for the management of non-alcoholic fatty liver disease: is universal screening appropriate? Diabetologia 2016;59(6):1141–4.

11. Rath MM, Panigrahi MK, Pattnaik K, et al. Histological evaluation of non-alcoholic fatty liver disease and its correlation with different noninvasive scoring systems with special reference to fibrosis: a single center experience. J Clin Exp Hepatol 2016;6(4):291–6.

12. Sterling RK, Lissen E, Clumeck N, et al, APRICOT clinical Investigators. Develop-
    ment of a simple noninvasive index to predict significant fibrosis in patients with
    HIV/HCV coinfection. Hepatology 2006;43(6):1317–25.
13. Luman W, Shaffer JL. Prevalence, outcome and associated factors of deranged
    liver function tests in patients on home parenteral nutrition. Clin Nutr 2002;21(4):
    337–43.
14. Sasdelli AS, Agostini F, Pazzeschi C, et al. Assessment of intestinal failure asso-
    ciated liver disease according to different diagnostic criteria. Clin Nutr 2018.
    https://doi.org/10.1016/j.clnu.2018.04.019.
15. Naini BV, Lassman CR. Total parenteral nutrition therapy and liver injury: a histo-
    pathologic study with clinical correlation. Hum Pathol 2012;43(6):826–33.
16. Buchman AL, Naini BV, Spilker B. The differentiation of intestinal-failure-
    associated liver disease from nonalcoholic fatty liver and nonalcoholic steatohe-
    patitis. Semin Liver Dis 2017;37(1):33–44.
17. Pironi L, Goulet O, Buchman A, et al, Home Artificial Nutrition and Chronic Intes-
    tinal Failure Working Group of ESPEN. Outcome on home parenteral nutrition for
    benign intestinal failure: a review of the literature and benchmarking with the Eu-
    ropean prospective survey of ESPEN. Clin Nutr 2012;31(6):831–45.
18. Beath S, Pironi L, Gabe S, et al. Collaborative strategies to reduce mortality and
    morbidity in patients with chronic intestinal failure including those who are
    referred for small bowel transplantation. Transplantation 2008;85:1378–84.
19. Van Gossum A, Pironi L, Messing B, et al. Transient elastography (FibroScan) is
    not correlated with liver fibrosis but with cholestasis in patients with long-term
    home parenteral nutrition. JPEN J Parenter Enteral Nutr 2015;39(6):719–24.
20. Hukkinen M, Kivisaari R, Lohi J, et al. Transient elastography and aspartate
    aminotransferase to platelet ratio predict liver injury in paediatric intestinal failure.
    Liver Int 2016;36(3):361–9.
21. Cahova M, Bratova M, Wohl P. Parenteral nutrition-associated liver disease: the
    role of the gut microbiota. Nutrients 2017;9(9). https://doi.org/10.3390/
    nu9090987.
22. Denton C, Price A, Friend J, et al. Role of the gut-liver axis in driving parenteral
    nutrition-associated injury. Children (Basel) 2018;5(10). https://doi.org/10.3390/
    children5100136.
23. Neelis E, de Koning B, Rings E, et al. The gut microbiome in patients with intes-
    tinal failure: current evidence and implications for clinical practice. JPEN J Paren-
    ter Enteral Nutr 2018. https://doi.org/10.1002/jpen.1423.
24. Just B, Messing B, Darmaun D, et al. Comparison of substrate utilization by indi-
    rect calorimetry during cyclic and continuous total parenteral nutrition. Am J Clin
    Nutr 1990;51:107–11.
25. Jensen AR, Goldin AB, Koopmeiners JS, et al. The association of cyclic nutrition
    and decreased incidence of cholestatic liver disease in patients with gastroschi-
    sis. J Pediatr Surg 2009;44:183–9.
26. Lee WS, Sokol RJ. Intestinal microbiota, lipids, and the pathogenesis of intestinal
    failure-associated liver disease. J Pediatr 2015;167(3):519–26.
27. Calkins KL, DeBarber A, Steiner RD, et al. Intravenous fish oil and pediatric intes-
    tinal failure-associated liver disease: changes in plasma phytosterols, cytokines,
    and bile acids and erythrocyte fatty acids. JPEN J Parenter Enteral Nutr 2017.
    https://doi.org/10.1177/0148607117709196.
28. Hukkinen M, Mutanen A, Nissinen M, et al. Parenteral plant sterols accumulate in
    the liver reflecting their increased serum levels and portal inflammation in children
    with intestinal failure. JPEN J Parenter Enteral Nutr 2017;41(6):1014–22.

29. Lichtman SN, Keku J, Schwab JH, et al. Hepatic injury associated with small bowel bacterial overgrowth in rats is prevented by metronidazole and tetracycline. Gastroenterology 1991;100(2):513–9.
30. Freund HR, Muggia-Sullam M, LaFrance R, et al. A possible beneficial effect of metronidazole in reducing TPN-associated liver function derangements. J Surg Res 1985;38(4):356–63.
31. Pironi L, Guidetti M, Verrastro O, et al. Functional lipidomics in patients on home parenteral nutrition: effect of lipid emulsions. World J Gastroenterol 2017;23(25):4604–14.
32. Vanek VW, Seidner DL, Allen P, et al, Novel Nutrient Task Force, Intravenous Fat Emulsions Workgroup, American Society for Parenteral and Enteral Nutrition (A.S.P.E.N.) Board of Directors. A.S.P.E.N. position paper: clinical role for alternative intravenous fat emulsions. Nutr Clin Pract 2012;27(2):150–92.
33. Bharadwaj S, Gohel T, Deen OJ, et al. Fish oil-based lipid emulsion: current updates on a promising novel therapy for the management of parenteral nutrition-associated liver disease. Gastroenterol Rep (Oxf) 2015;3(2):110–4.
34. Guthrie G, Premkumar M, Burrin DG. Emerging clinical benefits of new-generation fat emulsions in preterm neonates. Nutr Clin Pract 2017;32(3):326–36.
35. Pironi L, Agostini F, Guidetti M. Intravenous lipids in home parenteral nutrition. World Rev Nutr Diet 2015;112:141–9.
36. Klek S, Szczepanek K, Scislo L, et al. Intravenous lipid emulsions and liver function in adult chronic intestinal failure patients: results from a randomized clinical trial. Nutrition 2018;55-56:45–50.
37. Anez-Bustillos L, Dao DT, Fell GL, et al. Redefining essential fatty acids in the era of novel intravenous lipid emulsions. Clin Nutr 2018;37(3):784–9.
38. de Meijer VE, Gura KM, Meisel JA, et al. Parenteral fish oil monotherapy in the management of patients with parenteral nutrition-associated liver disease. Arch Surg 2010;145(6):547–51.
39. Nandivada P, Chang MI, Potemkin AK, et al. The natural history of cirrhosis from parenteral nutrition-associated liver disease after resolution of cholestasis with parenteral fish oil therapy. Ann Surg 2015;261(1):172–9.
40. Pironi L, Colecchia A, Guidetti M, et al. Fish oil-based emulsion for the treatment of parenteral nutrition associated liver disease in an adult patient. E Spen Eur E J Clin Nutr Metab 2010;5:e243–6.
41. Jurewitsch B, Gardiner G, Naccarato M, et al. Omega-3-enriched lipid emulsion for liver salvage in parenteral nutrition-induced cholestasis in the adult patient. J Parenter Enteral Nutr 2011;35(3):386–90.
42. Xu Z, Li Y, Wang J, et al. Effect of omega-3 polyunsaturated fatty acids to reverse biopsy-proven parenteral nutrition-associated liver disease in adults. Clin Nutr 2012;31(2):217–23.
43. Pironi L, Corcos O, Forbes A, et al, ESPEN Acute and Chronic Intestinal Failure Special Interest Groups. Intestinal failure in adults: recommendations from the ESPEN expert groups. Clin Nutr 2018. https://doi.org/10.1016/j.clnu.2018.07.036.

Hepatic Manifestations of Lymphoproliferative Disorders

Chalermrat Bunchorntavakul, MD[a,b], K. Rajender Reddy, MD[b,*]

KEYWORDS

- Lymphoproliferative disorders • Lymphoma • Hodgkin • Liver involvement
- Hepatitis • Vanishing bile duct syndrome

KEY POINTS

- Hepatic abnormalities in patients with lymphoproliferative disorders are common and can occur from direct infiltration by abnormal cells, bile duct obstruction by lymphadenopathy, paraneoplastic syndrome, hemophagocytic syndrome, drug-induced liver injury, opportunistic infections, and reactivation of viral hepatitis.
- Hepatic involvement by lymphoma is often in association with systemic disease and rarely as a primary hepatic disease.
- Vanishing bile duct syndrome is a well-known paraneoplastic manifestation of Hodgkin lymphoma, which typically presents as progressive jaundice, pruritus, and marked elevation of alkaline phosphatase.
- Antiviral prophylaxis for HBV reactivation is recommended for all HBsAg[+] patients undergoing chemotherapy and all resolved HBV patients (anti-HBc[+]) undergoing rituximab therapy and stem cell transplantation.

INTRODUCTION

Lymphoproliferative disorders (LPDs) are a heterogeneous group of disorders characterized by the abnormal proliferation of lymphocytes, mainly B lymphocytes, into a monoclonal lymphocytosis. Hepatic abnormalities are commonly seen in patients with LPDs. Because the liver contains multipotential cells that can differentiate into

Conflict of Interest: Dr K.R. Reddy serves on the Advisory Board for Abbvie, Merck, Gilead, Shionogi, and Dova. Research support (paid to the University of Pennsylvania): Abbvie, Gilead, Merck, Mallinckrodt, Intercept, Conatus. Dr C. Bunchorntavakul has nothing to disclose.

[a] Division of Gastroenterology and Hepatology, Department of Medicine, Rajavithi Hospital, College of Medicine, Rangsit University, Rajavithi Road, Ratchathewi, Bangkok 10400, Thailand; [b] Division of Gastroenterology and Hepatology, Department of Medicine, University of Pennsylvania, Philadelphia, PA 19104, USA

* Corresponding author. University of Pennsylvania, 2 Dulles, 3400 Spruce Street, Philadelphia, PA 19104.

E-mail address: rajender.reddy@uphs.upenn.edu

reticuloendothelial, myeloid, and lymphoid cells, it can be involved in malignant LPDs, such as lymphoma, often in association with systemic disease and rarely as a primary hepatic disease. Occasionally, clinical evidence of liver disease may be the first manifestation of LPDs. Apart from direct infiltration of abnormal cells, hepatic abnormalities in patients with LPDs can also occur from other causes, such as bile duct obstruction, paraneoplastic syndrome, hemophagocytic syndrome (HPS), drug-induced liver injury, opportunistic infections, and reactivation of viral hepatitis (**Fig. 1**).

PRIMARY HEPATIC LYMPHOMA

Primary hepatic lymphoma (PHL), defined as a liver-confined lymphoma without extrahepatic involvement, is a very rare malignancy that encompasses less than 1% of all lymphomas. It often occurs in men (in about two-thirds of cases) during the fifth to sixth decade of life (range 21–86 years).[1–4] Non-Hodgkin lymphoma (NHL) is the major histologic subtype of PHL, whereas Hodgkin histology is extremely rare. PHL may be of either T- or B-cell origin with diffuse large B-cell lymphoma (DLBCL) being the most common subtype and comprising 60% to 90% of cases.[1,2,5] Based on patterns of hepatic infiltration, PHL may present with nodules in the liver (70%–95%; single > multiple) or diffuse portal infiltration and sinusoidal spread (5%–30%).[5–8] Although the exact cause of PHL is unclear, chronic viral infection (eg, hepatitis B virus [HBV], hepatitis C virus [HCV], human immunodeficiency virus [HIV], or Epstein-Barr virus [EBV]) and/or immune dysfunction (eg, autoimmune disorders or immunosuppression) may play a role in its pathogenesis because these conditions are increasingly observed in patients with PHL than in the general population.[1–3,9–11]

PHL usually presents with right upper quadrant or epigastric pain/discomfort, hepatomegaly, palpable mass. Lymphoma-related B grade symptoms, including fever, night sweats, and weight loss, are present in about 50% of cases.[2,4,7] Physical

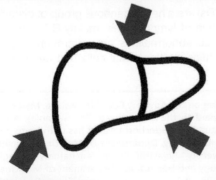

Related to lymphoma

- Direct infiltration of malignant cells
- Paraneoplastic syndrome (eg, vanishing bile duct syndrome)
- Bile duct obstruction from enlarged lymph nodes

Related to treatment

- Liver injury from chemotherapy, drugs and radiation
- Reactivation of viral hepatitis (HBV, HCV)
- Sinusoidal obstruction syndrome (SOS)
- Opportunistic infections

Miscellaneous

- Budd-Chiari syndrome
- Hemophagocytic syndrome
- Nodular regenerative hyperplasia

Fig. 1. Causes of liver abnormalities in patients with LPD.

examination frequently has revealed mild hepatomegaly (~80%), whereas jaundice has been an infrequent finding at presentation (~10%) and tended to be a late manifestation of disease progression.[2,4,7] Laboratory abnormalities associated with PHL include anemia, neutropenia, hypercalcemia, and variably elevated serum lactate dehydrogenase, bilirubin, alkaline phosphatase (ALP), and aminotransferase activities. Tumor markers of alpha fetoprotein and carcinoembryonic antigen are usually within normal range.[2,4,7] The severity of disease is variable, ranging from asymptomatic to rapidly progressing acute liver failure, encephalopathy, coma, or death.[2,4,7]

Although there are no pathognomonic features, radiological studies are the key in suspecting and diagnosing PHL, particularly in differentiating from other causes of liver disease. Imaging findings may show a solitary mass is most cases, whereas multiple masses or diffuse hepatomegaly (infiltrative type) may also be seen[2,8,12] (**Fig. 2**). Ultrasound often has noted a hypoechoic lesion with irregular margins.[2] Contrast-enhanced computed tomography (CT) scan often reveals slight perilesional enhancement (ringlike) in the arterial and venous phases, typically without lymphadenopathy, and morphologic changes of cirrhosis in the surrounding liver parenchyma.[2,8,12] MRI usually demonstrates hypointense lesion on the T1-weighted images and hyperintense lesion on the T2-weighted images; nonspecific dynamic enhancement has been noted after contrast administration, but in the hepatobiliary phase, PHL is mainly hypointense.[13] Although CT/MRI scan alone is inadequate to differentiate PHL from secondary hepatic lymphoma, PET with fludeoxyglucose F 18/CT can be more helpful by demonstrating the absence of pathologically hypermetabolic foci in any other nodes or organs.[2,14] The definite diagnosis of PHL requires a liver biopsy. However, the histologic diagnosis of PHL from a needle biopsy is often challenging because of its pleomorphic appearances so that a high index of suspicion for its diagnosis is important. Furthermore, immunophenotyping is always required for classification of lymphoma.[1,2]

In general, PHL is an aggressive disease associated with relatively poor prognosis. Early surgery and chemotherapy are treatment options for PHL, although only a minority are candidates for surgical resection. In a review of 84 cases of PHL, 10 patients were treated by surgical resection alone, and the median survival was 22 (1.5–120) months. The median survival was 13.6 (1.7–62) months, 6 (0.23–80) months, and 27.5 (3–42) months in patients treated by surgical resection with postoperative chemotherapy (n = 12), chemotherapy alone (n = 40), and a combination chemotherapy and radiotherapy (n = 9), respectively, whereas patients receiving only

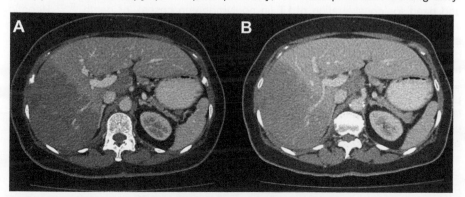

Fig. 2. CT findings in a patient with PHL: infiltrative pattern. (*A*) Late arterial phase. (*B*) Portal venous phase. (*Courtesy of* Sith Phongkitkarun, Associate Professor, Department of Diagnostic and Therapeutic Radiology, Ramathibodi Hospital, Mahidol University.)

supportive treatment (n = 11) had a median survival of 0.7 (0.06–18) months.[4] Nevertheless, a retrospective cohort of 24 patients with PHL treated by combination chemotherapy demonstrated a favorable outcome with the complete remission rate of 83%; the 5-year survival rate was 87%.[10] A combination of rituximab with cytotoxic treatment (especially for DLBCL) and the utilization of antiviral therapy (for HCV+ patients) have been shown to improve the clinical outcome of PHL significantly.[1,2,10]

LIVER INVOLVEMENT IN HODGKIN LYMPHOMA

Hodgkin lymphoma (HL) is a common type of lymphoma that is characterized by the presence of Reed-Sternberg cells in lymph nodes and by spread in a contiguous fashion via the lymphatic system.[5] It has a bimodal age distribution (20–40 years old and >55 years old) affecting about 574,000 people and causing about 23,900 deaths worldwide in 2015.[15] About half of HL cases are related to EBV infection, whereas other risk factors include a family history of HL and HIV/AIDS.[16] Patients with HL typically present with painless lymphadenopathy (cervical, supraclavicular, and mediastinal lymph nodes are most frequently involved), fever, night sweats, and weight loss. Splenomegaly is present in about 30% of cases. Liver infiltration by lymphoma cells has been reported in 15% of patients with HL, and hepatomegaly has been reported in 9% of patients with stage I/II and in 45% of patients with stage III/IV disease.[5,17] Jaundice is relatively common in patients with HL, which can occur from direct infiltration, extrahepatic biliary obstruction, vanishing bile duct syndrome (VBDS), hemolysis, viral hepatitis, or drug hepatotoxicity, and in approximately 3% to 13% of patients, jaundice is the presenting symptom.[5] Acute liver failure can occur due to ischemia secondary to compression of the hepatic sinusoids by infiltrating lymphoma cells and is often preceded by prodromal symptoms (eg, malaise, weight loss, right upper quadrant pain, and fever) about 2 to 4 weeks before the onset.[5,18]

VANISHING BILE DUCT SYNDROME

VBDS is an acquired condition characterized by progressive destruction and disappearance of the intrahepatic bile ducts (ductopenia) and, ultimately, cholestasis.[19–21] It is a final common pathologic pathway, resulting from multiple causes, including medications, infections, genetics, and autoimmune and neoplastic disorders.[20] Occasionally, progressive bile duct loss may lead to secondary biliary cirrhosis, liver failure, and need for consideration of LT (in nonlymphoma cases), or death.[19–21] Hepatic involvement with HL may be seen in up to 50% of patients and increases in frequency as the disease advances.[20] VBDS is a rare, but well-known complication of HL. It is defined histologically by loss of interlobular bile ducts in more than 50% of portal tracts in a pathologic specimen that is adequate for interpretation ($\geq$10 portal triads) and typically in the absence of direct infiltration by lymphoma cells.[20] Although a clear pathogenetic relationship between HL and VBDS has not yet been identified, VBDS is likely to be modulated by cytokine-mediated hepatic damage triggered by HL, so-called paraneoplastic manifestation. Histologically, hepatic sinusoidal dilatation (an early feature of VBDS) has been observed in up to 90% of HL patients with systemic symptoms (so-called B symptoms) but observed in only 20% in those without.[22] In addition, there has been some evidence that suggested that biliary epithelial cells express major histocompatibility complex antigens and intercellular adhesion molecules in response to cytokines produced by HL.[21,23] Notably, VBDS somewhat resembles a paraneoplastic cholestatic syndrome mediated partly by interleukin-6, so-called Stauffer syndrome, which has been described mostly in renal cell carcinoma.[24]

Patients with HL-related VBDS typically present with progressive jaundice, pruritus, and weight loss.[19,21] Marked elevations of serum ALP, bilirubin, and aminotransferases (in a lesser degree) are often observed. CT scan often reveals diffuse hepatomegaly without focal lesions or bile duct dilatation (**Fig. 3**). HL-related VBDS often develops at the same time or after the diagnosis of HL; however, in some patients, VBDS may precede the appearance of HL, even by several months.[25,26] Treatment of HL in those with VBDS is often challenging because appropriate therapy must often strike a balance between the need for aggressive chemoradiation, to achieve remission, and the degree of liver dysfunction. Based on greater than 40 case reports in the literature, liver failure is a major cause of death among patients with HL-related VBDS (up to 60% of cases), regardless of treatment.[19,21] Nevertheless, aggressive upfront chemotherapy can restore hepatic functions and achieved complete remission of HL in a significant proportion of patients. Of note, full-dose chemotherapy was used in most of these reports, whereas reduced-dose chemotherapy was used in some (doxorubicin and vinblastine are predominantly eliminated by the liver and there are recommendations for dose reduction in patients with significant hepatic insufficiency or cholestasis).[10,12] Strategies to treat cholestasis such as with ursodeoxycholic acid and cholestyramine may benefit patient symptoms, although limited data exist.[19,21]

LIVER INVOLVEMENT IN NON-HODGKIN LYMPHOMA

NHL is a large and heterogeneous group of malignancies involving mutations of B and T cells that basically include all lymphomas, other than HL. As compared with HL, NHL

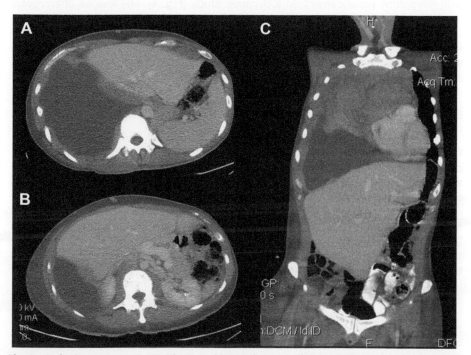

Fig. 3. CT findings in a patient with HL and VBDS showing a large mediastinal tumor invading chest wall, lymphadenopathy, massive right pleural effusion, and diffuse hepatomegaly and splenomegaly. (*A-B*) Portal venous phase, axial plane. (*C*) Portal venous phase, coronal plane).

is more common (affecting about 4.3 million people and causing 231,400 deaths worldwide in 2015), usually affects older patients (>60 year old), and spreads in a less contiguous fashion.[5,15] The most common high-grade NHL is a DLBCL, which is an aggressive malignancy that is curable in 60% to 70% of patients with combined immunochemotherapy.[27] The most common indolent NHL is follicular lymphoma, which is generally considered incurable and has a relapsing-remitting course with treatment required intermittently.[27]

Liver involvement and extrahepatic obstruction occur more commonly in NHL than in HL.[5,28] Liver infiltration by lymphoma cells is found in 16% to 27% of patients with NHL as evaluated by a percutaneous liver biopsy[29,30] and is found in up to 52% to 56% of patients when evaluated by staging laparotomy or autopsy.[31,32] Patterns of liver infiltration on histology may be distinct according to lymphoma subtypes: DLBCL and Burkitt lymphoma predominantly demonstrate tumor nodules deranging the normal hepatic architecture; chronic lymphocytic leukemia and HL mostly are characterized by infiltration of the portal fields; marginal zone B-cell lymphomas and HL may reveal lymphoepithelial lesions of bile ducts (~10% of cases).[6] Furthermore, liver infiltration tends to be more often in low-grade lymphomas than in those that are high grade.[5,28] However, it should be noted that hepatomegaly and mild to moderate elevations of serum ALP level commonly occur in NHL whether or not there is lymphomatous hepatic involvement.[5,28] Various presentations, mainly infiltrative and nodular patterns, can be seen on imaging studies in NHL patients with liver involvement, and there are no specific imaging characteristics for metastatic NHL.[8] Ultrasound may show hypoechoic/hyperechoic nodules of multiple small and large masses, or, rarely, may appear as a single large mass. CT scan often notes hypodense lesions with rim/patchy enhancement on a dynamic study (**Fig. 4**). MR images often reveal hypointense lesions on T1-weighted images and hyperintensity on T2-weighted images.[8] As in HL, acute liver failure and submassive hepatic necrosis can also occur in NHL and are associated with poor prognosis.[33–36] They share common clinical features that include hepatomegaly, lactic acidosis, and death shortly after the onset of symptoms.[33]

LYMPHOMA CAUSING BILIARY OBSTRUCTION AND PRIMARY LYMPHOMA OF THE BILE DUCT

Among all patients with malignant biliary obstruction, NHL accounts for 1% to 2% of all cases. Obstructive jaundice associated with lymphoma is mostly secondary to compression of the extrahepatic bile ducts by lymphadenopathy (periportal, perihepatic, or peripancreatic), and less commonly from primary bile duct lymphoma, or primary or secondary lymphoma of the pancreas.[37–39] Secondary pancreatic lymphoma can be seen in up to 30% of patients with advanced lymphoma, which is far more common than primary pancreatic lymphoma. The head of the pancreas is the most common location, and in the setting of a solitary pancreatic mass, key imaging findings highly suggestive of secondary pancreatic lymphoma and not of adenocarcinoma are the absence of vascular invasion, bile duct, and pancreatic duct obstruction, and the presence of lymphadenopathy below the level of the left renal vein.[38] Most of the cases of primary pancreatic lymphoma are large lesions with delayed homogeneous enhancement and often with peripancreatic fat stranding and vascular encasement, whereas vascular infiltration and pancreatic duct dilatation are rare.[40] Notably, DLBCL is the most common lymphoma type, accounting for 67% of all pancreatic lymphoma cases.[41]

Primary lymphoma of the bile duct is extremely rare and not uncommonly is preliminarily diagnosed as sclerosing cholangitis, Klatskin tumor, or pancreatic

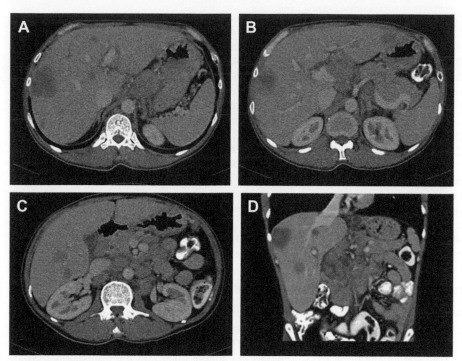

Fig. 4. CT findings in a patient with NHL and hepatic involvement: nodular pattern. (*A-C*) Portal venous phase, axial plane. (*D*) Portal venous phase, coronal plane. (*Courtesy of* Sith Phongkitkarun, Associate Professor, Department of Diagnostic and Therapeutic Radiology, Ramathibodi Hospital, Mahidol University.)

adenocarcinoma. The possibility for primary bile duct should be raised when cholangiography shows smooth, mild luminal narrowing of the extrahepatic ducts without mucosal irregularities, despite the diffuse thickening of the ductal wall noted on CT/MR images.[39] Endoscopic ultrasound-guided fine-needle aspiration biopsy has an important role in obtaining a tissue diagnosis of lymphoma-associated biliary obstruction, and treatment modalities included surgical resection, biliary drainage, chemotherapy, and radiotherapy.[37–39,41]

HEMOPHAGOCYTIC SYNDROME

HPS is a rare, but potentially life-threatening condition that is characterized by an uncontrolled immune response and a proliferation of macrophages.[42] The cytokine storm and infiltration of activated macrophages are responsible for features of persistent fever, hepatosplenomegaly, pancytopenia, hypertriglyceridemia, hyperferritinemia, and hemophagocytosis in the bone marrow, liver, and other organs.[43,44] Primary HPS typically occurs in infants and young children with a clear genetic susceptibility, whereas secondary HPS are triggered by various stimuli, including infections (eg, EBV, cytomegalovirus [CMV], and HIV), autoimmune disorders (eg, systemic lupus erythematosus, rheumatoid arthritis, and Still disease), malignancies, and immunosuppression.[42] Lymphoma is the most common underlying condition in malignancy-associated HPS and which may occur as an initial presentation, or as a complication at a relapse or an advanced stage of lymphoma.[43,44] Abnormal hepatic biochemical tests are common among patients with HPS and are supporting evidence for the diagnosis of HPS.[43] In a case series of 30 HPS patients (22 had lymphoma/leukemia), jaundice was present in 50% of patients, median ALT was 5 (0.3–125) times the upper limit of normal (xULN), median ALP was 2.7 (0.2–47.7) xULN, and median total bilirubin was 8 (0.2–39.8) mg/dL.[45] Kupffer cell hyperplasia, sinusoidal dilatation, and hemophagocytic histiocytosis were found in the biopsy specimen in all patients. High serum bilirubin and ALP levels were associated with a poorer prognosis.[45]

Lymphoma-associated HPS carries the worst prognosis among all secondary HPS types: with an overall 3-year survival of 8% to 48% (median survival 36–55 days) for B-cell lymphoma–associated HPS and 12% (median survival 28–40 days) for natural killer (NK)/T-cell lymphoma–associated HPS.[44,46,47] The treatment of lymphoma-associated HPS aims to treat underlying lymphoma and control the overactive immune system. Early diagnosis and appropriate immunosuppressive, chemotherapy, and hematopoietic stem cell transplantation are necessary to improve outcomes.[44,46,47] Rituximab and PEG-L-asparaginase–containing regimens are promising treatments for patients with B-cell and NK/T-cell lymphoma–associated HPS, respectively.[44]

POSTTRANSPLANT LYMPHOPROLIFERATIVE DISORDERS

Posttransplant lymphoproliferative disorders (PTLDs) are heterogeneous lymphoid disorders ranging from indolent polyclonal proliferations to aggressive lymphomas (~85% are B-cell origin) that complicate solid organ or hematopoietic transplantation.[48] The incidence of PTLD in adults is variable based on the transplanted organ: 2% to 5% in kidney or liver transplants (LT), 1% to 6% in heart transplants, 4% to 10% in lung transplants, and up to 20% in small intestine transplants.[48] In adult LT series, the cumulative incidence is 0.5% at 6 months, 1.1% at 18 months, 2.1% at 5 years, and 4.7% at 15 years after LT, with the highest incidence during the first 18 months.[49] The pathogenesis of PTLDs in most cases (60%–85%) relates to EBV-driven B-cell proliferations in the setting of chronic T-cell immunosuppression.[7,48,49] However, by unclear pathogenesis, EBV-negative tumors and T-cell tumors (~30% also positive for EBV) can also occur.[48,50] Risk factors for PTLDs include viral infections (eg, pretransplant EBV seronegativity, HCV infection, CMV mismatch), degree of immunosuppression (eg, intensive immunosuppression, anti-T-cell antibodies, such as OKT3, and antithymocyte globulins), recipient age (younger age), allograft type (small intestine), and host genetic variations.[7,48–52] The clinical manifestations of PTLDs can vary from asymptomatic state to localized signs (eg, lymphadenopathy, abdominal mass, swelling in the oral cavity), infectious mononucleosis-like syndrome (eg, fever, pharyngitis, cervical lymphadenopathy), and a very aggressive disease with rapid evolution to multiorgan failure.[48,51]

The 2017 World Health Organization classification of PTLDs includes 4 categories: (1) nondestructive PTLDs (plasmacytic hyperplasia, infectious mononucleosis, and follicular hyperplasia); (2) polymorphic PTLDs; (3) monomorphic PTLDs (classifying according to B-cell or T-cell lymphoma they resemble; DLBCL is the most common type); and (4) chronic HL PTLDs.[53] Localization patterns of PTLDs are variable according to the transplanted organ. For non–liver solid organ transplant recipients, PTLDs localized to the liver are uncommon and seen in 5% of PTLDs that occur after kidney and lung transplant, and in 9% of PTLDs that occur after heart transplant.[54] However, PTLDs in LT recipients have preference for localization to the liver. Posttransplant lymphomas are more likely than general lymphomas to have extranodal involvement, high-grade, aggressive clinical behavior, and poor outcomes.[51,55] Poor prognostic factors for PTLDs include high-grade histology, poor performance status, EBV nega-tivity, and graft involvement.[51,55] Based on the Collaborative Transplant Study including 165 LT recipients with posttransplant lymphomas, 21.8%, 12.1%, 9.7%, 4.2%, 4.2% had disease localized to the liver, gastrointestinal tract, lymph node, cen-tral nervous system, and lung, respectively, whereas 13.3% demonstrated multifocal disease. The 5-year survival rates were 33% for liver disease, 62% for nodal disease, and 21% for disseminated disease.[54]

A high index of suspicion and early diagnosis of PTLDs are important to facilitate prompt initiation of treatment and prevent evolution to more aggressive variants. Although diagnosis can be assumed based on clinical presentation and the measure-ment of quantitative EBV load in the peripheral blood, the gold standard for diagnosis remains tissue biopsy with histopathological and immunohistochemical examination. Notably, EBV load is highly sensitive for predicting PTLDs, but the specificity in LT re-cipients is only ~50%.[51] Once diagnosis of PTLDs is made, reduction in immunosup-pression to the lowest tolerated levels (usually by 25%–50% of baseline depending on the extension of disease and concern for graft rejection) should be initiated.[51,55] Early lesions and polymorphic PTLDs often respond well (typically seen in 2–4 weeks) to immunosuppression reduction. Late-onset, monomorphic PTLDs are less responsive and often need rituximab and/or chemotherapy with or without the need for local con-trol (eg, radiotherapy or surgery).[51,55]

REACTIVATION OF VIRAL HEPATITIS RELATED TO THE TREATMENT OF LYMPHOPROLIFERATIVE DISORDERS
Chronic Hepatitis B Virus

Although there is heterogeneity in the definitions of reactivation of HBV (HBVr), it is often defined as either the de novo detection of HBV-DNA, or a 10-fold (1 log) increase in HBV-DNA level when compared with the baseline, or sero-reversion to hepatitis B surface antigen (HBsAg) and/or hepatitis Be antigen positive status before chemo-therapy.[56–58] HBVr in patients receiving chemotherapy is often accompanied by a flare of hepatitis (often defined as 2- to 3-fold in ALT above the baseline), which can be associated with significant morbidity and mortality (up to 10%).[56,59] Notably, chemo-therapeutic regimens used for the treatment of lymphoma, such as high-dose cortico-steroids, CHOP, and rituximab, have most often been implicated in HBVr. The overall risk of HBVr in lymphoma patients receiving chemotherapy is 24.4% to 85% in HBsAg-positive patients and 4.1% to 41.5% in resolved HBV patients (HBsAg$^-$/anti-HBc$^+$).[60] Rituximab use is associated with an increased risk of HBVr (16.9%–25%) among resolved HBV patients.[58,61] Thus, in this setting, the presence of anti-HBs slightly reduced the risk of HBVr, but is not preventive, because HBVr developed in about 4% of anti-HBs$^+$ resolved HBV patients (HBsAg$^-$/anti-HBc$^+$/anti-HBs$^+$). Furthermore, there is the risk of HBVr even 12 months after the last dose of rituximab.[62]

Ideally, all patients should be screened for HBV (HBsAg and anti-HBc, followed by a sensitive HBV-DNA test if positive) before undergoing chemotherapy for lymphoma.[63] However, selective screening in higher-risk candidates with a baseline prevalence for HBV likely exceeding 2% (according to Centers for Disease Control and Prevention and US Preventive Services Task Force recommendations) may be a more cost-effective approach in a low prevalence area, such as in the United States.[58,59] In a meta-analysis of 11 studies (n = 620), lamivudine was shown to reduce the risk of HBVr (relative risk [RR] 0.13) and HBVr-related mortality (RR 0.30), and to reduce the delay/premature termination of chemotherapy (RR 0.41).[64] More recent studies have shown that entecavir is a more effective option for HBVr prophylaxis.[65–67] In a randomized controlled trial of 121 HBsAg[+] patients receiving R-CHOP, the rates of HBVr (0% vs 13.3%), HBVr-related hepatitis (13.3% vs 21.9%), and chemotherapy disruption (1.6% vs 18.3%) were significantly lower for the entecavir group versus the lamivudine group (all $P<.005$).[67]

Taken together, all HBsAg[+] patients should receive potent nucleos(t)ide analogues as treatment or prophylaxis before initiation of chemotherapy.[58,59,63] Patients with resolved HBV infection, regardless of anti-HBs status, should also receive prophylaxis if they are at high risk of HBV reactivation, such as those undergoing rituximab-based therapy or stem cell transplantation.[58,59,63] Prophylaxis should be continued for 6 to 12 months (12 months for rituximab-based regimens) after cessation of the chemotherapy and discontinued only if the underlying disease is under remission. Liver function tests and HBV-DNA should be tested every 3 to 6 months during prophylaxis and for at least 12 months after nucleos(t)ide analog (NA) withdrawal as a large proportion of HBV reactivations develop after NA discontinuation (**Fig. 5**).[58,59,63]

Chronic Hepatitis C Virus

Unlike HBVr, the incidence and outcomes of HCV reactivation (HCVr) during chemotherapy remain poorly described. HCVr appears to be less common and to have less severe consequences than HBVr, with only a few fatal cases of acute liver failure attributed to HCV being reported.[68–72] In a prospective observational study of 100 HCV[+] patients receiving chemotherapy (50 hematologic malignancies and 50 solid tumors), 23% of patients developed HCVr (defined as an increase in HCV-RNA ≥ 1 log[10] IU/mL over baseline and hepatitis flare as an increase in alanine aminotransferase to

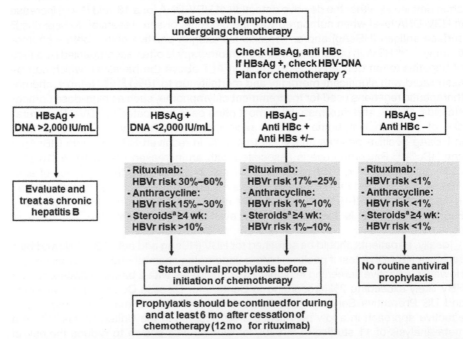

Fig. 5. Proposed algorithm for the prevention of HBV reactivation in patients with lymphoma undergoing chemotherapy. [a] Dose: $\geq$10–20 mg prednisolone daily or equivalent.

≥3 xULN), 10% developed hepatitis flare, and 6% required discontinuation or dose reduction of chemotherapy.[72] In multivariate analysis, the 2 statistically significant predictors of HCVr were use of rituximab (odds ratio [OR] 9.52) and high-dose steroids (OR 5.05), which paralleled the observation that HCVr was more common (22%–50%) in hematologic malignancies, particularly lymphoma, for which these regimens are used.[72] Taken together, it appears that HCVr is quite common in lymphoma patients undergoing chemotherapy, but does not detrimentally impact short-term hepatic or hematologic outcomes, although long-term consequences remain unclear.[73]

Recently, several reports have highlighted the safety and efficacy of direct acting antivirals (DAA) therapy for HCV along with chemotherapy.[72,74,75] In a prospective historically matched cohort of genotype 1b HCV-infected DLBCL patients treated concurrently with sofosbuvir/ledipasvir for 12 weeks and chemotherapy (70% of whom received rituximab), sustained virological response (SVR) was achieved in 100% of patients.[76] Although there was no difference in overall survival, disease-free survival was significantly improved in DAA-treated patients when compared with untreated historical controls (95% vs 67% at 48 weeks).[76] Similarly, a strong correlation of SVR and lymphoma regression in HCV⁺ lymphoma patients was previously observed with interferon-based therapy supporting a hypothesis of a causal relationship of HCV and lymphomagenesis.[77] In addition, remission of cryoglobulinemic vasculitis has increasingly been reported in HCV⁺ patients who achieved SVR by DAA.[78–80] Unlike HBVr, there has been no international guideline for managing HCV⁺ patients undergoing chemotherapy. Preemptive DAA therapy before or concurrent with chemotherapy in HCV⁺ lymphoma patients is an attractive option to prevent HCVr and to improve long-term hepatic or hematologic outcomes.[73]

SUMMARY

LPDs are a heterogeneous group of disorders with variable prognosis. Hepatic abnormalities in patients with LPDs are common in clinical practice and require special attention. Liver involvement from systemic lymphoma is quite common. PHL presenting as a mass is rare but needs to be promptly differentiated from other liver mass lesions due to differences in management. Apart from direct lymphoma infiltration, hepatic dysfunction in patients with LPDs can also occur from bile duct obstruction, paraneoplastic syndrome, HPS, drug-induced liver injury, opportunistic infections, and reactivation of viral hepatitis. Of note, all patients undergoing chemotherapy should be screened for current and past HBV infection, and antiviral prophylaxis is recommended in appropriate patients.

REFERENCES

1. Choi WT, Gill RM. Hepatic lymphoma diagnosis. Surg Pathol Clin 2018;11(2): 389–402.

2. Mastoraki A, Stefanou MI, Chatzoglou E, et al. Primary hepatic lymphoma: dilemmas in diagnostic approach and therapeutic management. Indian J Hematol Blood Transfus 2014;30(3):150–4.

3. Yang XW, Tan WF, Yu WL, et al. Diagnosis and surgical treatment of primary hepatic lymphoma. World J Gastroenterol 2010;16(47):6016–9.

4. Lei KI. Primary non-Hodgkin's lymphoma of the liver. Leuk Lymphoma 1998; 29(3–4):293–9.

5. Singh MM, Pockros PJ. Hematologic and oncologic diseases and the liver. Clin Liver Dis 2011;15(1):69–87.

6. Baumhoer D, Tzankov A, Dirnhofer S, et al. Patterns of liver infiltration in lympho-proliferative disease. Histopathology 2008;53(1):81–90.

7. Pieri G, Theocharidou E, Burroughs AK. Liver in haematological disorders. Best Pract Res Clin Gastroenterol 2013;27(4):513–30.

8. Abe H, Kamimura K, Kawai H, et al. Diagnostic imaging of hepatic lymphoma. Clin Res Hepatol Gastroenterol 2015;39(4):435–42.

9. Kikuma K, Watanabe J, Oshiro Y, et al. Etiological factors in primary hepatic B-cell lymphoma. Virchows Arch 2012;460(4):379–87.

10. Page RD, Romaguera JE, Osborne B, et al. Primary hepatic lymphoma: favorable outcome after combination chemotherapy. Cancer 2001;92(8):2023–9.

11. De Renzo A, Perna F, Persico M, et al. Excellent prognosis and prevalence of HCV infection of primary hepatic and splenic non-Hodgkin's lymphoma. Eur J Haematol 2008;81(1):51–7.

12. Foschi FG, Dall'Aglio AC, Marano G, et al. Role of contrast-enhanced ultrasonog-raphy in primary hepatic lymphoma. J Ultrasound Med 2010;29(9):1353–6.

13. Colagrande S, Calistri L, Grazzini G, et al. MRI features of primary hepatic lym-phoma. Abdom Radiol (NY) 2018;43(9):2277–87.

14. Gota VS, Purandare NC, Gujral S, et al. Positron emission tomography/computer-ized tomography evaluation of primary Hodgkin's disease of liver. Indian J Cancer 2009;46(3):237–9.

15. GBD 2015 Mortality and Causes of Death Collaborators. Global, regional, and na-tional life expectancy, all-cause mortality, and cause-specific mortality for 249 causes of death, 1980-2015: a systematic analysis for the Global Burden of Dis-ease Study 2015. Lancet 2016;388(10053):1459–544.

16. Punnett A, Tsang RW, Hodgson DC. Hodgkin lymphoma across the age spec-trum: epidemiology, therapy, and late effects. Semin Radiat Oncol 2010;20(1): 30–44.

17. Brinckmeyer LM, Skovsgaard T, Thiede T, et al. The liver in Hodgkin's disease–I. Clinico-pathological relations. Eur J Cancer Clin Oncol 1982;18(5):421–8.

18. Rowbotham D, Wendon J, Williams R. Acute liver failure secondary to hepatic infiltration: a single centre experience of 18 cases. Gut 1998;42(4):576–80.

19. Bakhit M, McCarty TR, Park S, et al. Vanishing bile duct syndrome in Hodgkin's lymphoma: a case report and literature review. World J Gastroenterol 2017; 23(2):366–72.

20. Reau NS, Jensen DM. Vanishing bile duct syndrome. Clin Liver Dis 2008;12(1): 203–17, x.

21. Rota Scalabrini D, Caravelli D, Carnevale Schianca F, et al. Complete remission of paraneoplastic vanishing bile duct syndrome after the successful treatment of Hodgkin's lymphoma: a case report and review of the literature. BMC Res Notes 2014;7:529.

22. Bruguera M, Caballero T, Carreras E, et al. Hepatic sinusoidal dilatation in Hodg-kin's disease. Liver 1987;7(2):76–80.

23. Reynoso-Paz S, Coppel RL, Ansari AA, et al. Vanishing bile duct syndromes: con-siderations of the immunobiology of autoimmune biliary diseases. Isr Med Assoc J 1999;1(1):37–44.

24. Fontes-Sousa M, Magalhaes H, da Silva FC, et al. Stauffer's syndrome: a compre-hensive review and proposed updated diagnostic criteria. Urol Oncol 2018;36(7): 321–6.

25. Pass AK, McLin VA, Rushton JR, et al. Vanishing bile duct syndrome and Hodgkin disease: a case series and review of the literature. J Pediatr Hematol Oncol 2008; 30(12):976–80.

26. Yeh P, Lokan J, Anantharajah A, et al. Vanishing bile duct syndrome and immunodeficiency preceding the diagnosis of Hodgkin lymphoma. Intern Med J 2014;44(12a):1240–4.
27. Bowzyk Al-Naeeb A, Ajithkumar T, Behan S, et al. Non-Hodgkin lymphoma. BMJ 2018;362:k3204.
28. Shimizu Y. Liver in systemic disease. World J Gastroenterol 2008;14(26):4111–9.
29. Kolaric K, Roth A, Dominis M, et al. The diagnostic value of percutaneus liver biopsy in patients with non Hodgkin's lymphoma - a preliminary report. Acta hepato-gastroenterologica 1977;24(6):440–3.
30. Roth A, Cerlek S, Dominis M, et al. Histologic and cytologic liver changes induced by cytostatic drugs in 32 patients with non-Hodgkin's lymphomas. Acta Med Iugosl 1979;33(1):13–20.
31. Bagley CM Jr, Thomas LB, Johnson RE, et al. Diagnosis of liver involvement by lymphoma: results in 96 consecutive peritoneoscopies. Cancer 1973;31(4): 840–7.
32. Scheimberg IB, Pollock DJ, Collins PW, et al. Pathology of the liver in leukaemia and lymphoma. A study of 110 autopsies. Histopathology 1995;26(4):311–21.
33. Lettieri CJ, Berg BW. Clinical features of non-Hodgkins lymphoma presenting with acute liver failure: a report of five cases and review of published experience. Am J Gastroenterol 2003;98(7):1641–6.
34. Morali GA, Rozenmann E, Ashkenazi J, et al. Acute liver failure as the sole manifestation of relapsing non-Hodgkin's lymphoma. Eur J Gastroenterol Hepatol 2001;13(10):1241–3.
35. Salo J, Nomdedeu B, Bruguera M, et al. Acute liver failure due to non-Hodgkin's lymphoma. Am J Gastroenterol 1993;88(5):774–6.
36. Ohtani H, Komeno T, Koizumi M, et al. Submassive hepatocellular necrosis associated with infiltration by peripheral T-cell lymphoma of cytotoxic phenotype: report of two cases. Pathol Int 2008;58(2):133–7.
37. Lokich JJ, Kane RA, Harrison DA, et al. Biliary tract obstruction secondary to cancer: management guidelines and selected literature review. J Clin Oncol 1987; 5(6):969–81.
38. Blouhos K, Boulas KA, Paraskeva A, et al. Obstructive jaundice as primary presentation of a stage IIE Non-Hodgkin lymphoma: a decision making process between advanced lymphoma and locally advanced/metastatic pancreatic adenocarcinoma. Int J Surg Case Rep 2018;44:226–9.
39. Zakaria A, Al-Obeidi S, Daradkeh S. Primary non-Hodgkin's lymphoma of the common bile duct: a case report and literature review. Asian J Surg 2017; 40(1):81–7.
40. Boninsegna E, Zamboni GA, Facchinelli D, et al. CT imaging of primary pancreatic lymphoma: experience from three referral centres for pancreatic diseases. Insights Imaging 2018;9(1):17–24.
41. Ramesh J, Hebert-Magee S, Kim H, et al. Frequency of occurrence and characteristics of primary pancreatic lymphoma during endoscopic ultrasound guided fine needle aspiration: a retrospective study. Dig Liver Dis 2014;46(5):470–3.
42. Zhang L, Zhou J, Sokol L. Hereditary and acquired hemophagocytic lymphohistiocytosis. Cancer Control 2014;21(4):301–12.
43. Wang H, Xiong L, Tang W, et al. A systematic review of malignancy-associated hemophagocytic lymphohistiocytosis that needs more attentions. Oncotarget 2017;8(35):59977–85.
44. Chang Y, Cui M, Fu X, et al. Lymphoma associated hemophagocytic syndrome: a single-center retrospective study. Oncol Lett 2018;16(1):1275–84.

45. de Kerguenec C, Hillaire S, Molinie V, et al. Hepatic manifestations of hemophagocytic syndrome: a study of 30 cases. Am J Gastroenterol 2001;96(3):852–7.
46. Han AR, Lee HR, Park BB, et al. Lymphoma-associated hemophagocytic syndrome: clinical features and treatment outcome. Ann Hematol 2007;86(7):493–8.
47. Han L, Li L, Wu J, et al. Clinical features and treatment of natural killer/T cell lymphoma associated with hemophagocytic syndrome: comparison with other T cell lymphoma associated with hemophagocytic syndrome. Leuk Lymphoma 2014; 55(9):2048–55.
48. Al-Mansour Z, Nelson BP, Evens AM. Post-transplant lymphoproliferative disease (PTLD): risk factors, diagnosis, and current treatment strategies. Curr Hematol Malig Rep 2013;8(3):173–83.
49. Kremers WK, Devarbhavi HC, Wiesner RH, et al. Post-transplant lymphoproliferative disorders following liver transplantation: incidence, risk factors and survival. Am J Transplant 2006;6(5 Pt 1):1017–24.
50. Inayat F, Hassan GU, Tayyab GUN, et al. Post-transplantation lymphoproliferative disorder with gastrointestinal involvement. Ann Gastroenterol 2018;31(2):248–51.
51. Kamdar KY, Rooney CM, Heslop HE. Posttransplant lymphoproliferative disease following liver transplantation. Curr Opin Organ Transplant 2011;16(3):274–80.
52. Lo RC, Chan SC, Chan KL, et al. Post-transplant lymphoproliferative disorders in liver transplant recipients: a clinicopathological study. J Clin Pathol 2013;66(5): 392–8.
53. Swerdlow SH, Webber SA, Chadburn A, et al. Post-transplant lymphoproliferative disorders. In: Swerdlow SH, Campo E, Harris NL, et al, editors. WHO classification of tumors of haematopoietic and lymphoid tissues. Lyon (France): International Agency for Research on Cancer; 2017. p. 453–62.
54. Opelz G, Dohler B. Lymphomas after solid organ transplantation: a collaborative transplant study report. Am J Transplant 2004;4(2):222–30.
55. Parker A, Bowles K, Bradley JA, et al. Management of post-transplant lymphoproliferative disorder in adult solid organ transplant recipients - BCSH and BTS Guidelines. Br J Haematol 2010;149(5):693–705.
56. Gonzalez SA, Perrillo RP. Hepatitis B virus reactivation in the setting of cancer chemotherapy and other immunosuppressive drug therapy. Clin Infect Dis 2016;62(Suppl 4):S306–13.
57. Di Bisceglie AM, Lok AS, Martin P, et al. Recent US Food and Drug Administration warnings on hepatitis B reactivation with immune-suppressing and anticancer drugs: just the tip of the iceberg? Hepatology 2015;61(2):703–11.
58. Perrillo RP, Gish R, Falck-Ytter YT. American Gastroenterological Association Institute technical review on prevention and treatment of hepatitis B virus reactivation during immunosuppressive drug therapy. Gastroenterology 2015;148(1): 221–44.e3.
59. Reddy KR, Beavers KL, Hammond SP, et al. American Gastroenterological Association Institute guideline on the prevention and treatment of hepatitis B virus reactivation during immunosuppressive drug therapy. Gastroenterology 2015; 148(1):215–9 [quiz: e216–7].
60. Gentile G, Andreoni M, Antonelli G, et al. Screening, monitoring, prevention, prophylaxis and therapy for hepatitis B virus reactivation in patients with haematologic malignancies and patients who underwent haematologic stem cell transplantation: a systematic review. Clin Microbiol Infect 2017;23(12):916–23.
61. Yeo W, Chan TC, Leung NW, et al. Hepatitis B virus reactivation in lymphoma patients with prior resolved hepatitis B undergoing anticancer therapy with or without rituximab. J Clin Oncol 2009;27(4):605–11.

62. Nakaya A, Fujita S, Satake A, et al. Delayed HBV reactivation in rituximab-containing chemotherapy: how long should we continue anti-virus prophylaxis or monitoring HBV-DNA? Leuk Res 2016;50:46–9.

63. EASL 2017 Clinical Practice Guidelines on the management of hepatitis B virus infection. J Hepatol 2017;67(2):370–98.

64. Martyak LA, Taqavi E, Saab S. Lamivudine prophylaxis is effective in reducing hepatitis B reactivation and reactivation-related mortality in chemotherapy patients: a meta-analysis. Liver Int 2008;28(1):28–38.

65. Chen FW, Coyle L, Jones BE, et al. Entecavir versus lamivudine for hepatitis B prophylaxis in patients with haematological disease. Liver Int 2013;33(8): 1203–10.

66. Li HR, Huang JJ, Guo HQ, et al. Comparison of entecavir and lamivudine in preventing hepatitis B reactivation in lymphoma patients during chemotherapy. J Viral Hepat 2011;18(12):877–83.

67. Huang H, Li X, Zhu J, et al. Entecavir vs lamivudine for prevention of hepatitis B virus reactivation among patients with untreated diffuse large B-cell lymphoma receiving R-CHOP chemotherapy: a randomized clinical trial. JAMA 2014; 312(23):2521–30.

68. Mahale P, Kontoyiannis DP, Chemaly RF, et al. Acute exacerbation and reactivation of chronic hepatitis C virus infection in cancer patients. J Hepatol 2012;57(6): 1177–85.

69. Vento S, Cainelli F, Longhi MS. Reactivation of replication of hepatitis B and C viruses after immunosuppressive therapy: an unresolved issue. Lancet Oncol 2002;3(6):333–40.

70. Vento S, Cainelli F, Mirandola F, et al. Fulminant hepatitis on withdrawal of chemotherapy in carriers of hepatitis C virus. Lancet 1996;347(8994):92–3.

71. Zuckerman E, Zuckerman T, Douer D, et al. Liver dysfunction in patients infected with hepatitis C virus undergoing chemotherapy for hematologic malignancies. Cancer 1998;83(6):1224–30.

72. Torres HA, Hosry J, Mahale P, et al. Hepatitis C virus reactivation in patients receiving cancer treatment: a prospective observational study. Hepatology 2018;67(1):36–47.

73. Kriss M, Burchill M. HCV and nonhepatic malignancy: is pre-emptive direct-acting antiviral therapy indicated prior to treatment? Hepatology 2018;67(1):4–6.

74. Economides MP, Mahale P, Kyvernitakis A, et al. Concomitant use of direct-acting antivirals and chemotherapy in hepatitis C virus-infected patients with cancer. Aliment Pharmacol Ther 2016;44(11–12):1235–41.

75. Kyvernitakis A, Mahale P, Popat UR, et al. Hepatitis C virus infection in patients undergoing hematopoietic cell transplantation in the era of direct-acting antiviral agents. Biol Blood Marrow Transplant 2016;22(4):717–22.

76. Persico M, Aglitti A, Caruso R, et al. Efficacy and safety of new direct antiviral agents in hepatitis C virus-infected patients with diffuse large B-cell non-Hodgkin's lymphoma. Hepatology 2018;67(1):48–55.

77. Peveling-Oberhag J, Arcaini L, Bankov K, et al. The anti-lymphoma activity of antiviral therapy in HCV-associated B-cell non-Hodgkin lymphomas: a meta-analysis. J Viral Hepat 2016;23(7):536–44.

78. Bunchorntavakul C, Mitrani R, Reddy KR. Advances in HCV and cryoglobulinemic vasculitis in the era of DAAs: are we at the end of the road? J Clin Exp Hepatol 2018;8:81–94.

79. Gragnani L, Visentini M, Fognani E, et al. Prospective study of guideline-tailored therapy with direct-acting antivirals for hepatitis C virus-associated mixed cryoglobulinemia. Hepatology 2016;64(5):1473–82.
80. Saadoun D, Pol S, Ferfar Y, et al. Efficacy and safety of sofosbuvir plus daclatasvir for treatment of HCV-associated cryoglobulinemia vasculitis. Gastroenterology 2017;153(1):49–52.e5.

Liver Disease in Human Immunodeficiency Virus Infection

Katerina G. Oikonomou, MD, PhD*, Eugenia Tsai, MD,
Dost Sarpel, MD, Douglas T. Dieterich, MD

KEYWORDS

- Liver • HIV • Hepatitis • ART

KEY POINTS

- Liver disease in human immunodeficiency virus (HIV) can be a result of multiple factors and can present with liver enzyme abnormalities.
- HIV can have direct effects on the liver; however, opportunistic infections and viral hepatitides remain major causes of liver dysfunction.
- Alcohol abuse and nonalcoholic steatohepatitis are more common in the era of highly active antiretroviral treatment, and are increasing in prevalence in patients with HIV.

INTRODUCTION

Liver disease in patients with human immunodeficiency virus (HIV) infection represents a significant cause of morbidity and mortality, and includes the spectrum of abnormal liver tests to fulminant hepatic failure and necrosis. Cirrhosis and hepatocellular carcinoma are terminal complications in patients with HIV and viral hepatitis coinfection, alcohol abuse, or other underlying liver processes.[1-3]

In patients living with HIV (PLWH), there are several distinct scenarios in which liver damage can occur. The virus itself has direct effect on hepatocytes. The sequelae of advanced immunosuppression in acquired immunodeficiency syndrome (AIDS) also can lead to liver disease. In addition, effects of highly acting antiretroviral therapy (ART), opportunistic infections, liver steatosis, and HIV coinfection with viral hepatitis all can be considered manifestations of HIV-related effects on the liver.

Liver disease in HIV patients can manifest as isolated elevation in liver enzymes or with fever, hepatomegaly, and right upper quadrant abdominal pain. Management of liver disease in HIV-infected patients requires recognition of underlying conditions and

The authors have nothing to disclose.
Icahn School of Medicine at Mount Sinai, 1 Gustav L. Levy Place, New York, NY 10029-6574, USA
* Corresponding author.
E-mail address: katerina.oikonomou@mountsinai.org

a systematic approach to targeted diagnosis and treatment to reduce morbidity and mortality, and to improve quality of life and life expectancy.

DIRECT EFFECTS OF HUMAN IMMUNODEFICIENCY VIRUS IN THE LIVER

The interactions between HIV and the liver occur through direct and indirect mechanisms. Indirectly, HIV causes depletion of CD4 T cells. Directly, HIV can infect Kupffer cells, which represent a distinct macrophage population of the liver, hepatic stellate cells (HSC), and hepatocytes.

Hepatocytes may act as an HIV reservoir and promote CD4 T-cell infection by cell-to-cell contact.[4,5] HSC infected with HIV show increased activation and fibrogenesis, with alpha-smooth muscle actin, and collagen production and increased levels of monocyte chemotactic protein-1.[4] Reduction of gastrointestinal (GI) CD4 T cells is thought to lead to impaired permeability of the GI tract, which may cause exposure to endotoxins. This in turn can induce hepatocytes, Kupffer cells, and HSC to produce proinflammatory cytokines and chemokines, such as tumor necrosis factor-α, transforming growth factor-β, and interleukins, which promote fibrosis.[6]

HIV has also been shown to suppress the activity of peroxisome proliferator-activated receptors, which play an important role in glucose and lipid metabolism, inflammation, and fibrosis. This is yet another potential mechanism by which HIV contributes to liver disease progression.[7]

HUMAN IMMUNODEFICIENCY VIRUS AND VIRAL HEPATITIDES COINFECTIONS

Liver disease among HIV-infected individuals is most commonly due to coinfection with hepatitis C virus (HCV) and/or hepatitis B virus (HBV) owing to shared risk factors. These include injection drug use (IDU), vertical mother-to-child transmission during pregnancy or birth, and sexual contact.[8,9] Although less common, acute hepatitis A virus (HAV) and both acute and chronic hepatitis E virus (HEV) infections are emerging issues in patients with HIV.[10–13]

HUMAN IMMUNODEFICIENCY VIRUS–HEPATITIS C VIRUS COINFECTION

Chronic liver disease has been among the leading causes of morbidity and mortality in HIV-HCV coinfected patients since the introduction of ART.[14] One-quarter of HIV-positive individuals are coinfected with HCV, which translates to approximately 7 million persons worldwide have HIV-HCV coinfection.[15,16] HIV and HCV have similar transmission risks (**Table 1**).[17,18]

The primary method of HCV transmission remains via parenteral transmission. There has been an increasing epidemic of HCV infection among the younger population due to the opioid crisis. The coinfection rate among HIV patients who are intravenous drug users is greater than 75%.[17] During the recent HIV epidemic in Scott County, Indiana, 99% of the people diagnosed with HIV were coinfected with HCV.[18]

Table 1		
Incidence of human immunodeficiency virus and hepatitis C virus		
	HIV (%)	HCV (%)
Intravenous drug users	31	60
Men who have sex with men (MSM)	47	Unclear
Men who have sex with women	10	20

HIV-positive men who have sex with men (MSM) are another emerging risk factor for HCV coinfection, as well as reinfection. Risk of transmission is due to HCV in semen, as well as in the rectum.[19,20] In 2017, a study with HIV-positive MSM with HCV infection demonstrated rectal HCV shedding as the mode of transmission risk in almost half of the patients.[20] In this era of successful eradication with direct-acting antiviral (DAA) therapy, a subsequent high incidence of reinfection with HCV has been reported in patients with IDU and in MSM.[21,22] In a German HCV cohort, the HCV reinfection rate was higher in MSM when compared with those with IDU.[23] Prevention measures are needed in both of these high-risk groups if HCV-elimination targets are to be realized.

HIV infection alters the natural history of HCV through a multitude of mechanisms via the direct and indirect effects of HIV. These include increasing HCV replication and HCV-induced inflammation, as well as impaired HCV-specific immune responses.[24,25] Coinfected patients have been shown to have accelerated rates of hepatic fibrosis progression, hepatic decompensation, hepatocellular carcinoma, and ultimately higher rates of liver-related mortality.[26–29]

The impact of HCV on the natural history of HIV disease progression is unclear. Studies show faster HIV progression in coinfected patients and, conversely, lower HIV progression and non–liver-related mortality in HCV-treated HIV-infected patients who achieved a sustained virologic response (SVR).[30] However, other studies demonstrate no impact.[31]

Due to the high prevalence of HCV in PLWH, screening should be performed using third-generation enzyme immunoassays for hepatitis C antibody, which has a sensitivity of 92% to 97%.[32] If positive, chronic HCV infection should be confirmed by HCV RNA polymerase chain reaction.[33] In those in whom acute infection is suspected or in those with significant risk factors, HCV RNA should be checked along with HCV antibody. In addition, patients who are severely immunocompromised should be monitored with HCV RNA because they do not frequently develop an antibody. Patients infected with HIV should be counseled on avoiding risk factors for contracting HCV infection. HIV-positive MSM successfully treated for HCV infection should be tested for reinfection every 3 to 6 months.

With the development of DAA therapy, the paradigm for treatment of HCV has changed dramatically in the last decade.[34,35] A summary of the DAAs studied and associated SVR at week 12 is shown in **Table 2**. In all studies, common reported side effects included fatigue, headache, and nausea. Side effects were mild and did not lead to any treatment discontinuations.

HUMAN IMMUNODEFICIENCY VIRUS–HEPATITIS B VIRUS COINFECTION

HIV-HBV coinfection is estimated at 3 million persons worldwide. In the United States, 1 in 10 HIV-positive individuals are also infected with HBV.[15] As with HIV-HCV coinfection, HIV can affect the natural history of HBV. Those with HIV infection are at higher risk for developing chronic HBV after an acute exposure and clinical illness than those without HIV infection.[42] HIV-infected patients with higher CD4 cell counts were more likely to clear hepatitis B surface antigen.[43] All PLWH should be screened for HBV infection. Evaluation should be done with 3 serologic tests[44]:

- Hepatitis B surface antigen indicates hepatitis B infection
- Hepatitis B core antibody total indicates prior exposure
- Hepatitis B surface antibody indicates immunity to infection, natural or from vaccination.

Table 2
Sustained virologic response rates in treatment-naive adults with human immunodeficiency virus–hepatitis C virus coinfection

	HCV Genotype	DAA	SVR at 12 Weeks
TURQUOISE-I Sulkowski et al,[36] 2015	1	Ombitasvir + paritaprevir + ritonavir + dasabuvir	94%
C-EDGE Coinfection Rockstroh et al,[37] 2015	1, 4, or 6	Daclatasvir + sofosbuvir	95%
ION-4 Naggie et al,[38] 2015	1 or 4	Ledipasvir + sofosbuvir	96%
ALLY-2 Luetkemeyer et al,[39] 2016	Pangenotypic	Daclatasvir + sofosbuvir	97%
ASTRAL-5 Wyles et al,[40] 2017	1–4	Sofosbuvir + velpatasvir	95%
EXPEDITION-2 Rockstroh et al,[41] 2018	Pangenotypic	Glecaprevir + pibrentasvir	98%

HBV vaccination or combined HAV-HBV vaccination should be provided to those without immunity. However, studies have demonstrated a poor response to vaccination in those whose CD4 cell count is less than 200 cells/mm^3.[45] Therefore, patients should be counseled to avoid risk factors for HBV transmission.

All patients with HIV-HBV coinfection should receive ART, regardless of HBV viremia and serum alanine aminotransferase (ALT) levels. ART should contain tenofovir-based therapy: tenofovir disoproxil fumarate (TDF) or tenofovir alafenamide (TAF). In 2 randomized clinical trials, TAF has been shown to be noninferior to TDF in the treatment of HBV infection.[46,47] Due to TDF's side effects of nephrotoxicity and effect on bone mineral density, TAF is preferred.[48] In those in whom tenofovir is contraindicated, entecavir should be used for HBV treatment owing to its demonstrated high efficacy and high genetic barrier to resistance.[49]

HEPATITIS A

Acute hepatitis A infection has a prolonged viremia and higher serology titers in patients who have HIV than in patients who are HIV-negative.[50,51] This increases the window of opportunity for transmission of HAV to those patients following high-risk behaviors.[52,53] Several outbreaks of acute HAV infection among MSM have been reported worldwide.[10,11,54–57] In 2017, a 10-fold increase in hepatitis A among MSM was reported by the New York City Department of Health in MSM who did not have a history of international travel.[58,59] These outbreaks outline the importance of HAV vaccination in high-risk individuals, including those with HIV.

HEPATITIS E

Although less common, HEV can cause abnormal liver tests results.[60,61] It does not often cause significant liver disease in HIV patients[61]; however, severe immunosuppression, defined by a decrease in CD4 T cells to less than 100 to 200/mm^3, is the most important risk factor associated with hepatitis E in HIV patients.[12,62] Although hepatitis E can become chronic in patients with solid organ or bone marrow transplants, not much is known about the chronicity of hepatitis E in HIV/AIDS patients. Past studies found increased prevalence of positive hepatitis E serologies in HIV patients; however, chronic detection of HEV RNA in these samples was very limited.[63,64]

Additionally, in a recent study in HIV-infected patients in the United States, including about 3000 samples of hepatitis E in HIV-infected patients, only 1 case was found with chronic hepatitis E infection.[13]

OTHER INFECTIOUS CAUSES: LIVER DISEASE IN HUMAN IMMUNODEFICIENCY VIRUS

Several infectious agents, including common and opportunistic pathogens, are commonly associated with abnormal liver enzymes in patients with HIV (**Box 1**). Cytomegalovirus (CMV) commonly affects the liver and can present with fever, malaise, weight loss, hepatomegaly, and pancytopenias. CMV hepatitis is characterized by mild elevation in transaminases and mild cholestasis. Liver biopsy demonstrates liver necrosis, typically with a portal and periportal mononuclear cell infiltrates, and large intranuclear and small cytoplasmic inclusions, forming the characteristic owl's eye appearance. Rarely, CMV in the liver can present as mass lesions similar to neoplasia or with granulomatous disease.[65,66]

Herpes simplex virus (HSV) can also affect the liver in HIV patients, particularly in disseminated disease in patients with low CD4 T-cell counts. AIDS patients with HSV hepatitis present with severe aminotransferase elevations. On histology, hepatocytes contain Cowdry type A intranuclear inclusion bodies and immunopathologic staining is needed to distinguish this entity from CMV. HSV hepatitis may result in acute liver failure and necrosis with coagulopathy, encephalopathy, and shock.[67] In a study by Remis and colleagues,[68] viral infections, including HBV, HCV, HSV-2, and CMV, were most common in MSM living with HIV, in comparison with MSM without HIV. Varicella-zoster virus and Epstein-Barr virus infections can also be associated with elevations in aminotransferases; however, most commonly, the liver dysfunction is self-limited, rarely leading to hepatocellular necrosis.[69]

Granulomatous inflammation is a common histologic finding associated with liver infectious processes. It is characterized by elevated alkaline phosphatase levels due to obstruction of the terminal of branches of the biliary tree. Granulomatous inflammation

---

Box 1
Infections with hepatic involvement in human immunodeficiency virus

Hepatitis
  Hepatitis A
  Hepatitis B plus or minus delta
  Hepatitis C
  Hepatitis E
  Other viral infections
  CMV
  HSV
  Varicella-zoster virus
  Epstein-Barr virus

Granulomatous infections
  Mycobacterium avium complex
  Mycobacterium tuberculosis

Fungal infections
  Histoplasma capsulatum
  Cryptococcus neoformans
  Coccidioides immitis
  Candida spp

can be a result of mycobacterial infections, such as disseminated *Mycobacterium avium* complex or extrapulmonary tuberculosis (TB). Extrapulmonary TB has been reported in about 60% of AIDS patients with concomitant lung disease. Fifty percent of HIV and TB coinfected patients present with extrapulmonary involvement, most commonly hepatic TB.[70] Liver biopsy in these cases can show noncaseating granulomas. Ziehl-Neelsen stain and tissue culture can aid in the establishment of diagnosis of mycobacterial infections. Hepatic involvement of *M tuberculosis*, including liver abscesses, has been reported in patients with extrapulmonary TB and HIV infection.[71,72] Less commonly, other nontuberculous mycobacteria, such as *M xenopi* or *M kansasii*, are associated with hepatic granulomatosis.[73]

Fungal hepatitis or fungal liver abscesses are less common and can be rarely observed in HIV patients with advanced immunosuppression and AIDS. Common fungal pathogens include *Cryptococcus neoformans*, *Histoplasma capsulatum*, *Candida albicans*, and *Coccidioides immitis*. Hepatic pneumocystis is rare and may present with mild abdominal pain, transaminitis, and elevated alkaline phosphatase. Liver biopsy demonstrates foamy nodules that are periportal or diffuse and *Pneumocystis* cysts stain with methenamine silver stain.[65] Of note, in HIV patients trimethoprim-sulfamethoxazole for treatment or prophylaxis for *Pneumocystis* is another cause of elevated liver enzymes in HIV patients, and aerosolized pentamidine prophylaxis has been reported as a risk factor for extrapulmonary pneumocystis infection.[71]

HIV-related cholangiopathy was first described in 1983 by Pitlik and colleagues[74] and Guarda and colleagues.[75] It is a clinical entity related to biliary obstruction due to opportunistic pathogens in HIV patients. In the era of ART, the prevalence of HIV-related cholangiopathy is decreasing and is mostly seen in patients without access to health care and medication nonadherence. In the pre-ART era, the estimated prevalence of this entity was 26% to 46%.[76] *Cryptosporidium parvum* the most common pathogen associated with AIDS cholangiopathy.[77] Although the exact effect of *Cryptosporidium parvum* in the biliary tree is not entirely clear, it seems that active HIV replication and *Cryptosporidium parvum* infection synergistically increase apoptosis of cholangiocytes leading to HIV-related cholangiopathy.[78] There are several other pathogens implicated in AIDS cholangiopathy, such as CMV, microsporidia, isospora, and histoplasma.[79] The most serious complications of AIDS-related cholangiopathy are development of cholangiocarcinoma and progression to sclerosing cholangitis, which are irreversible and do not respond to ART.[80]

ANTIRETROVIRAL THERAPY EFFECTS

One of the most common complications of HIV treatment is elevation of liver enzymes.[81,82] Hepatotoxicity is frequently observed with combination medications and multidrug regimens add synergistic toxicities. The range of hepatotoxicity due to ART ranges from asymptomatic elevation of liver enzymes to severe and fulminant hepatic failure.[83] Retrospective studies have shown that severe hepatic failure due to ART was observed in approximately 10% of HIV patients, with life-threatening events appearing at a rate of 2.6 per 100 person years.[84] In randomized controlled trials, the incidence of significant, grade 3 (defined as >5 times the upper limit of normal) and grade 4 (>10 times the upper limit of normal) elevations in levels of liver enzymes that were associated with the use of combination ART was between 1% and 14%.[1]

The 4 primary pathways of ART-associated liver damage include mitochondrial toxicity, hypersensitivity reactions, direct hepatocellular toxicity, and immune reconstitution in the presence of HCV or HBV[1,83] (**Box 2**).

| Box 2 |
| Effects of antiretroviral therapy on liver |
| Direct toxicity |
| Mitochondrial toxicity |
| Hypersensitivity reactions |
| Immune reconstitution inflammatory syndrome |

Mitochondrial Toxicity

Nucleoside reverse transcriptase inhibitors (NRTIs) can directly cause mitochondrial toxicity. The main mechanism is the inhibition of mitochondrial polymerase and increase in lipids of cell membranes. This leads to impaired oxidative phosphorylation and fatty acid oxidation, with accumulation of microvesicular steatosis in liver cells. This in turn causes endoplasmic reticulum and mitochondrial dysfunction, leading to hepatic steatosis and hyperlactatemia–lactic acidosis.[85,86]

Apart from the liver injury, mitochondrial toxicity is also manifested clinically as myopathy, neuropathy, and pancreatitis.[87]

Protease Inhibitors (PIs) are also related to drug-induced unconjugated or indirect hyperbilirubinemia due to impairment of bilirubin uridine diphosphate–glucuronosyltransferase activity.[87,88] This indirect hyperbilirubinemia is not associated with liver injury and does not require treatment discontinuation.[88]

Hypersensitivity Reactions

Hypersensitivity reactions usually occur within the first 8 to 12 weeks of treatment. They are typically associated with rash and are most common in women with low CD4 T-cell counts and in patients taking abacavir or nevirapine. The estimated incidence of symptomatic reactions is up to 4.9%.[1,89] Abacavir can cause hypersensitivity reactions in patients with positive Human Leukocyte Antigen B-5701. Additionally, maraviroc, a C-C chemokine receptor type 5 inhibitor can cause hepatotoxicity as a result of hypersensitivity.[85]

Direct Toxicity

Because many drugs are metabolized in the liver by the cytochrome P-450, liver injury may be due to supratherapeutic serum levels of PIs in patients with HCV or HBV coinfection, or with preexisting liver disease. Integrase strand transfer inhibitors and NRTIs are also associated with the development of ART-associated hepatotoxicity.[90,91]

Immune Reconstitution Inflammatory Syndrome

Immune reconstitution inflammatory syndrome (IRIS) is the paradoxic worsening of infectious processes as a result of rapid immune reconstitution after ART initiation. IRIS is usually observed 6 to 8 weeks after ART initiation and it is associated with decline in HIV RNA and an increase in CD4 count. IRIS in patients coinfected with viral hepatitides has been reported most commonly as hepatitis flares and transition from normal liver enzymes to liver injury, fibrosis, and active hepatitis. In HIV-HCV coinfection, treatment with ART may precipitate flares of hepatitis in up to 18% of patients, and less commonly to acute decompensation in preexisting cirrhosis.[1,92–94]

In HIV-HBV coinfected patients, regimens such as lamivudine, emtricitabine, and tenofovir can lead to HBV reactivation and severe acute hepatitis if stopped abruptly or if resistance develops. In previous reports, prolonged use of the older NRTI didanosine has been associated with portal hypertension, esophageal varices, and bleeding.[1,85,95,96]

Steatosis-lipodystrophy

Fatty liver disease is associated with increased risk of cardiovascular events and related mortality. Both alcoholic liver disease (ALD) and nonalcoholic fatty liver disease (NAFLD) are seen in increasing prevalence in both the HIV-infected and general populations.

Alcoholic liver disease Alcohol use disorder (AUD) encompasses both alcohol abuse and alcohol dependence. The diagnostic criteria for AUD, as defined by the *Diagnostic and Statistical Manual of Mental Health Disorders*, 5th edition, are listed in **Box 3**. AUD is associated with significant disease burden in the Western world.[97]

Almost 9% of adults in the United States meet AUD criteria and alcohol is responsible for 4% of deaths annually.[98,99] Alcohol use is prevalent among individuals with and without HIV[100] and can often lead to ALD, which encompasses a spectrum of liver injuries, including simple steatosis, alcoholic hepatitis, fibrosis, and cirrhosis.

Box 3
Alcohol use disorder: DSM-5

Diagnosis of AUD requires meeting any 2 of the 11 criteria during the same 12-month period.

In the past year:

1. Alcohol is often taken in larger amounts or over a longer period than was intended.

2. There is a persistent desire or unsuccessful efforts to cut down or control alcohol use.

3. A great deal of time is spent in activities necessary to obtain alcohol, use alcohol, or recover from its effects.

4. Craving, or a strong desire or urge to use alcohol.

5. Recurrent alcohol use resulting in a failure to fulfill major role obligations at work, school, or home.

6. Continued alcohol use despite having persistent or recurrent social or interpersonal problems caused or exacerbated by the effects of alcohol.

7. Important social, occupational, or recreational activities are given up or reduced because of alcohol use.

8. Recurrent alcohol use in situations in which it is physically hazardous.

9. Alcohol use is continued despite knowledge of having a persistent or recurrent physical or psychological problem that is, likely to have been caused or exacerbated by alcohol.

10. Tolerance, as defined by either of the following:
    a. A need for markedly increased amounts of alcohol to achieve intoxication or desired effect.
    b. A markedly diminished effect with continued use of the same amount of alcohol.

11. Withdrawal, as manifested by either of the following:
    a. The characteristic withdrawal syndrome for alcohol (refer to Criteria A and B of the criteria set for alcohol withdrawal, pp. 499–500).
    b. Alcohol (or a closely related substance, such as a benzodiazepine) is taken to relieve or avoid withdrawal symptoms.

Reprinted with permission from the Diagnostic and Statistical Manual of Mental Disorders, Fifth Edition, (Copyright ©2013). American Psychiatric Association. All Rights Reserved.

Moderate alcohol intake, defined as 10 to 80 g alcohol per day, or 4 alcoholic drinks for men or 3 alcoholic drinks for women in any single day, or a maximum of 14 drinks for men or 7 drinks for women per week, can lead to fatty liver changes in up to 40% of patients.[101] Although there is no direct linear correlation between amount of alcohol use and severity of liver disease, higher levels of consumption are associated with increased risk of developing liver injury.[102,103] Heavy alcohol use is associated with accelerated liver fibrosis and increased liver-related mortality in PLWH.[104]

AUD is common in PLWH, with reported rates of almost 50%.[105] The prevalence of heavy drinking in this population is almost double that of the general population.[106] Studies suggest that in PLWH, any amount of drinking is associated with medication nonadherence and a dose-dependent relationship between alcohol use and number of missed pills.[107] Heavy alcohol use leads to lower CD4 counts and increased viral burden among PLWH on ART.[108]

The pathophysiology of alcohol and HIV infection's effects on the immune system is not well understood. However, recent data suggest that both share common targets and thus synergistically contribute to liver disease. Although intoxicating doses of alcohol are immunosuppressive, chronic alcohol use is immune-activating and leads to chronic inflammation and oxidative stress, which involves the same pathway as ALD.[109] Furthermore, both HIV infection and chronic alcohol have adverse effects on the integrity and immunology of the GI tract.[110] Mechanisms lead to increased gut permeability, which in turn can lead to increased transfer of endotoxin from intestine to liver, triggering inflammation in the liver.[111,112]

Nonalcoholic fatty liver disease Since the advent of effective ART for HIV, the life expectancy for individuals with HIV on ARV is improving and approaching that of the general population.[113] As the number of older HIV-positive patients increases, the rates of comorbidities, in particular cardiovascular complications, also increases.[114]

NAFLD is the excess accumulation of fat in the liver. It is an increasing cause of liver injury in the Western world and the incidence of fatty liver disease is growing.[115,116] The data on prevalence, predictors, and natural history of NAFLD among HIV-infected persons remain limited; however, studies have demonstrated that almost half of HIV patients who undergo evaluation for unexplained liver test abnormalities have NAFLD.[117,118] In a cross-sectional study of 216 HIV-monoinfected subjects, 31% had NAFLD diagnosed by ultrasonography.[119] This mirrors the prevalence of NAFLD in the general adult population, which is estimated at one-third of adults.[116,119,120] Metabolic derangements are common in PLWH on ARV, especially those on NRTI-PI combination medications.[121] These derangements include insulin resistance, dyslipidemia, hypertriglyceridemia, and lipodystrophy, peripheral fat distribution leading to lipodystrophy and visceral adiposity.

NAFLD encompasses a spectrum of diseases ranging from mild steatosis to severe fibrosis and cirrhosis.(IMAGE). Risk factors for NAFLD are generally similar in individuals with or without HIV[119] and are associated with features of metabolic syndrome (MetS) central obesity, insulin resistance, type 2 diabetes mellitus dyslipidemia[122]: Examination of liver histology in unexplained transaminase elevation in patients with HIV on ARV revealed varying stages of NAFLD in 18 of 30 patients and correlated with high fasting glycemic levels and insulin resistance.[123]

In addition to the traditional risk factors, other factors such as HIV infection itself and use of ART may contribute to NAFLD. In a study of 26 subjects with HIV, the subjects had statistically lower body mass index, lower percentage of fat mass, higher physical activity, and higher blood triglycerides.[124] Although the pathophysiology is not yet clearly understood, individuals with HIV are at higher risk for new-onset diabetes mellitus type 2, a strong risk factor for NAFLD.[125,126] Evaluation and diagnosis is often based on clinical history and biochemical and/or radiographic data. Risk factors for NAFLD are included in **Box 4**.

Although measurement of liver chemistries can aid in the diagnosis of NAFLD, up to 80% of patients can have normal ALT levels.[127] Routine ultrasonography is the most widely used modality for assessment of steatosis and NAFLD. However, sensitivity (approximately 61%) is limited owing to its inability to detect mild steatosis, or less than 20% fat in the liver.[128,129]

The gold standard for diagnosis and staging of NAFLD remains histologic evaluation; however, liver biopsy is fraught with limitations, including sampling variability and complications such as pain, bleeding, and (although rare) death.[130] Newer technologies, such as transient elastography, magnetic resonance elastography, and acoustic radiation force impulse, are allowing for noninvasive methods for the diagnosis and staging of NAFLD.[131,132]

Currently, there are no FDA-approved pharmacologic treatments for NAFLD. The mainstay of treatment is lifestyle changes that include healthy diet, physical exercise, and weight loss. Studies have shown that moderate weight loss of up to 5% to 10% of body weight can reduce liver steatosis and improve insulin resistance.[133,134] Several drugs targeting the various pathophysiological pathways of NAFLD are currently in phase 2 and 3 clinical trials. Their efficacy as therapeutic options for treating fatty liver and reversing fibrosis remain to be seen.

NONCIRRHOTIC PORTAL HYPERTENSION

Noncirrhotic portal hypertension (NCPH) is a rare condition observed in less than 1% of patients.[17] It is possible that NCPH is underrecognized owing to the limited availability of liver biopsy.[135] It is characterized by the presence of intrahepatic portal hypertension in the absence of known risk factors of liver disease and histologic absence of cirrhosis.[136] Patients with portal hypertension may have splenomegaly and/or thrombocytopenia and usually present with ascites or bleeding varices.[137,138] HIV and ARV treatment, in addition to other conditions, have been associated with NCPH.[139,140] Histologically, NCPH is marked by

- Periportal or perisinusoidal fibrosis with portal tract remnants
- Fibrotic degeneration of the venous wall
- Nodular regeneration.

Box 4
Components of clinical history for assessment of nonalcoholic fatty liver disease

Age greater than or equal to 50

Body mass index greater than or equal to 30 kg/m^2

Diabetes mellitus type 2

Hypertension

Elevated fasting insulin

Postmenopausal woman

Hispanic ethnicity

Fig. 1 demonstrates histologic findings in NCPH compared with normal liver histology.

Portal vein occlusion with focal fibrous obliteration of small portal veins or portal venopathy in the setting of nodular regenerative hyperplasia is often seen.[135] Also described is more nodular regeneration observed in HIV-associated NCPH than in those without.[135]

NCPH has a relatively benign disease course; however, in rare instances, liver failure can occur including hepatic encephalopathy and hepatopulmonary syndrome. These are considered indications for liver transplantation.[137]

INITIAL DIAGNOSTIC APPROACH IN LIVER DISORDERS IN HUMAN IMMUNODEFICIENCY VIRUS

The initial diagnostic approach in an HIV patient who presents with elevated liver enzymes includes a thorough history and physical examination as a first step. Important elements include previous history of opportunistic infections, hepatotoxic medications or alcohol, recent travel, and other exposures. Initial laboratory tests should include absolute CD4 T-cell count and percentage, and HIV viral load, which can lead to potential diagnosis based on level of immunosuppression as defined by CD4 and viral load.

There are 2 distinct patterns of liver-associated enzyme abnormalities, hepatocellular and cholestatic; although most patients present with a mixed picture. Hepatocellular patterns with predominantly elevated transaminases usually are characteristic of hepatocellular disease and appropriate workup for viral, autoimmune, and metabolic diseases is warranted. Laboratory evaluation includes HAV, HBV, or HCV serologies, and viral load in cases of HIV-viral hepatitides coinfection and alpha-fetoprotein. Ceruloplasmin, antinuclear antibodies, iron and total iron binding capacity, and antimitochondrial and antismooth muscle antibodies can reveal many non-AIDS-related liver diseases, such as Wilson disease, hemochromatosis, or autoimmune liver diseases.

Cholestatic disease is characterized by predominantly elevated alkaline phosphatase and gamma-glutamyl transferase. Imaging with ultrasound is essential to identify intrahepatic and extrahepatic biliary obstruction. Computerized tomography scan is indicated for better delineation of focal lesions and presence of splenomegaly and intraabdominal lymphadenopathy. Endoscopic retrograde cholangiopancreatography

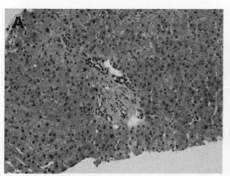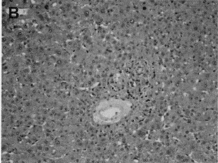

Fig. 1. (*A*) Normal portal area with a large central portal vein, bile duct, and accompanying hepatic artery. (*B*) Portal area showing small attenuated, branched herniating portal veins and obliterated or absent large portal vein. (*Courtesy of* Dr Madhavi Rayapudi, Icahn School of Medicine at Mount Sinai, New York, USA.)

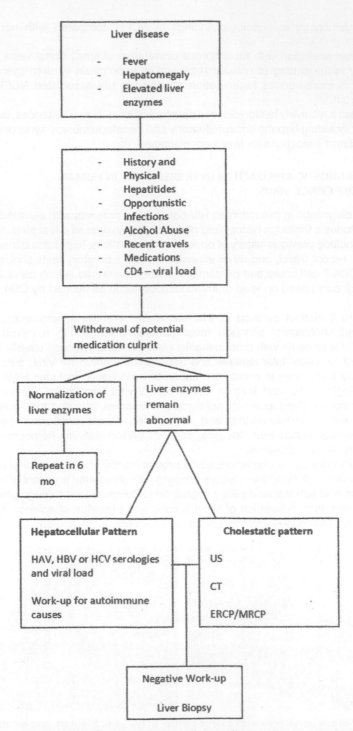

Fig. 2. Diagnostic algorithm for HIV patients with liver disease. CT, computerized tomography; ERCP, endoscopic retrograde cholangiopancreatography; MRCP, magnetic resonance cholangiopancreatography; US, ultrasound.

and magnetic resonance cholangiopancreatography are the studies of choice for HIV-related cholangiopathy. If the initial workup is negative, liver function tests should follow every 6 months. If they are not normalized, liver biopsy should be considered. Tissue sampling with liver biopsy is indicated when a diagnosis is not achieved after less invasive workup and liver enzymes remain elevated after removal of reversible causes, such as discontinuation of hepatotoxic medications.[62]

In patients on ART, baseline liver function tests should be obtained and should be repeated at 4 to 6 weeks following initiation of ART and at least every 3 months thereafter if the values are within normal limits. In patients on treatment with nevirapine or abacavir because of the possibility of hypersensitivity reaction, ART must be withheld completely in case of liver enzyme elevation within the first 4 to 6 weeks after treatment initiation (**Fig. 2**).

Similarly, in cases of serum lactate level elevation, NRTI must be withdrawn. Elevations in liver enzymes greater than 10 times the upper limit of normal can be a sign of liver failure and warrant prompt withdrawal of ART, particularly if no other cause of liver injury is identified. A careful medication review can reveal other hepatotoxic medications that can act synergistically with ART and intensify liver damage, such as isoniazid, rifampin, or statins.[82]

In HIV-coinfected patients with viral hepatitides, use of transient elastography is indicated for evaluation of liver fibrosis and progression to cirrhosis, whereas monitoring of albumin and coagulation studies can be an easy first tool to assess liver synthetic function.

SUMMARY

Liver-related complications are an important cause of hospitalizations and deaths in HIV-infected patients. Causes include a variety of factors, including coinfection with HCV or HBV, alcohol abuse, toxic effects of ARV medications, and fatty liver disease. With current available therapies, coinfection with HBV and HCV is treatable and curable, respectively. Increased risk for severe liver disease in coinfected patients renders timely diagnosis and consideration of treatment paramount. Additionally, management of liver disease in the era of ART requires recognizing and understanding that the landscape of liver disease in PLWH has evolved dramatically, changing from complications of opportunistic infections to sequelae of medication side effects and fatty liver disease.

REFERENCES

1. Sulkowski MS. Management of hepatic complications in HIV-infected persons. J Infect Dis 2008;197(Suppl 3):S279–93.
2. Sherman KE, Peters MG, Thomas D. Human immunodeficiency virus and liver disease: a comprehensive update. Hepatol Commun 2017;1(10):987–1001.
3. Smith CJ, Ryom L, Weber R, et al, D:A:D Study Group. Trends in underlying causes of death in people with HIV from 1999 to 2011 (D:A:D): a multicohort collaboration. Lancet 2014;384:241–8.
4. Crane M, Iser D, Lewin SR. Human immunodeficiency virus infection and the liver. World J Hepatol 2012;4(3):91–8.
5. Fromentin R, Tardif MR, Tremblay MJ. Human hepatoma cells transmit surface bound HIV-1 to CD4+ T cells through an ICAM-1/LFA-1-dependent mechanism. Virology 2010;398:168–75.
6. Schwabe RF, Seki E, Brenner DA. Toll-like receptor signaling in the liver. Gastroenterology 2006;130:1886–900.

7. Lemoine M, Capeau J, Serfaty L. PPAR and liver injury in HIV-infected patients. PPAR Res 2009;2009:906167.

8. Weber R, Sabin CA, Friis-Moller N, et al. Liver-related deaths in persons infected with the human immunodeficiency virus: the D:A:D study. Arch Intern Med 2006; 166(15):1632–41.

9. Thio CL, Nolt KR, Astemborski J, et al. Screening for hepatitis C virus in human immunodeficiency virus-infected individuals. J Clin Microbiol 2000;38(2):575–7.

10. Freidl GS, Sonder GJ, Bovee LP, et al. Hepatitis A outbreak among men who have sex with men (MSM) predominantly linked with the EuroPride, The Netherlands, 2017. Euro Surveill 2017;22 [pii:30468].

11. Beebeejaun K, Degala S, Balogun K, et al. Outbreak of hepatitis A associated with men who have sex with men (MSM), England, 2017. Euro Surveill 2017; 22 [pii:30454].

12. Debes JD, Pisano MB, Lotto M, et al. Hepatitis E virus infection in the HIV-positive patient. J Clin Virol 2016;80:102–6 [Erratum appears in J Clin Virol 2016;82: 181-182].

13. Kuniholm MH, Ong E, Hogema BM, et al. Acute and chronic hepatitis E virus infection in human immunodeficiency virus-infected U.S. women. Hepatology 2016;63:712–20.

14. Palella FJ Jr, Baker RK, Moorman AC, et al. Mortality in the highly active antiretroviral therapy era: changing causes of death and disease in the HIV outpatient study. J Acquir Immune Defic Syndr 2006;43:27–34.

15. Soriano V, Vispo E, Fernandez-Montero JV, et al. Update on HIV/HCV coinfection. Curr HIV/AIDS Rep 2013;10(3):226–34.

16. Platt L, Easterbrook P, Gower E, et al. Prevalence and burden of HCV coinfection in people living with HIV: a global systematic review and meta-analysis. Lancet Infect Dis 2016;16(7):797–808.

17. Puoti M, Moioli MC, Travi G, et al. The burden of liver disease in human immunodeficiency virus-infected patients. Semin Liver Dis 2012;32(2):103–13.

18. Conrad C, Bradley HM, Broz D, et al. Community outbreak of HIV infection linked to injection drug use of oxymorphone – Indiana, 2015. MMWR Morb Mortal Wkly Rep 2015;64(16):443–4.

19. Falade-Nwulia O, Sulkowski MS, Merkow A, et al. Understanding and addressing hepatitis C reinfection in the oral direct-acting antiviral era. J Viral Hepat 2018;25(3):220–7.

20. Foster AL, Gaisa MM, Hijdra RM, et al. Shedding of hepatitis C virus into the rectum of HIV-infected men who have sex with men. Clin Infect Dis 2017; 64(3):284–8.

21. Young J, Rossi C, Walmsley S, et al. Risk factors for hepatitis C virus reinfection after sustained virologic response in patients coinfected with HIV. Clin Infect Dis 2017;64(9):1154–62.

22. Inglitz P, Martin T, Rodger A, et al. HCV reinfection incidence and spontaneous clearance rates in HIV-positive men who have sex with men in Western Europe. J Hepatol 2017;66(2):282–7.

23. Inglitz P, Wehmeyer M, Christensen S, et al. High Incidence of HCV Reinfection in MSM in the DAA Era. Conference on Retroviruses and Opportunistic infections, Boston, March 4–7, 2018, Poster 612.

24. Jordan AE, Perlman DC, Neurer J, et al. Prevalence of hepatitis C virus infection among HIV+ men who have sex with men: a systematic review and meta-analysis. Int J STD AIDS 2016;28(2):145–59.

25. Chen JY, Feeney ER, Chung RT. HCV and HIV co-infection: mechanisms and management. Nat Rev Gastroenterol Hepatol 2014;11(6):362–71.

26. Abutaleb A, Sherman KE. A changing paradigm: management and treatment of the HCV/HIV-co-infected patient. Hepatol Int 2018;12(6):500–9.

27. Soto B, Sanchez-Quijano A, Rodrigo L, et al. Human immunodeficiency virus infection modifies the natural history of chronic parenterally-acquired hepatitis C with an unusually rapid progression to cirrhosis. J Hepatol 1997;26(1):1–5.

28. Benhamou Y, Bochet M, Di Martino V, et al. Liver fibrosis progression in human immunodeficiency virus and hepatitis C virus coinfected patients. The Multivirc Group. Hepatology 1999;30(4):1054–8.

29. Klein MB, Althoff KN, Jing Y, et al. North American AIDS cohort collaboration on research and design of IeDEA; North American AIDS cohort collaboration on research and design (NA-ACCORD) of IeDEA. Risk of end-stage liver disease in HIV-viral hepatitis coinfected persons in North America from the early to modern antiretroviral therapy eras. Clin Infect Dis 2016;63(9):1160–7.

30. Dieterich DT. Hepatitis C virus and human immunodeficiency virus: clinical issues in coinfection. Am J Med 1999;107:79S–84S.

31. Causse X, Payen JL, Izopet J, et al. Does HIV-infection influence the response of chronic hepatitis C to interferon treatment? A French multicenter prospective study. French Multicenter Study Group. J Hepatol 2000;32:1003 10.

32. Smith BD, Morgan RL, Beckett GA, et al. Recommendations for the identification of chronic hepatitis C virus infection among persons born during 1945-1965. MMWR Recomm Rep 2012;61:1–32.

33. Kwo PY, Cohen SM, Lim JK. ACG clinical guideline: evaluation of abnormal liver chemistries. Am J Gastroenterol 2017;112(1):18–35.

34. Thomas DL. The challenge of hepatitis C in the HIV-infected person. Annu Rev Med 2008;59:473–85.

35. Bischoff J, Rockstron JK. Are there any challenges left in hepatitis C virus therapy of HIV infected patients? Int J Antimicrob Agents 2018. [Epub ahead of print].

36. Sulkowski MS, Eron JJ, Wyles DL, et al. Ombitasvir, paritaprevir co-dosed with ritonavir, dasabuvir, and ribavirin for hepatitis C in patients co-infected with HIV-1: a randomized trial. JAMA 2015;313(12):1223–31.

37. Rockstroh JK, Nelson M, Katlama C, et al. Efficacy and safety of grazoprevir (MK-5172) and elbasvir (MK-8742) in patients with hepatitis C virus and HIV co-infection (C-EDGE CO-INFECTION): a non-randomised, open-label trial. Lancet HIV 2015;2(8):e319–27.

38. Naggie S, Cooper C, Saag M, et al. Ledipasvir and sofosbuvir for HCV in patients coinfected with HIV-1. N Engl J Med 2015;373(8):705–13.

39. Luetkemeyer AF, McDonald C, Ramgopal M, et al. 12 weeks of daclatasvir in combination with Sofosbuvir for HIV-HCV coinfection (ALLY-2 Study): efficacy and safety by HIV combination antiretroviral regimens. Clin Infect Dis 2016; 62(12):1489–96.

40. Wyles D, Bräu N, Kottilil S, et al. Sofosbuvir and Velpatasvir for the treatment of hepatitis C virus in patients coinfected with human immunodeficiency virus type 1: an open-label, phase 3 study. Clin Infect Dis 2017;65(1):6–12.

41. Rockstroh JK, Lacombe K, Viani RM, et al. Efficacy and safety of glecaprevir/pibrentasvir in patients coinfected with hepatitis C virus and human immunodeficiency virus type 1: the EXPEDITION-2 study. Clin Infect Dis 2018;67(7):1010–7.

42. Hadler SC, Judson FN, O'Malley PM, et al. Outcome of hepatitis B virus infection in homosexual men and its relation to prior human immunodeficiency virus infection. J Infect Dis 1991;163(3):454–9.

43. Bodsworth NJ, Cooper DA, Donovan B. The influence of human immunodeficiency virus type 1 infection on the development of the hepatitis B virus carrier state. J Infect Dis 1991;163(5):1138–40.

44. Lok AS, McMahon BJ. Chronic hepatitis B: update 2009. Hepatology 2009;50: 661–2.

45. Kim HN, Harrington RD, Van Rompaey SE, et al. Independent clinical predictors of impaired response to hepatitis B vaccination in HIV-infected persons. Int J STD AIDS 2008;19(9):600–4.

46. Buti M, Gane E, Seto WK, et al. Tenofovir alafenamide versus tenofovir disoproxil fumarate for the treatment of patients with HBeAg-negative chronic hepatitis B virus infection: a randomised, double-blind, Phase 3, non-inferiority trial. Lancet Gastroenterol Hepatol 2016;1:196–206.

47. Chan HLY, Fung S, Seto WK, et al. Tenofovir alafenamide versus tenofovir disoproxil fumarate for the treatment of HBeAg-positive chronic hepatitis B virus infection: a randomised, double-blind, Phase 3, non-inferiority trial. Lancet Gastroenterol Hepatol 2016;1:185–95.

48. Seto W, Asahina Y, Peng C, et al. Reduced changes in bone mineral density in chronic HBV (CHB) patients receiving tenofovir alafenamide (TAF) compared with tenofovir disoproxil fumarate (TDF). Hepatology 2016;64(1 Suppl):35A.

49. Dimou E, Papadimitropoulos V, Hadziyannis SJ. The role of entecavir in the treatment of chronic hepatitis B. Ther Clin Risk Manag 2007;3(6):1077–86.

50. Davoudi S, Rasoolinejad M, Jafari S, et al. Prevalence of hepatitis A virus infection in a HIV positive community. Acta Med Iran 2010;48(3):192–5.

51. Gallego M, Robles M, Palacios R, et al. Impact of acute hepatitis A virus (HAV) infection on HIV viral load in HIV-infected patients and influence of HIV infection on acute HAV infection. J Int Assoc Physicians AIDS Care (Chic) 2011;10(1): 40–2.

52. Lin KY, Chen GJ, Lee YL, et al. Hepatitis A virus infection and hepatitis A vaccination in human immunodeficiency virus-positive patients: a review. World J Gastroenterol 2017;23(20):3589–606.

53. DeGroote NP, Mattson CL, Tie Y, et al. Hepatitis A virus immunity and vaccination among at-risk persons receiving HIV medical care. Prev Med Rep 2018;11: 139–44.

54. Werber D, Michaelis K, Hausner M, et al. Ongoing outbreaks of hepatitis A among men who have sex with men (MSM), Berlin, November 2016 to January 2017 - linked to other German cities and European countries. Euro Surveill 2017; 22(5):30457.

55. Boucher A, Meybeck A, Alidjinou K, et al. Clinical and virological features of acute hepatitis A during an ongoing outbreak among men who have sex with men in the North of France. Sex Transm Infect 2019;95(1):75–7.

56. Yoshimura Y, Horiuchi H, Sawaki K, et al. Hepatitis A outbreak among men who have sex with men, Yokohama, Japan, January to May 2018. Sex Transm Dis 2019;46(3):e26–7.

57. Cheng CY, Wu HH, Zou H, et al. Epidemiological characteristics and associated factors of acute hepatitis A outbreak among HIV-coinfected men who have sex with men in Taiwan, June 2015-December 2016. J Viral Hepat 2018;25(10): 1208–15.

58. Gozlan Y, Bar-Or I, Rakovsky A, et al. Ongoing hepatitis A among men who have sex with men (MSM) linked to outbreaks in Europe in Tel Aviv area, Israel, December 2016 – June 2017. Euro Surveill 2017;22(29) [pii:30575].

59. Bassett MT. 2017 DOHMH Alert #34: UPDATE: Increase in Cases of Hepatitis A among Men Who Have Sex with Men. NYC Dept of Health and Mental Hygiene. 2017.

60. Crum-Cianflone NF, Curry J, Drobeniuc J, et al. Hepatitis E virus infection in HIV-infected persons. Emerg Infect Dis 2012;18(3):502–6.

61. Merchante N, Parra-Sanchez M, Rivero-Juarez A, et al. High prevalence of antibodies against hepatitis E virus in HIV-infected patients with unexplained liver disease. Enferm Infecc Microbiol Clin 2015;33(8):532–5.

62. Neukam K, Barreiro P, Macias J, et al. Chronic hepatitis E in HIV patients: rapid progression to cirrhosis and response to oral ribavirin. Clin Infect Dis 2013; 57(3):465–8.

63. Feldt T, Sarfo FS, Zoufaly A, et al. Hepatitis E virus infections in HIV-infected patients in Ghanaand Cameroon. J Clin Virol 2013;58:18–23.

64. Scotto G, Martinelli D, Centra M, et al. Epidemiological and clinical features of HEV infection: a survey in the district of Foggia (Apulia, Southern Italy). Epidemiol Infect 2014;142(2):287–94.

65. Poles MA, Lew EA, Dieterich DT. Diagnosis and treatment of hepatic disease in patients with HIV. Gastroenterol Clin North Am 1997;26(2):291–321.

66. Albaadania A, Alhumaidib S, Asiric S. Cytomegalovirus hepatitis in HIV infection. J Med Cases 2016;7(9):403–5.

67. Erdmann N, Hewitt BA, Atkinson TP, et al. Disseminated primary herpes simplex virus type 2 infection in a 22-year-old male. Open Forum Infect Dis 2015;2(3): ofv092.

68. Remis RS, Liu J, Loutfy MR, et al. Prevalence of sexually transmitted viral and bacterial infections in HIV-positive and HIV-negative men who have sex with men in Toronto. PLoS One 2016;11(7):e0158090.

69. Brewer EC, Hunter L. Acute liver failure due to disseminated varicella zoster infection. Case Rep Hepatol 2018;2018:1269340.

70. Hickey AJ, Gounder L, Moosa MY, et al. A systematic review of hepatic tuberculosis with considerations in human immunodeficiency virus co-infection. BMC Infect Dis 2015;15:209.

71. Dey J, Gautam H, Venugopal S, et al. Tuberculosis as an etiological factor in liver abscess in adults. Tuberc Res Treat 2016;2016:8479456.

72. Hoffmann CJ, Hoffmann JD, Kensler C, et al. Tuberculosis and hepatic steatosis are prevalent liver pathology findings among HIV-infected patients in South Africa. PLoS One 2015;10(2):e0117813.

73. Karam MB, Mosadegh L. Extra-pulmonary *Pneumocystis jiroveci* infection: a case report. Braz J Infect Dis 2014;18(6):681–5.

74. Pitlik SD, Fainstein V, Garza D, et al. Human cryptosporidiosis: spectrum of disease. Report of six cases and review of the literature. Arch Intern Med 1983;143: 2269–75.

75. Guarda LA, Stein SA, Cleary KA, et al. Human cryptosporidiosis in the acquired immune deficiency syndrome. Arch Pathol Lab Med 1983;107:562–6.

76. Enns R. AIDS cholangiopathy: "an endangered disease". Am J Gastroenterol 2003;98:2111–2.

77. Sharma A, Duggal L, Jain N, et al. AIDS cholangiopathy. JIACM 2006;7(1): 49–55.

78. De Angelis C, Mangone M, Bianchi M, et al. An update on AIDS-related cholangiopathy. Minerva Gastroenterol Dietol 2009;55(1):79–82.

79. Kapelusznik L, Arumugam V, Caplivski D, et al. Disseminated histoplasmosis presenting as AIDS cholangiopathy. Mycoses 2011;54(3):262–4.

80. Naseer M, Dailey FE, Juboori AA, et al. Epidemiology, determinants, and management of AIDS cholangiopathy: a review. World J Gastroenterol 2018;24(7): 767–74.

81. Soriano V, Barreiro P, Sherman KE. The changing epidemiology of liver disease in HIV patients. AIDS Rev 2013;15(1):25–31.

82. Jones M, Núñez M. Liver toxicity of antiretroviral drugs. Semin Liver Dis 2012; 32(2):167–76.

83. Sherman KE, Thomas DL, Chung RT. Human immunodeficiency virus and liver disease forum 2010: conference proceedings. Hepatology 2011;54(6):2245–53.

84. Massimo P, Nasta P, Gatti F, et al. HIV-related liver disease: ARV drugs, coinfection, and other risk factors. J Int Assoc Physicians AIDS Care (Chic) 2009;8(1): 30–2.

85. Price JC, Thio CL. Liver disease in the HIV-infected individual. Clin Gastroenterol Hepatol 2010;8:1002–12.

86. Cengiz C, Park JS, Saraf N, et al. HIV and liver diseases: recent clinical advances. Clin Liver Dis 2005;9(4):647–66.

87. Lankisch TO, Behrens G, Ehmer U, et al. Gilbert's syndrome and hyperbilirubinemia in protease inhibitor therapy–an extended haplotype of genetic variants increases risk in indinavir treatment. J Hepatol 2009;50(5):1010–8.

88. Lankisch TO, Moebius U, Wehmeier M, et al. Gilbert's disease and atazanavir: from phenotype to UDP glucuronosyltransferase haplotype. Hepatology 2006; 44:1324–32.

89. Sulkowski MS, Mehta SH, Chaisson RE, et al. Hepatotoxicity associated with protease inhibitor based antiretroviral regimens with or without concurrent ritonavir. AIDS 2004;18:2274–84.

90. Spengler U, Lichterfeld M, Rockstroh JK. Antiretroviral drug toxicity—a challenge for the hepatologist? J Hepatol 2002;36:283–94.

91. Gonzalez de Requena D, Nunez M, Jimenez-Nacher I. Liver toxicity caused by nevirapine. AIDS 2002;16:290–1.

92. Colonno RJ, Rose R, Baldick CJ, et al. Entecavir resistance is rare in nucleoside naive patients with hepatitis B. Hepatology 2006;44:1656–65.

93. Drake A, Mijch A, Sasadeusz J. Immune reconstitution hepatitis in HIV and hepatitis B coinfection, despite lamivudine therapy as part of ART. Clin Infect Dis 2004;39:129–32.

94. Kim HN, Harrington RD, Shuhart MC, et al. Hepatitis C virus activation in HIV-infected patients initiating highly active antiretroviral therapy. AIDS Patient Care STDS 2007;21(10):718–23.

95. Maida I, Nunez M, Rios MJ, et al. Severe liver disease associated with prolonged exposure to antiretroviral drugs. J Acquir Immune Defic Syndr 2006; 42:177–82.

96. Kovari H, Ledergerber B, Peter U, et al. Association of noncirrhotic portal hypertension in HIV-infected persons and antiretroviral therapy with didanosine: a nested case-control study. Clin Infect Dis 2009;49:626–35.

97. Fuster D, Sanvisens A, Bolao F, et al. Alcohol use disorder and its impact on chronic hepatitis C virus and human immunodeficiency virus infections. World J Hepatol 2016;8(31):1295–308.

98. Rehm J, Mathers C, Popova S, et al. Global burden of disease and injury and economic cost attributable to alcohol use and alcohol-use disorders. Lancet 2009;373:2223–33.

99. Friedmann PD. Clinical practice. Alcohol use in adults. N Engl J Med 2013;368: 365–73.

100. Chander G, Lau B, Moore RD. Hazardous alcohol use: a risk factor for non-adherence and lack of suppression in HIV infection. J Acquir Immune Defic Syndr 2006;43:411–7.

101. Savolainen VT, Liesto K, Männikkö A, et al. Alcohol consumption and alcoholic liver disease: evidence of a threshold level of effects of ethanol. Alcohol Clin Exp Res 1993;17(5):1112–7.

102. Torruellas C, French SW, Medici V. Diagnosis of alcoholic liver disease. World J Gastroenterol 2014;20(33):11684–99.

103. Chaudhry AA, Sulkowski MS, Chander G, et al. Hazardous drinking is associated with an elevated aspartate aminotransferase to platelet ratio index in an urban HIV-infected clinical cohort. HIV Med 2009;10:133–42.

104. Lim JK, Tate JP, Fultz SL, et al. Relationship between alcohol use categories and noninvasive markers of advanced hepatic fibrosis in HIV-infected, chronic hepatitis C virus-infected, and uninfected patients. Clin Infect Dis 2014;58:1449–58.

105. Sacco P, Bucholz KK, Spitznagel EL. Alcohol use among older adults in the National Epidemiologic Survey on Alcohol and Related Conditions: a latent class analysis. J Stud Alcohol Drugs 2009;70(6):829–38.

106. Galvan FH, Bing EG, Fleishman JA, et al. The prevalence of alcohol consumption and heavy drinking among people with HIV in the United States: results from the HIV cost and services utilization study. J Stud Alcohol 2002;63:179–86.

107. Parsons JT, Rosof E, Mustanski B. The temporal relationship between alcohol consumption and HIV-medication adherence: a multilevel model of direct and moderating effects. Health Psychol 2008;27:628–37.

108. Miguez MJ, Shor-Posner G, Morales G, et al. HIV treatment in drug abusers: impact of alcohol use. Addict Biol 2003;8(1):33–7.

109. Molina PE, Happel KI, Zhang P, et al. Focus on: alcohol and the immune system. Alcohol Res Health 2010;33:97–108.

110. Bagby GJ, Amedee AM, Siggins RW, et al. Alcohol and HIV effects on the immune system. Alcohol Res 2015;37(2):287–97.

111. Purohit V, Bode JC, Bode C, et al. Alcohol, intestinal bacterial growth, intestinal permeability to endotoxin, and medical consequences: summary of a symposium. Alcohol 2008;42(5):349–61.

112. Brenchley JM, Douek DC. HIV infection and the gastrointestinal immune system. Mucosal Immunol 2008;1(1):23–30.

113. Rodger AJ, Lodwick R, Schechter M, et al. INSIGHT SMART, ESPRIT Study Groups. Mortality in well controlled HIV in the continuous antiretroviral therapy arms of the SMART and ESPRIT trials compared with the general population. AIDS 2013;27(6):973–9.

114. Guaraldi G, Orlando G, Squillace N, et al. Multidisciplinary approach to the treatment of metabolic and morphologic alterations of HIV-related lipodystrophy. HIV Clin Trials 2006;7:97–106.

115. Vallet-Pichard A, Mallet V, Pol S. Nonalcoholic fatty liver disease and HIV infection. Semin Liver Dis 2012;32(2):158–66.

116. Do A, Lim JK. Epidemiology of nonalcoholic fatty liver disease: a primer. Clin Liver Dis 2016;7(5):106–8.

117. Crum-Cianflone N, Collins G, Medina S, et al. Prevalence and factors associated with liver test abnormalities among human immunodeficiency virus-infected persons. Clin Gastroenterol Hepatol 2010;8(2):183–91.
118. Guaraldi G, Squillace N, Stentarelli C, et al. Nonalcoholic fatty liver disease in HIV-infected patients referred to a metabolic clinic: prevalence, characteristics, and predictors. Clin Infect Dis 2008;47(2):250–7.
119. Crum-Cianflone N, Dilay A, Collins G, et al. Nonalcoholic fatty liver disease among HIV-infected persons. J Acquir Immune Defic Syndr 2009;50:464–73.
120. Loomba R, Sanyal A. The global NAFLD epidemic. Nat Rev Gastroenterol Hepatol 2013;10:686–90.
121. Michelotti GA, Machado MV, Diehl AM. NAFLD, NASH and liver cancer. Nat Rev Gastroenterol Hepatol 2013;10:656–65.
122. Angulo P. Nonalcoholic fatty liver disease. N Engl J Med 2002;346(16):1221–31.
123. Ingiliz P, Valantin MA, Duvivier C, et al. Liver damage underlying unexplained transaminase elevation in human immunodeficiency virus-1 mono-infected patients on antiretroviral therapy. Hepatology 2009;49(2):436–42.
124. Mohammed SS, Aghdassi E, Salit IE, et al. HIV-positive patients with nonalcoholic fatty liver disease have a lower body mass index and are more physically active than HIV-negative patients. J Acquir Immune Defic Syndr 2007;45:432–8.
125. Samaras K. The burden of diabetes and hyperlipidemia in treated HIV infection and approaches for cardiometabolic care. Curr HIV/AIDS Rep 2012;9:206–17.
126. Kasturiratne A, Weerasinghe S, Dassanayake AS, et al. Influence of nonalcoholic fatty liver disease on the development of diabetes mellitus. J Gastroenterol Hepatol 2013;28(1):142–7.
127. Dyson JK, Anstee QM, McPherson S. Non-alcoholic fatty liver disease: a practical approach to treatment. Frontline Gastroenterol 2014;5(4):277–86.
128. Dasarathy S, Dasarathy J, Khiyami A, et al. Validity of real time ultrasound in the diagnosis of hepatic steatosis: a prospective study. J Hepatol 2009;51(6):1061–7.
129. Bril F, Ortiz-Lopez C, Lomonaco R, et al. Clinical value of liver ultrasound for the diagnosis of nonalcoholic fatty liver disease in overweight and obese patients. Liver Int 2015;35(9):2139–46.
130. Myers RP, Fong A, Shaheen AAM. Utilization rates, complications and costs of percutaneous liver biopsy: a population-based study including 4275 biopsies. Liver Int 2008;28(5):705–12.
131. Frulio N, Trillaud H, Perez P, et al. Acoustic radiation force impulse (ARFI) and transient elastography (TE) for evaluation of liver fibrosis in HIV-HCV co-infected patients. BMC Infect Dis 2014;14:405.
132. Njei B, McCarty TR, Luk J, et al. Use of transient elastography in patients with HIV-HCV coinfection: a systematic review and meta-analysis. J Gastroenterol Hepatol 2016;31(10):1684–93.
133. Cusi K. Role of obesity and lipotoxicity in the development of nonalcoholic steatohepatitis: pathophysiology and clinical implications. Gastroenterology 2012;142(4):711–25.e6.
134. Wong VW, Chan RS, Wong GL, et al. Community-based lifestyle modification programme for non-alcoholic fatty liver disease: a randomized controlled trial. J Hepatol 2013;59(3):536–42.
135. Verheij J, Schouten JNL, Komuta M, et al. Histological features in western patients with idiopathic non-cirrhotic portal hypertension. Histopathology 2013;62:1083–91.

136. Schouten JN, Verheij J, Seijo S. Idiopathic non-cirrhotic portal hypertension: a review. Orphanet J Rare Dis 2015;10:67.
137. Schouten JNL, García-Pagán JC, Valla DC, et al. Idiopathic noncirrhotic portal hypertension. Hepatology 2011;54:1071–81.
138. Siramolpiwat S, Seijo S, Miquel R, et al. Idiopathic portal hypertension: natural history and long-term outcome. Hepatology 2014;59:2276–85.
139. Chang P-E, Miquel R, Blanco J-L, et al. Idiopathic portal hypertension in patients with HIV infection treated with highly active antiretroviral therapy. Am J Gastroenterol 2009;104:1707–14.
140. Schouten JNL, Van der Ende ME, Koëter T, et al. Risk factors and outcome of HIV-associated idiopathic noncirrhotic portal hypertension. Aliment Pharmacol Ther 2012;36(9):875–85.

Sarcoidosis and the Liver

Manoj Kumar, MD, MPH, Jorge L. Herrera, MD*

KEYWORDS

- Sarcoidosis • Granuloma • Hepatitis • Liver

KEY POINTS

- Up to 90% of patients with systemic sarcoidosis have hepatic granulomas, most are asymptomatic.
- Elevated liver enzymes, in particular alkaline phosphatase, is the most common presentation of hepatic sarcoidosis.
- The diagnosis of hepatic sarcoidosis is a diagnosis of exclusion; careful attention is necessary to exclude other causes of liver granuloma.
- Only a minority of patients require therapy. It is not clear if therapy alters the natural course of the disease.
- Hepatic sarcoidosis can cause noncirrhotic presinusoidal portal hypertension. Once cirrhosis develops, clinically significant portal hypertension is common, but synthetic liver dysfunction is rare.

INTRODUCTION

Sarcoidosis is a systemic disease affecting multiple organ systems and histologically characterized by noncaseating granulomas.[1] It was first described by Sir Jonathan Hutchinson in 1877 as a skin disease, presented as "'Case of Livid Papillary Psoriasis."[2] In 1899, Caesar Boeck[3] observed extremely slow-growing skin nodules in one of his patients resembling sarcoma, and coined the condition as "multiple benign sarcoid of the skin."

Sarcoidosis occurs worldwide; however, its highest prevalence is reported from Nordic countries and among African American individuals in the United States.[4,5] In the United States, the reported prevalence of sarcoidosis has been between 1 and 40 per 100,000, with incidence rates of 5.9 in male and 6.3 in female individuals per 100,000 person-years. The age-adjusted and sex-adjusted incidence has been reported as 6.1 per 100,000 person-years.[6] In general, the disease affects women

Disclosure Statements: The authors have nothing to disclose.
Division of Gastroenterology, University of South Alabama College of Medicine, UCOM 6000, 75 University Boulevard South, Mobile, AL 36688, USA
* Corresponding author.
E-mail address: jherrera18@gmail.com

Clin Liver Dis 23 (2019) 331–343
https://doi.org/10.1016/j.cld.2018.12.012
1089-3261/19/© 2018 Elsevier Inc. All rights reserved.

more than men, but men tend to have a younger age onset as compared with women, with peak age at onset between 20 and 50 years.[4,6–10] A second age peak (>50 years) also has been described.[11] Among African American individuals, for both men and women, peak incidence usually occurs in fourth decade and they are more likely to have extrathoracic lymph node, liver, and bone marrow involvement than the white population.[4,12]

The most commonly affected organ in sarcoidosis is the lung; however, 50% of cases have extrapulmonary involvement.[12–14] Liver involvement is found in 11% to 80% of cases, with lower rates reported among symptomatic cases and higher rates from random liver biopsy findings.[15] The diagnosis of hepatic sarcoidosis (HS) can be difficult. Most patients are asymptomatic, there is no single definite laboratory test to establish the diagnosis, and radiologic imaging studies are usually unremarkable. Hepatic granulomas seen on histopathology usually forms the foundation for the definite diagnosis. Based on the type of granulomas present on histopathology, HS can be essentially distinguished from its most common differentials, such as primary biliary cholangitis (PBC) and primary sclerosing cholangitis (PSC).[16,17] Management of HS involves either clinical observation or pharmacologic treatment, depending on presence of symptoms or the severity of liver involvement.

PATHOGENESIS OF SARCOIDOSIS

Despite advancements, the exact cause of sarcoidosis remains unknown, however pathogenesis is believed to be multifactorial, including immunologic, genetic, and environmental factors.[11,18]

Immunologic Factors

The aggregation of CD4+ T cells of the Th1 type and macrophages at the sites of ongoing inflammation marks the immunologic response in sarcoidosis. These cells produce cytokines, including interleukin (IL)-1, IL-6, and tumor necrosis factor (TNF)-α, which facilitate further macrophage aggregation leading to granuloma formation.[19,20] These activated macrophages also secrete fibroblast growth factors and contribute in the development of fibrosis in sarcoidosis.[21]

Genetic Factors

The risk for sarcoidosis has been linked with class I and II HLA molecules and a role of genes within the major histocompatibility complex (MHC) locus has been suggested.[22–24] Specific MHC alleles and gene variations have been implicated to determine the progression of disease, susceptibility, and prognosis. Berlin and colleagues[25] investigated the correlation between HLA class II alleles and the clinical outcome in white patients with sarcoidosis. In this 10-year study, 122 Scandinavian patients with sarcoidosis were typed for HLA-DR, HLA-DQA1, and HLA-DQB1 alleles using polymerase chain reaction amplification and were compared with 250 healthy Swedish volunteers as controls. The study showed strong association between HLA-DR17(3) with good prognosis, and between DR15(2) and DR14(6) with chronic form of the disease. Another study confirmed a genetic predisposition based on allelic variation at the HLA-DRB1 locus.[26] Five DRB1 alleles, 1 DRB3 allele, and 1 DPB1 amino acid residue were established as risk factors for sarcoidosis and DRB1 amino acid residue was determined as protective. Genomic studies have conferred strong roles of gene butyrophilin-like 2 (BTNL2) and ANXA11 (annexin A11; gene on chromosome 10q22.3) in sarcoidosis predisposition.[27,28] These genomic findings suggest genetic susceptibility for the disease.

Environmental Factors

Numerous occupational and environmental exposures have been reported in association with sarcoidosis.[29–33] Newman and colleagues[34] in their multicenter case control study compared 706 newly diagnosed patients with sarcoidosis with an equal number of control subjects matched for age, race, and sex. Data regarding occupational and nonoccupational exposures were collected and analyzed. The study could not demonstrate a single environmental or occupational etiology of sarcoidosis. However, a role for multiple environmental factors setting up the granulomatous response was suspected. Insecticides, agricultural employment, moldy musty environments, and bioaerosol exposure showed a positive association with sarcoidosis. On the other hand, tobacco smoking had a negative association with sarcoidosis risk.

Infectious etiology also has been suggested to play a possible role. The mycobacterial antigen, *Mycobacterium tuberculosis* catalase-peroxidase (mKatG), was detected in 5 (55%) of 9 sarcoidosis tissues and none in 14 control tissues ($P = .0037$). mKatG was suggested to be one of the targets of the immune response in sarcoidosis pathogenesis.[35] *Propionibacterium acnes* (now *Cutibacterium acnes*) have been found in patients with sarcoidosis. Nevertheless, it is not clear if this has any causal relationship.[36]

Several other chemicals have been studied in association with sarcoidosis. Kveim reagent and vimentin were found to induce a proinflammatory cytokine secretion from sarcoidosis peripheral blood mononuclear cells; however, further investigation is needed.[37] Serum amyloid A has been suggested as a constituent and innate regulator of granulomatous inflammation in sarcoidosis.[38]

Hepatic Sarcoidosis Histo-Pathogenesis

After lung and lymph nodes, sarcoidosis commonly involves the liver.[39] Up to 90% of patients with systemic sarcoidosis demonstrate liver granulomas.[40] Sarcoid liver involvement is more common in patients with sarcoid changes in lung parenchyma rather than in those with only bilateral hilar adenopathy.[16] Even though finding of hepatic granuloma suggests a diagnosis of hepatic sarcoidosis, an array of other systemic conditions also exhibit liver granulomas and must be considered in the differential diagnosis. Hepatic granulomas typically have 4 histologic variants, including noncaseating, caseating, fibrin ring, and lipogranulomas. Noncaseating (epithelioid granuloma) is characteristic of sarcoidosis. In contrast, tuberculosis is associated with caseating type. Fibrin ring granulomata can be seen in a variety of infections, such as Q fever, cytomegalovirus, Epstein-Barr virus, hepatitis A, and leishmaniosis. Medications such as allopurinol and check-point inhibitor, malignancy such as Hodgkin and non-Hodgkin lymphoma, and autoimmune conditions like giant cell arteritis can also cause fibrin ring hepatic granulomas.[41,42] Hepatic lipogranuloma is seen in people who use mineral oil; however, it also can be found in patients with hepatic steatosis, hepatitis C, and fatty liver disease.[43] An accurate diagnosis of HS requires the presence of other histopathological features typical of HS, laboratory evaluation to exclude other causes of granulomatous liver disease, and the proper clinical context.

The histologic characteristics of sarcoid granulomas are shown in **Box 1**. The granulomas are characterized by aggregates of epithelioid histiocytic and multinucleated giant cells with lymphocytes and fibrin deposits mostly at the periphery. These lesions are small, abundant, and evenly dispersed in the liver parenchyma (although favor periportal and portal regions) and display identical stage of maturation.[44,45] Necrosis is typically absent; however, some atypical cases may show small areas of necrosis.

Box 1
Histologic characteristics of sarcoid liver granuloma

Histologic variant: Well-differentiated, noncaseating granuloma

Cellular components:
   Epithelioid histiocytes
   Multinucleated giant cells and lymphocytes
   Peripheral fibrin deposit

Location:
   Evenly dispersed in hepatic parenchyma, favor portal and peri-portal regions

Fibrosis:
   Cuffs of fibrosis may mimic primary sclerosing cholangitis

---

Older lesions show reticulin fibers within the granulomas and sometimes a prominent cuff of fibrosis. Large confluent granulomas may lead to hyalinized scar formation.[45–47] These changes, along with chronic intrahepatic cholestasis, may lead to micronodular biliary cirrhosis.[17] HS may present with intrahepatic or extrahepatic cholestasis. Histologically, the intrahepatic cholestasis in HS mimics PBC as well as lesions of PSC.[16,47] Adenopathy at liver hilum can lead to extrahepatic cholestasis due to external compression of the common hepatic duct, sometimes leading to cholangitis.[48,49] Other histologic changes include sinusoidal dilatation, particularly around zone 3, and nodular regenerative hyperplasia.

Patients with HS may develop noncirrhotic presinusoidal portal hypertension.[50] Valla and colleagues[51] found perisinusoidal block and portal flow obstruction secondary to hepatic granulomas in the absence of cirrhosis as a cause for portal hypertension in 35 of 47 patients with HS.

Clinical Presentation

Patients with HS are usually asymptomatic (50%–80%); however, the clinical spectrum of symptomatic hepatic sarcoidosis can be broad, as shown in **Table 1**. Pruritus from chronic cholestasis and abdominal pain secondary to stretching of Glisson's capsule are reported in approximately 15%.[52] Jaundice is rare, but may reflect

Table 1
Clinical spectrum of hepatic sarcoidosis

Feature	Presentation, %
Asymptomatic	50–80
Abnormal liver enzymes	30
Hepatomegaly or splenomegaly	50 on radiologic examination, <15–20 detected clinically
Symptoms	Abdominal pain 15, pruritus and jaundice <5
Cirrhosis	6–8
Portal hypertension • Severe liver dysfunction • Esophageal varices	3–18 Rare Up to 78% of cases with portal hypertension
Advanced disease requiring transplantation	0.012% of all transplants in the United States

Adapted from Tadros M, Forouhar F, Wu GY. Hepatic sarcoidosis. J Clin Transl Hepatol 2013;1:89, with permission.

intrahepatic or extrahepatic cholestasis,[52] fever is reported among 3% to 28% of patients,[53] and fatigue is common. Hepatomegaly and splenomegaly are noted in 5% to 10%, especially if portal hypertension is present.[54] Even in the presence of portal hypertension, severe liver dysfunction is uncommon, although esophageal varices can be seen in up to 78% of patients. Local inflammation causing obliteration of small portal veins can result in portal vein thrombosis, and extrinsic compression of hepatic veins due to granulomas can lead to Budd-Chiari syndrome.[55,56] Elevated liver enzymes can be seen in HS; however, the degree of elevation does not always correlate with the severity of the liver involvement. A predominant elevation of alkaline phosphatase, often 5 to 10 times the upper limit of normal (ULN) is the usual pattern. A retrospective study of 837 patients with sarcoidosis by Cremers and colleagues[57] showed liver-test abnormalities in 24% of patients, among whom 15% were suspected to have hepatic involvement. Liver biopsy was performed in 22 of these 127 subjects; all except one biopsy was found to be consistent with HS. Moderate and severe liver test abnormalities were associated with advanced histopathological disease. Thus, the investigators suggested liver biopsy should be considered among patients with moderate to severe liver test abnormalities. Because HS is a chronic disease, 6% to 8% of patients progress to cirrhosis, and a few develop liver failure requiring liver transplantation.[58–60]

Differential Diagnosis

Lacking a single diagnostic test, the diagnosis of hepatic sarcoidosis requires a careful evaluation to exclude other conditions that can mimic the histologic findings of HS. Important differential features are shown on **Table 2**. One of the key differential diagnoses of hepatic sarcoidosis is PBC characterized by noncaseating granulomas within portal tracts; however, these granulomas are poorly differentiated in comparison with HS. Another differentiating feature is presence of antimitochondrial antibody in most patients with PBC. Pulmonary hilar adenopathy, frequently present in sarcoidosis, is not a feature of PBC. A few case reports have reported overlap of sarcoidosis and PBC; however, such occurrence is very rare.[46,61] PSC can simulate hepatic sarcoidosis histologically when periductal fibrosis is present. However, clinically, differences can be appreciated due to absence of inflammatory bowel disease association and absence of perinuclear anti-neutrophil cytoplasmic antibody in HS, as well by observing typical PSC-related endoscopic retrograde cholangiopancreatography and magnetic resonance cholangiopancreatography findings that are absent in HS. Sarcoidlike granulomas also have been reported in patients with chronic hepatitis

Table 2
Main differential diagnosis of hepatic sarcoidosis

Condition	Histology	Associated Findings
Sarcoidosis	Well-differentiated noncaseating granuloma	Pulmonary adenopathy Pulmonary interstitial disease
Primary biliary cholangitis	Poorly differentiated noncaseating granuloma	Positive antimitochondrial antibody No pulmonary hilar adenopathy
Primary sclerosing cholangitis	"Onion-skin" periductal fibrosis	Association with inflammatory bowel disease Typical magnetic resonance cholangiography findings
Drug-induced hepatic granulomas	Variable, depending on drug; presence of eosinophils in granulomas suggests diagnosis	Medication history

C. Some patients treated with interferon and ribavirin for hepatitis C before the era of direct-acting antiviral agents reported a sarcoid-like illness, and withdrawal of the medications resulted in spontaneous remission in approximately 85% of patients.[62] Drugs, such as sulfonamides, allopurinol, carbamazepine, quinine, and phenylbutazone, among others, also can cause noncaseating liver granulomas involving portal tracts and hepatic lobules. Careful medication history is thus essential during initial workup.[63]

Diagnosis

The diagnosis of hepatic sarcoidosis is usually suspected when patients present with elevated liver tests. Because of the infiltrative nature of the disease, patients with liver sarcoidosis have elevated alkaline phosphatase and/or gamma glutamyl-transpeptidase (more than 3 times the ULN) aspartate aminotransferase and alanine aminotransferase can be elevated as well; however, usually less than 2 times of ULN.[64] Hyperglobulinemia can be seen. Serum angiotensin-converting enzyme level is elevated in 60% of patients with HS but carries poor sensitivity and specificity, and low positive and negative predictive value.[65] Unfortunately, there is no single serologic test that is diagnostic of HS.

Hepatic sarcoidosis has no specific features on radiologic imaging. Ultrasound can show heterogeneous and coarse echo pattern of the liver parenchyma. Computed tomography (CT) and MRI abdominal findings are also nonspecific in most patients. Warshauer and colleagues[66] studied abdominal CT examination findings in 59 patients with sarcoidosis and evaluated them for adenopathy, liver and spleen size, and discrete lesions within the liver or spleen. Only 10% of patients had extensive adenopathy. Marked hepatic and splenic enlargement was seen in only 8% and 6%, respectively. Splenic nodules were seen in 15%, and 5% had nodules in their liver. Abdominal CT findings did not correlate with chest radiographic findings. MRI also does not show any characteristic signal intensity changes adequate enough to specifically identify liver sarcoidosis.[67] However, it is a useful modality to distinguish liver sarcoidosis from lesions due to infections or neoplasms on the basis of signal intensity.[68,69] If multiple nodules are found, careful differentiation from other granulomatous disease and metastatic lesions should be done. In the event of unexplained elevated alkaline phosphatase and if suspicion of sarcoidosis remains high, histopathological findings from liver biopsy assists in establishing the definite diagnosis.

Management

As most patients with HS are asymptomatic, most do not require specific medical therapy; however, in patients with symptoms due to liver involvement or those with severe disease at risk of liver complications or significant cholestasis, pharmacologic treatment can be considered. A suggested approach to patients with hepatic sarcoidosis is shown in **Fig. 1**. A number of pharmacologic treatment options have been reported with corticosteroids and ursodeoxycholic acid most often used.[70,71]

Corticosteroids

The role of corticosteroids in HS is supported only by data from retrospective analysis and no randomized controlled trials have been done with respect to efficacy and its long-term benefits in the HS population. In contrast with the role of corticosteroids in the treatment of pulmonary sarcoidosis, the role of corticosteroids in HS is imprecise. Patients with mild disease often spontaneously achieve remission. Thus, for patients with mild or no symptoms, treatment with corticosteroids is not recommended due to steroid-related adverse events and lack of proven efficacy of therapy in these

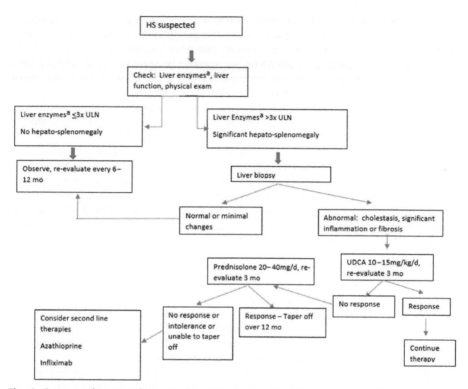

Fig. 1. Suggested approach to HS. [a] In HS, alkaline phosphatase is typically elevated to a higher degree than ALT and AST.

groups. Among symptomatic patients, such as those with significant abdominal pain due to hepatomegaly and ongoing inflammation, or for those with acute or chronic cholestasis and pruritus, corticosteroids have been shown to decrease the number of hepatic granulomas and liver size resulting in improvement of symptoms.[71,72] After initiating therapy with corticosteroids, liver enzyme levels may improve despite no improvement in liver histology, thus treatment may not alter the natural course of the disease.[13] In patients with advanced liver disease and cirrhosis secondary to HS with or without portal hypertension, no consistent clinical or pathologic benefits of corticosteroids could be demonstrated.[50] Steroid therapy may be particularly useful in cases of HS with marked porta hepatis adenopathy causing biliary obstruction; steroid therapy has been reported to shrink lymph node volume with resolution of hyperbilirubinemia.[48,73] There is no definite consensus on the optimal dosage, but most experts initiate therapy at 20 to 40 mg/d for severe disease, after 4 to 6 weeks steroids are tapered by 5-mg to 10-mg decrements every 4 to 8 weeks followed by maintenance at lowest effective dose.[14,71,74,75] Discontinuation of treatment may result in relapse necessitating close monitoring.

Ursodeoxycholic Acid

Chronic cholestasis associated with HS can be treated with ursodeoxycholic acid (UDCA).[76–78] UDCA protects the cholangiocytes against cytotoxicity of hydrophobic bile acids, resulting from modulation of the composition of mixed phospholipid-rich micelles, reduction of bile acid cytotoxicity of bile, and decrease of the concentration of hydrophobic bile acids in the cholangiocytes. It also stimulates hepatobiliary secretion by insertion of transporter molecules into the canalicular membrane of the hepatocyte and protects the hepatocytes against bile acid–induced apoptosis.[79] UDCA also decreases HLA class I and class II on hepatic and biliary duct epithelial cell membranes, thus modulating the immune response and preventing cellular injury. Randomized controlled trials of UDCA for HS have not been performed; however, UDCA is widely used in clinical practice for this indication. There are data demonstrating improvement in liver tests with the use of UDCA,[76–78] but no evidence that it affects long-term prognosis.

In a retrospective cohort study, Bakker and colleagues[80] analyzed the effects of UDCA, prednisolone, or no treatment on liver-related symptoms and liver biochemistries of 17 patients with HS. They noted that treatment with UDCA resulted in a greater improvement in fatigue, pruritus, and liver aminotransferases compared with corticosteroids or no treatment. Given the favorable safety profile of UDCA, it could be considered as the empirical first-line therapy for symptomatic HS.[80] The typical dosage is 10 to 15 mg/kg orally per day.[14,70]

Other Treatment Options

Among patients with HS who are either steroid dependent or did not respond well to other therapies, several other treatment options have been tried. Kennedy and colleagues[13] reported 2 patients with HS with normalization of liver enzymes after treatment with azathioprine (AZA). Standard dosage is 50 to 150 mg/d.[14] Blood counts and hepatic function should be monitored frequently. Thiopurine methyltransferase enzyme activity should be measured in all patients before starting AZA.

Methotrexate (MTX) also has been reported to normalize liver enzymes in patients with HS.[13] The starting dosage of MTX is 10 mg/wk with maximum dosage of 15 mg/wk and should be adjusted based on any evidence of toxicity. Blood count and renal function and hepatic function should be monitored every 8 weeks and folic acid 1 mg/d should be considered for gastrointestinal toxicity. Potential liver toxicity of MTX should be considered and monitored carefully. Other medications, such as cyclosporine, cyclophosphamide, thalidomide, pentoxifylline, and infliximab, have been successfully used to treat HS as secondary or tertiary line of treatments, but supporting evidence of efficacy and safety is lacking for these medications.[70,81,82] There may be a role for anti-TNF-α therapy in patients with necrotizing sarcoid granulomatosis of the liver, a variant of "classic" sarcoidosis. A recent case report illustrated dramatic response to infliximab therapy[83]

Liver Transplantation

Liver transplantation for advanced HS accounts for only 0.012% of liver transplants in the United States. Through the United Network for Organ Sharing/Organ Procurement and Transplantation Network database, Vanatta and colleagues[63] evaluated patient and graft survival after orthotopic liver transplantation for sarcoidosis. The results indicated that the patient and allograft survival rates for HS were satisfactory (1-year and 5-year survival rates for the patients with sarcoidosis were 78% and 61%, respectively) but worse in comparison with the rates for other cholestatic liver diseases. However, another long-term outcome study from a single-center experience (retrospective, case control) of patients undergoing liver transplantation for HS revealed statistically comparable graft and patient survival for such patients with end-stage liver disease secondary to sarcoidosis when compared with other cholestatic diseases. In this study, the 1, 3, 5, and 10-year patient survival rates were 84.6%, 76.9%, 61.1%, and 51.3%, respectively, for the sarcoidosis group and

82.1%, 78.6%, 78.6%, and 61.9%, respectively, for the matched PSC/PBC group (*P* = .739).[84] Recurrence of sarcoidosis in transplanted liver has been reported and can occur anywhere between 8 months to 5 years after transplantation.[13,85] Cost-effectiveness of liver transplantation in hepatic sarcoidosis is unknown.

SUMMARY

In many cases, the diagnosis of hepatic sarcoidosis remains a diagnosis of exclusion. A thorough clinical assessment and careful patient evaluation to exclude pertinent differential diagnoses is necessary for accurate diagnosis. Liver histopathology demonstrating typical noncaseating granulomata provides important supporting evidence for the diagnosis of HS. Most patients remain asymptomatic and do not require therapy for HS. Although progression to severe liver disease is uncommon, monitoring for disease progression and identification of complications is crucial. Corticosteroids and UDCA can be used as primary treatment modality for symptomatic patients, recognizing that therapy may improve symptoms and liver chemistries but not alter the long-term outcome of the disease. Other secondary or tertiary line of treatments should only be considered in special circumstances after pertinent discussion regarding potential efficacy and expected side effects with patients. Prognosis of hepatic sarcoidosis is overall good, but can be more aggressive among African American individuals, individuals with advanced age, and those with concomitant advanced pulmonary disease. Liver transplantation should be reserved for advanced cases with significant compromise of liver function.

REFERENCES

1. Judson MA. Extrapulmonary sarcoidosis. Semin Respir Crit Care Med 2007;28: 83–101.
2. Hutchinson J. Case of livid papillary psoriasis. In: Illustrations of clinical surgery vol. 1. London: J & A Churchill; 1875. p. 42.
3. Boeck C. Multiple benign sarcoid of the skin. Journal of cutaneous and genitourinary diseases 1899;17:543–50.
4. Hillerdal G, Nou E, Osterman K, et al. Sarcoidosis: epidemiology and prognosis. A 15-year European study. Am Rev Respir Dis 1984;130:29–32.
5. Rybicki BA, Major M, Popovich J Jr, et al. Racial differences in sarcoidosis incidence: a 5-year study in a health maintenance organization. Am J Epidemiol 1997;145:234–41.
6. Henke CE, Henke G, Elveback LR, et al. The epidemiology of sarcoidosis in Rochester, Minnesota: a population-based study of incidence and survival. Am J Epidemiol 1986;123:840–5.
7. Byg KE, Milman N, Hansen S. Sarcoidosis in Denmark 1980–1994. A registry-based incidence study comprising 5536 patients. Sarcoidosis Vasc Diffuse Lung Dis 2003;20:46–52.
8. Deubelbeiss U, Gemperli A, Schindler C, et al. Prevalence of sarcoidosis in Switzerland is associated with environmental factors. Eur Respir J 2010;35: 1088–97.
9. Selroos O. The frequency, clinical picture and prognosis of pulmonary sarcoidosis in Finland. Acta Med Scand Suppl 1969;503:3–73.
10. Kowalska M, Niewiadomska E, Zejda JE. Epidemiology of sarcoidosis recorded in 2006–2010 in the Silesian voivodeship on the basis of routine medical reporting. Ann Agric Environ Med 2014;21:55–8.

11. Iannuzzi MC, Rybicki BA, Teirstein AS. Sarcoidosis. N Engl J Med 2007;357: 2153–65.
12. Baughman RP, Teirstein AS, Judson MA, et al. Clinical characteristics of patients in a case control study of sarcoidosis. Am J Respir Crit Care Med 2001;164: 1885–9.
13. Kennedy PT, Zakaria N, Modawi SB, et al. Natural history of hepatic sarcoidosis and its response to treatment. Eur J Gastroenterol Hepatol 2006;18:721–6.
14. Ayyala US, Padilla ML. Diagnosis and treatment of hepatic sarcoidosis. Curr Treat Options Gastroenterol 2006;9:475–83.
15. Available at: https://www.stopsarcoidosis.org/wp-content/uploads/FSR-Physicians-Protocol1.pdf. Accessed August 26, 2018.
16. Alam I, Levenson SD, Ferrell LD, et al. Diffuse intrahepatic biliary strictures in sarcoidosis resembling sclerosing cholangitis: case report and review of the literature. Dig Dis Sci 1997;42:1295–301.
17. Rudzki C, Ishak KG, Zimmerman HJ. Chronic intrahepatic cholestasis of sarcoidosis. Am J Med 1975;59:373–87.
18. Culver DA. Sarcoidosis. Immunol Allergy Clin North Am 2012;32:487–511.
19. Zissel G, Prasse A, Muller-Quernheim J. Immunologic response of sarcoidosis. Semin Respir Crit Care Med 2010;31:390–403.
20. Chesnutt MS, Gifford AH, Prendergast TJ. Pulmonary disorders. In: McPhee SJ, Papadakis MA, editors. 2010 Current medical diagnosis and treatment. New York: McGraw-Hill; 2010.
21. Costabel U. Sarcoidosis: clinical update. Eur Respir J 2001;18(32 suppl): 56s–68s.
22. Luisetti M, Beretta A, Casali L. Genetic aspects in sarcoidosis. Eur Respir J 2000; 16:768–80.
23. Schurmann M, Reichel P, Muller-Myhsok B, et al. Results from a genome-wide search for predisposing genes in sarcoidosis. Am J Respir Crit Care Med 2001;164(5):840–6.
24. Iannuzzi MC, Iyengar SK, Gray-McGuire C, et al. Genome-wide search for sarcoidosis susceptibility genes in African Americans. Genes Immun 2005;6: 509–18.
25. Berlin M, Fogdell-Hahn A, Olerup O, et al. HLA-DR predicts the prognosis in Scandinavian patients with pulmonary sarcoidosis. Am J Respir Crit Care Med 1997;156:1601–5.
26. Rossman MD, Thompson B, Frederick M, et al. HLA-DRB1*1101: a significant risk factor for sarcoidosis in blacks and whites. Am J Hum Genet 2003;73:720–35.
27. Valentonyte R, Hampe J, Huse K, et al. Sarcoidosis is associated with a truncating splice site mutation in BTNL2. Nat Genet 2005;37:357–64.
28. Hofmann S, Franke A, Fischer A, et al. Genome-wide association study identifies ANXA11 as a new susceptibility locus for sarcoidosis. Nat Genet 2008;40: 1103–6.
29. Bresnitz EA, Strom BL. Epidemiology of sarcoidosis. Epidemiol Rev 1983;5: 124–56.
30. Kucera GP, Rybicki B, Kirkey KL, et al. Occupational risk factors for sarcoidosis in African-American siblings. Chest 2003;123:1527–35.
31. Parkes SA, Baker SBdC, Bourdillon RE, et al. Epidemiology of sarcoidosis in the Isle of Man—1: a case controlled study. Thorax 1987;42:420–6.
32. Bresnitz EA, Stolley PD, Israel HL, et al. Possible risk factors for sarcoidosis: a case-control study. Ann N Y Acad Sci 1986;465:632–42.

33. Keller AZ. Hospital, age, racial, occupational, geographical, clinical, and survivorship characteristics in the epidemiology of sarcoidosis. Am J Epidemiol 1971;94:222–30.

34. Newman LS, Rose CS, Bresnitz EA, et al. A case control etiologic study of sarcoidosis: environmental and occupational risk factors. Am J Respir Crit Care Med 2004;170:1324–30.

35. Song Z, Marzilli L, Greenlee BM, et al. Mycobacterial catalase-peroxidase is a tissue antigen and target of the adaptive immune response in systemic sarcoidosis. J Exp Med 2005;201:755–67.

36. Eishi Y, Suga M, Ishige I, et al. Quantitative analysis of mycobacterial and propionibacterial DNA in lymph nodes of Japanese and European patients with sarcoidosis. J Clin Microbiol 2002;40:198–204.

37. Eberhardt C, Thillai M, Parker R, et al. Proteomic analysis of Kveim reagent identifies targets of cellular immunity in sarcoidosis. PLoS One 2017;12(01): e0170285.

38. Chen ES, Song Z, Willett MH, et al. Serum amyloid A regulates granulomatous inflammation in sarcoidosis through Toll-like receptor-2. Am J Respir Crit Care Med 2010;181:360–73.

39. Kahi CJ, Saxena R, Temkit M, et al. Hepatobiliary disease in sarcoidosis. Sarcoidosis Vasc Diffuse Lung Dis 2006;23:117–23.

40. Vatti R, Sharma OP. Course of asymptomatic liver involvement in sarcoidosis: role of therapy in selected cases. Sarcoidosis Vasc Diffuse Lung Dis 1997;14:73–6.

41. Evandro Sobroza Mello, Venancio Avancini Ferreira Alves. Hepatic granulomas. Practical Hepatic Pathology: A Diagnostic Approach, 2011.p. 291–302

42. Tjwa M, De Hertogh G, Neuville B, et al. Hepatic fibrin-ring granulomas in granulomatous hepatitis: report of four cases and review of the literature. Acta Clin Belg 2001;56(6):341–8.

43. Zhu H, Bodenheimer HC Jr, Clain DJ, et al. Hepatic lipogranulomas in patients with chronic liver disease: association with hepatitis C and fatty liver disease. World J Gastroenterol 2010;16(40):5065–9.

44. Karagiannidis A, Karavalaki M, Koulaouzidis A. Hepatic sarcoidosis. Ann Hepatol 2006;5:251–6.

45. Hercules HD, Bethlem NM. Value of liver biopsy in sarcoidosis. Arch Pathol Lab Med 1984;108:831–4.

46. Valla DC, Benhamou JP. Hepatic granulomas and hepatic sarcoidosis. Clin Liver Dis 2000;4:269–85.

47. Murphy JR, Sjogren MH, Kikendall JW, et al. Small bile duct abnormalities in sarcoidosis. J Clin Gastroenterol 1990;12:555.

48. Bloom R, Sybert A, Mascatello VJ. Granulomatous biliary tract obstruction due to sarcoidosis. Am Rev Respir Dis 1978;117:783–7.

49. Rezeig MA, Fashir BM. Biliary tract obstruction due to sarcoidosis: a case report. Am J Gastroenterol 1996;92:527–8.

50. Maddrey WC, Johns CJ, Boitnott JK, et al. Sarcoidosis and chronic hepatic disease: a clinical and pathologic study of 20 patients. Medicine 1970;49:375–95.

51. Valla D, Pessegueiro-Miranda H, Degott C, et al. Hepatic sarcoidosis with portal hypertension. A report of seven cases with a review of the literature. Q J Med 1987;63:531–44.

52. Dulai PS, Rothstein RI. Disseminated sarcoidosis presenting as granulomatous gastritis: a clinical review of the gastrointestinal and hepatic manifestations of sarcoidosis. J Clin Gastroenterol 2012;46:367–74.

53. Nolan JP, Klatskin G. The fever of sarcoidosis. Ann Intern Med 1964;61:455–61.

54. Israel HL, Kataria YP. Clinical aspects of sarcoidosis. In: Lieberman J, editor. Sarcoidosis. Orlando (FL): Grune and Stratton; 1985. p. 7–23.
55. Moreno-Merlo F, Wanless IR, Shimamatsu K, et al. The role of granulomatous phlebitis and thrombosis in the pathogenesis of cirrhosis and portal hypertension in sarcoidosis. Hepatology 1997;26:554–60.
56. Russi EW, Bansky G, Pfaltz M, et al. Budd-Chiari syndrome in sarcoidosis. Am J Gastroenterol 1986;81:71–5.
57. Cremers J, Drent M, Driessen A, et al. Liver-test abnormalities in sarcoidosis. Eur J Gastroenterol Hepatol 2012;24:17–24.
58. Blich M, Edoute Y. Clinical manifestations of sarcoid liver disease. J Gastroenterol Hepatol 2004;19:732–7.
59. Malhotra A, Naniwadekar A, Sood G. Hepatobiliary and pancreatic: cirrhosis secondary to hepatic sarcoidosis. J Gastroenterol Hepatol 2008;23:1942.
60. Gupta S, Faughnan ME, Prud'homme GJ, et al. Sarcoidosis complicated by cirrhosis and hepatopulmonary syndrome. Can Respir J 2008;15:124–6.
61. Stanca CM, Fiel MI, Allina J, et al. Liver failure in an antimitochondrial antibody-positive patient with sarcoidosis: primary biliary cirrhosis or hepatic sarcoidosis? Semin Liver Dis 2005;25:364–70.
62. Ramos-Casals M, Mana J, Nardi N, et al. Sarcoidosis in patients with chronic hepatitis C virus infection: analysis of 68 cases. Medicine (Baltimore) 2005;84:69–80.
63. Vanatta JM, Modanlou KA, Dean AG, et al. Outcomes of orthotopic liver transplantation for hepatic sarcoidosis: an analysis of the United Network for Organ Sharing/Organ Procurement and Transplantation Network data files for a comparative study with cholestatic liver disease. Liver Transpl 2011;17:1027–34.
64. Ungprasert P, Crowson CS, Simonetto DA, et al. Clinical characteristics and outcome of hepatic sarcoidosis: a population-based study 1976–2013. Am J Gastroenterol 2017;112:1556–63.
65. Studdy PR, Bird R. Serum angiotensin converting enzyme in sarcoidosis—its value in present clinical practice. Ann Clin Biochem 1989;26:13–8.
66. Warshauer DM, Dumbleton SA, Molina PL, et al. Abdominal CT findings in sarcoidosis: radiologic and clinical correlation. Radiology 1994;192:93–8.
67. Mergo PJ, Ros PR, Buetow PC, et al. Diffuse disease of the liver: radiologic-pathologic correlation. Radiographics 1994;14:1291–307.
68. Karaosmanoğlu AD, Onur MR, Saini S, et al. Imaging of hepatobiliary involvement in sarcoidosis. Abdom Imaging 2015;40:3330–7.
69. Gezer NS, Başara I, Altay C, et al. Abdominal sarcoidosis: cross-sectional imaging findings. Diagn Interv Radiol 2015;21:111–7.
70. Cremers JP, Drent M, Baughman RP, et al. Therapeutic approach of hepatic sarcoidosis. Curr Opin Pulm Med 2012;18:472–82.
71. Tadros M, Forouhar F, Wu GY. Hepatic sarcoidosis. J Clin Transl Hepatol 2013;1: 87–93.
72. Moller DR. Treatment of sarcoidosis–from a basic science point of view. J Intern Med 2003;253:31–40.
73. Baughman RP. Sarcoidosis. Usual and unusual manifestations. Chest 1988;94: 165–70, 58.
74. Denys BG, Bogaerts Y, Coenegrachts KL, et al. Steroid-resistant sarcoidosis: is antagonism of TNF-alpha the answer? Clin Sci (Lond) 2007;112:281–9.
75. Wu JJ, Schiff KR. Sarcoidosis. Am Fam Physician 2004;70:312–22.
76. Becheur H, Dall'osto H, Chatellier G, et al. Effect of ursodeoxycholic acid on chronic intrahepatic cholestasis due to sarcoidosis. Dig Dis Sci 1997;42:789–91.

77. Alenezi B, Lamoureux E, Alpert L, et al. Effect of ursodeoxycholic acid on granulomatous liver disease due to sarcoidosis. Dig Dis Sci 2005;50:196–200.
78. Baratta L, Cascino A, Delfino M, et al. Ursodeoxycholic acid treatment in abdominal sarcoidosis. Dig Dis Sci 2000;45:1559–62.
79. Paumgartner G, Beuers U. Ursodeoxycholic acid in cholestatic liver disease: mechanisms of action and therapeutic use revisited. Hepatology 2002;36: 525–31.
80. Bakker GJ, Haan YCL, Maillette de Buy LJ, et al. Sarcoidosis of the liver: to treat or not to treat? Neth J Med 2012;70:349–56.
81. Baughman RP. Methotrexate for sarcoidosis. Sarcoidosis Vasc Diffuse Lung Dis 1998;15:147–9.
82. Doty JD, Mazur JE, Judson MA. Treatment of sarcoidosis with infliximab. Chest 2005;127:1064–71.
83. Sebode M, Weidemann S, Wehmeyer M, et al. Anti-TNF-α for necrotizing sarcoid granulomatosis of the liver. Hepatology 2017;65:1410.
84. Bilal M, Satapathy SK, Ismail MK, et al. Long-term outcomes of liver transplantation for hepatic sarcoidosis: a single center experience. J Clin Exp Hepatol 2016; 6(02):94–9.
85. Cengiz C, Rodriguez-Davalos M, deBoccardo G, et al. Recurrent hepatic sarcoidosis post-liver transplantation manifesting with severe hypercalcemia: a case report and review of the literature. Liver Transpl 2005;11:1611–4.

Liver Diseases During Pregnancy

Karen Ma, MD[a], Daniel Berger, MD[a], Nancy Reau, MD[b],*

KEYWORDS

- Liver tests pregnancy • Intrahepatic cholestasis of pregnancy • HELLP syndrome
- Acute fatty liver of pregnancy • Autoimmune • Liver transplantation • Cirrhosis
- Hepatitis

KEY POINTS

- All pregnant women presenting with abnormal liver tests should undergo evaluation.
- Pregnancy-associated liver disease is rare but recognition is important because it has the potential to affect maternal and fetal morbidity and mortality.
- Most chronic liver diseases have limited impact on pregnancy if managed proactively.
- Vertical transmission of viral hepatitis is the leading cause of hepatitis B virus worldwide and the leading cause of pediatric hepatitis C virus infection. Recognition is important to disrupt transmission.

INTRODUCTION

Liver diseases during pregnancy pose a unique clinical challenge as they can affect the lives of both the mother and unborn child. Although severe liver disease is rare, pregnancy-related liver disease affects approximately 3% of pregnancies and can be fatal. Timely recognition and diagnosis are essential in order to institute appropriate management strategies. These challenging cases are best approached in a multidisciplinary model with consultant hepatologists and obstetricians, often necessitating high-risk specialists. This article provides an overview of liver diseases during pregnancy and is divided into 2 sections: (1) liver diseases specific to pregnancy, and (2) preexisting or coincident liver diseases during pregnancy.

Disclosure: The authors have nothing to disclose.
[a] Section of Gastroenterology, Division of Digestive Diseases, Department of Internal Medicine, Rush University Medical Center, 1725 West Harrison Street, Suite 207, Chicago, IL 60612, USA;
[b] Section of Hepatology, Division of Digestive Diseases, Department of Internal Medicine, Rush University Medical Center, 1725 West Harrison Street, Suite 319, Chicago, IL 60612, USA
* Corresponding author.
E-mail address: Nancy_reau@rush.edu

Clin Liver Dis 23 (2019) 345–361
https://doi.org/10.1016/j.cld.2018.12.013
1089-3261/19/© 2018 Elsevier Inc. All rights reserved.

LIVER DISEASES SPECIFIC TO PREGNANCY
Physiologic Changes in Liver During Pregnancy

Several important physiologic changes occur during pregnancy and need to be considered when evaluating women with suspected liver disease. Pregnancy is associated with a hyperdynamic circulatory status, because maternal cardiac output is increased by 40% to 45% along with an increase in heart rate.[1,2] Although there is increased blood supply to the renal, uterine, and skin systems, the liver's blood flow remains fairly constant.[3] The hyperestrogenic state during pregnancy leads to the presence of spider angiomata and palmar erythema in up to 70% of women, which usually disappear after delivery.[4] Gallbladder motility is decreased, which increases the incidence of cholelithiasis in pregnant women.

Fig. 1 shows the biochemical laboratory fluctuations that can be expected during a normal pregnancy. In general, most liver tests remain in the normal range during pregnancy, except those produced by the placenta or affected by hemodilution.[5–7] Alkaline phosphatase (ALP) level is increased secondary to placental origin resultant from fetal bone development. Alpha fetoprotein (AFP) levels are also increased because it is produced by the fetal liver. Albumin and hemoglobin levels are decreased in all trimesters secondary to hemodilution. Other liver biochemical tests, including total bilirubin, serum aspartate transaminase (AST), alanine transaminase (ALT), gamma glutamyl transpeptidase (GGT), and total bile acid concentrations, remain unaffected during a normal pregnancy after accounting for hemodilution. Pregnancy is a procoagulant state in which levels of clotting factors (I, II, V, VII, X, and XII) and fibrinogen are increased, whereas the ranges for prothrombin time (PT) and activated partial thromboplastin time (APTT) are within normal values. Thus, increases in levels of transaminases, bilirubin, fasting total bile acids, or the PT above the normal range during pregnancy are abnormal and warrant further investigation.

Hyperemesis Gravidarum

Hyperemesis gravidarum (HG) is defined as nausea and intractable vomiting that result in dehydration, ketosis, and weight loss of greater than 5%.[8] The symptoms can be severe and it often leads to electrolyte disturbances, fluid depletion, and nutritional deficiencies that necessitate hospital admission.[1] HG is uncommon, because it is reported to affect 0.3% to 2% of pregnancies. HG typically starts early in the first trimester (before the ninth week of gestation) and resolves by the twentieth week; however, some patients experience symptoms throughout pregnancy. Risk factors include multiple gestations, molar pregnancy, HG during prior pregnancies, increased body mass index, and preexisting diabetes.[5] Common electrolyte abnormalities

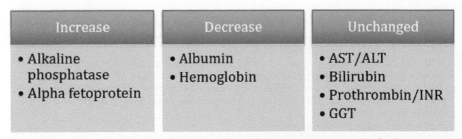

Increase	Decrease	Unchanged
• Alkaline phosphatase • Alpha fetoprotein	• Albumin • Hemoglobin	• AST/ALT • Bilirubin • Prothrombin/INR • GGT

Fig. 1. Physiologic changes in laboratory values during pregnancy. ALT, alanine transaminase; AST, aspartate transaminase; GGT, gamma glutamyl transpeptidase; INR, international normalized ratio.

include increased serum urea and creatinine levels, hypophosphatemia, hypomagnesemia, and hypokalemia. Abnormal liver aminotransferase levels can occur in 50% of cases, because aminotransferase levels may increase up to 200 U/L with associated mild hyperbilirubinemia (usually up to bilirubin of 4 mg/dL).[9] It is important to obtain an abdominal ultrasonography scan to rule out biliary obstruction as well as an obstetric ultrasonography scan to exclude hydatidiform mole and multiple gestation pregnancy. The laboratory changes often return to normal within days after the resumption of adequate nutrition.

Management of HG is supportive and includes correction of electrolyte disturbances, intravenous fluids, antiemetic treatment, and thiamine supplementation to prevent Wernicke encephalopathy.[5] Antiemetics such as dopamine agonists (metoclopramide), phenothiazines (prochlorperazine), antihistamines (promethazine), and ondansetron have all been shown to be safe. Dietary modifications, including avoiding trigger food items and eating small, frequent, low-fat meals, may help as well. Enteric nutrition via nasogastric access or parenteral nutrition may be needed in cases of severe malnutrition and prolonged inability to tolerate oral nutrition.

Intrahepatic Cholestasis of Pregnancy

The most common liver disease unique to pregnancy is intrahepatic cholestasis of pregnancy (ICP), with a reported prevalence of 0.3% to 5.6%.[10–12] ICP typically presents in the second and third trimesters and is characterized by persistent pruritus, typically worst in the palms and soles, and more severe overnight. Serologically, ICP is characterized by increased bile acid and/or transaminase levels, particularly ALT.[13] Bile acid concentrations can be 1.5 to 15 times the upper limit of normal, whereas aminotransferase levels may be increased to values greater than 1000 U/L.[14] Symptoms and serologic abnormalities typically resolve within 4 to 6 weeks after pregnancy; otherwise, evaluation for alternate causes of cholestasis should be pursued.

For pregnant women with ICP, the disease usually follows a benign course, although quality of life may be affected by itching, jaundice, and fat malabsorption. Postpartum bleeding may be exacerbated in patients because of a decreased absorption of vitamin K. In contrast, there are risks to the fetus of premature birth, fetal distress, and intrauterine demise. Therefore, early delivery at 37 weeks is encouraged.[6,15] Maternal bile acid levels greater than or equal to 40 μmol/L have been associated with a higher probability of fetal complications.[16,17]

Once the diagnosis of ICP is made based on a combination of symptoms and increased serum bile acid concentrations, treatment should be considered. The first-line therapy for ICP is ursodeoxycholic acid (UDCA), which has been shown to improve maternal symptoms, improve liver enzymes, and possibly improve fetal outcomes.[18] Treatment with UDCA at 10 to 15 mg/kg is well tolerated and considered safe for both the mother and fetus, with a US Food and Drug Administration pregnancy category B.[18–20] In women who do not respond to UDCA alone, addition of rifampicin may be considered, because the combination of rifampicin with UDCA may have a synergistic effect and lead to improvement in symptoms and biochemical derangements.[21]

Long-term considerations for women who have ICP are several. Note that ICP has a high recurrence rate in subsequent pregnancies. Women with ICP may also have an increased risk of hepatobiliary disease later in life, most commonly cholelithiasis. Higher prevalence of hepatobiliary malignancy and hepatitis C has also been reported.[22,23]

Preeclampsia, Eclampsia, and HELLP Syndrome

Preeclampsia is a pregnancy-specific systemic disorder characterized by new-onset hypertension (systolic blood pressure ≥140 mm Hg or diastolic blood pressure ≥90 mm Hg) and proteinuria (≥300 mg/d) after 20 weeks of gestation.[24] Severe preeclampsia occurs when there is evidence of end-organ dysfunction, such as the presence of pulmonary edema, renal insufficiency, or hepatocellular injury.[25] The presence of grand mal seizures in addition to signs of preeclampsia is the defining feature of eclampsia.

The HELLP (hemolysis, elevated liver enzymes, and low platelet count) syndrome is considered to be a complication of preeclampsia and occurs in approximately 10% to 20% of women with severe preeclampsia.[26–28] This syndrome is characterized by hemolytic anemia, increased liver enzyme levels, and low platelet count. Risk factors include advanced maternal age, nulliparity, and multiparity.[29] HELLP typically presents between 28 and 36 weeks of gestation; however, up to 30% of patients do not manifest symptoms until the first week postpartum.[24,30]

HELLP can be diagnosed based on clinical features and laboratory findings. However, it is important to recognize that there are no pathognomonic clinical signs and the diagnosis is often difficult to distinguish from other hypertension-related liver diseases. Laboratory findings of hemolytic anemia (with increased unconjugated bilirubin and lactate dehydrogenase levels), thrombocytopenia with platelet count less than 100,000/μL, and increased AST/ALT levels are suggestive of HELLP. Renal impairment is common. Because HELLP is a complication of preeclampsia, hypertension and proteinuria are often present too. A liver biopsy is not necessary but, when performed, shows histologic features of periportal changes with hemorrhage, sinusoidal fibrin deposition, and hepatocyte necrosis.[1,31]

Symptomatically, patients may describe epigastric or right upper quadrant pain related to hepatomegaly and stretching of the Glisson capsule.[32] Liver injury occurs as a result of vasoconstriction and fibrin precipitation leading to sinusoidal obstruction and hepatic ischemia. Biochemically, this often manifests with increases in aminotransferase levels, which can occur in 30% of cases.[33] However jaundice is rarely seen. Complications of liver injury in preeclampsia include subcapsular hematoma, hepatic infarction, hepatic rupture, and even fulminant hepatic failure. Abdominal imaging should be considered in women who have symptoms of right upper quadrant pain, right shoulder pain, or hypotension to evaluate for potential subcapsular hematoma, hepatic rupture, or infarction.

The management of preeclampsia, eclampsia, and HELLP syndrome is primarily supportive. Delivery of the fetus and the placenta should be accomplished as soon as possible, especially if after 34 weeks' gestation, or if there is evidence of maternal decompensation or fetal distress. If gestation is less than 34 weeks and only mild preeclampsia is present, conservative management can be considered with close monitoring for evidence of disease progression. With conservative management, hypertension should be treated with antihypertensives such as intravenous labetalol or hydralazine, which are considered safe in pregnancy. Magnesium sulfate should be given to women with severe preeclampsia or HELLP syndrome to reduce risk of progression to eclampsia.[25] Corticosteroids can also be considered to promote fetal lung maturity.[34]

In pregnant women with a high risk for preeclampsia, the US Preventive Services Task Force recommends the use of low-dose aspirin (81 mg/d) after 12 weeks of gestation as a preventive measure.[35] Low-dose aspirin has been shown to reduce the risk for preeclampsia by 24% in clinical trials and reduced the risk for preterm birth by 14% and intrauterine growth retardation by 20%.[35,36]

Acute Fatty Liver of Pregnancy

Acute fatty liver of pregnancy (AFLP) is an emergent, life-threatening condition characterized by microvesicular fatty infiltration of the liver that can precipitate fulminant liver failure without early recognition and appropriate management.[37] This rare complication of pregnancy usually occurs in the third trimester and affects approximately 1 in 7000 to 1 in 20,000 pregnancies.[38–40] Key risk factors for AFLP include twin pregnancies, low body mass index, and nulliparity.[39]

The pathophysiology of AFLP is still not completely understood, although defects in fatty acid metabolism are likely implicated.[41] Long-chain 3-hydroxyacyl coenzyme A (CoA) dehydrogenase (LCHAD) deficiency is another known cause of AFLP. LCHAD is an enzyme that catalyzes beta oxidation of mitochondrial fatty acids. When a fetus is homozygous for LCHAD deficiency, intermediate products of fatty acid metabolism accumulate in maternal circulation and can cause hepatotoxicity in the maternal liver. Children born to mothers with AFLP should be tested for LCHAD deficiency, because a diagnosis could potentially be lifesaving for the newborn.[42]

Initial presenting symptoms of AFLP are often nonspecific and may include abdominal pain, nausea, vomiting, headache, and generalized malaise. Up to half of women with AFLP may also have concomitant preeclampsia.[39] Biochemical derangements are characterized by increases in aminotransferase levels, usually 5 to 10 times the upper limit of normal, along with hyperbilirubinemia.[43] In addition, serum ammonia, lactic acid, and amino acid levels may be increased, reflecting underlying mitochondrial dysfunction.

The diagnosis of AFLP is often a clinical diagnosis based on a combination of factors, including presenting symptoms and laboratory abnormalities. Although liver biopsy provides the gold standard in diagnosis of AFLP, it is rarely performed because of the need to stabilize women and provide delivery of the fetus. The Swansea criteria (**Box 1**) are a diagnostic tool that has been created and validated for AFLP and have allowed improved diagnosis of AFLP without the need for liver biopsy.[44]

Box 1
Swansea criteria

- Nausea/emesis
- Abdominal pain
- Polydipsia/polyuria
- Encephalopathy
- Ascites or bright liver on ultrasonography
- Renal dysfunction (serum creatinine level >150 μmol/L)
- Microvesicular steatosis on liver biopsy
- Leukocytosis (>11 × 10^6 cells/L)
- Increased ammonia level (>47 μmol/L)
- Increased transaminase levels (>42 IU/L)
- Increased bilirubin level (>14 μmol/L)
- Hypoglycemia (<4 mmol/L)
- Increased uric acid level (>340 μmol/L)
- Coagulopathy (PT>14 seconds or APTT >34 seconds)

Diagnosis of AFLP requires the presence of 6 or more criteria in the absence of another cause. In cases in which a liver biopsy is performed, the characteristic histologic feature of AFLP is microvesicular steatosis, as shown in **Fig. 2**.

Although there is significant overlap between severe preeclampsia, HELLP syndrome, and AFLP, the management of these three conditions is the same and focuses on maternal support and delivery of the fetus. After delivery, liver injury related to AFLP often resolves within 1 to 2 weeks.[40] If liver function does not rapidly improve, evaluation for liver transplant should be considered because this may provide the best chance for survival.

PREEXISTING OR COINCIDENT LIVER DISEASES DURING PREGNANCY
Hepatitis B Infection

It is recommended that all pregnant women be screened for hepatitis B virus (HBV) by testing for the presence of hepatitis B surface antigen (HBsAg) on initial encounter.[45] Chronic HBV infection is more likely in the newborn of an HBsAg-positive mother. Risk factors for vertical transmission include the presence of hepatitis B e antigen (HBeAg) and the maternal viral load.[46] It is critical that active-passive immunoprophylaxis with hepatitis B immunoglobulin and HBV vaccination series both be administered to all infants born to HBV-infected mothers within 12 hours after birth. This practice has been shown to reduce the risk of vertical transmission from greater than 90% to less than 10% in these infants with HBsAg-positive mothers.[45–47]

The risk of immunoprophylaxis failure increases with increased maternal viral load.[1,5] Therefore, in pregnant women with a high viral load, guidelines recommend antiviral therapy in the third trimester in HBsAg-positive pregnant women with HBV DNA greater than,200,000 IU/mL to reduce the risk of perinatal HBV transmission.[6,46] Women who meet other standard indications for HBV therapy, such as for immune-active hepatitis B, should be treated based on recommendations for nonpregnant women.

Telbivudine and tenofovir are both pregnancy category B agents, whereas lamivudine is category C. Of these studied antiviral agents, tenofovir seems to be preferred, owing to its antiviral potency, better resistance profile, and safety during pregnancy. A recent analysis of the Antiretroviral Pregnancy Registry found no increased risk of major birth defects in pregnant women exposed to lamivudine or tenofovir disoproxil fumarate.[48,49]

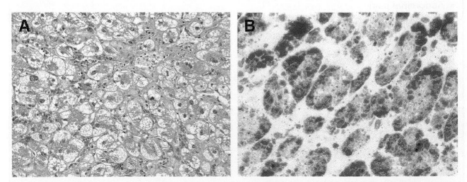

Fig. 2. (A) View of liver showing extensive microvesicular steatosis with centrally placed hepatocellular nuclei and surrounding microvesicles expanding the cytoplasm (hematoxylin-eosin, original magnification ×200). (B) Frozen section liver biopsy highlighting the fatty microvesicles (oil red O, original magnification ×400). (Courtesy of Shriram Jakate, MD, Rush University, Chicago, IL.)

Most studies initiate antiviral therapy at 28 to 32 weeks of gestation and discontinue antiviral therapy between birth and 3 months postpartum. After discontinuation of treatment, women should be monitored for HBV flares every 3 months for 6 months.[46] A hepatitis B flare, with or without HBeAg seroconversion, can occur in around 25% of women within the first months after delivery.[46,50] Most cases are mild and resolve spontaneously, although cases of acute liver failure have been described. Extending the duration of antiviral prophylaxis in the peripartum period was not found to be effective in one study.[51]

Cesarean sections should not be performed electively in HBV-positive mothers to prevent fetal infection.[6] In breastfeeding women with hepatitis B infection, the American Association for the Study of Liver Diseases (AASLD) does not consider antiviral therapy as a contraindication to breastfeeding. Antivirals are minimally excreted in breast milk and unlikely to cause significant toxicity. Mothers should be informed of the insufficient longitudinal follow-up safety data regarding breastfeedings while on antiviral therapy.

Hepatitis C Infection

The prevalence of hepatitis C virus (HCV) infection among US women giving birth nearly doubled from 1.8 to 3.4 per 1000 live births during 2009 to 2014, based on a recent Morbidity and Mortality Weekly Report.[52] Because of inconsistent screening and underreporting, these estimates likely underestimate the prevalence of disease burden in pregnant women. The HCV guidelines jointly published by the AASLD and Infectious Diseases Society of America (IDSA) recommend universal screening for HCV infection at the initiation of prenatal care.[53] Other societies, such as the American College of Gastroenterology (ACG) and Society for Maternal-Fetal Medicine, recommend risk-based assessment and limiting screening to women with risk factors for HCV acquisition.[6,54] Women should be screened with an HCV-antibody test and, if positive, followed with testing for HCV RNA.

In women with preexisting chronic HCV, pregnancy does not seem to adversely affect the clinical course of HCV infection. Most pregnant anti-HCV–positive women are asymptomatic. Pregnant women with HCV have 20-fold higher odds of developing ICP.[55] A decrease in serum ALT levels along with an increase in HCV RNA levels during the second and third trimesters is often observed,[56,57] and these typically return to prepregnancy levels after delivery. These effects are suspected to be secondary to the immunosuppressive effects of pregnancy. There is a possibility of spontaneous viral clearance postpartum, and thus it is recommended that HCV RNA levels be reevaluated after delivery.[53]

Mother-to-child transmission of HCV is reported to occur in 3% to 15% of cases, with around 3% to 5% progressing to chronic infection.[5,53,58,59] Coexistent human immunodeficiency virus (HIV) infection increases risk of transmission, and the suppression of HIV replication can help to reduce transmission rates.[60] Avoiding invasive procedures such as amniocentesis, instrumented vaginal delivery, fetal scalp electrodes, and birth trauma can help to minimize the risk of perinatal HCV transmission.[5,6] There are no data to support elective cesarean delivery for HCV-infected women.

HCV therapy is not currently recommended during pregnancy to treat HCV or decrease the risk for perinatal transmission because the safety and efficacy data are still lacking.[6,53,61] The safety of direct-acting antivirals in pregnancy is unknown. Breastfeeding is not contraindicated except when the mother has cracked or bleeding nipples.

Autoimmune Hepatitis

Maternal and fetal outcomes in pregnant women with underlying autoimmune hepatitis (AIH) primarily depend on the level of disease control in the preconception period. Pregnancy outcomes are often favorable in women who reach disease remission before pregnancy without any evidence of cirrhosis or portal hypertension. Thus, it is prudent for women to achieve good control of AIH before conceiving. Poor disease control during the year before pregnancy has been associated with poor pregnancy outcomes.[1,61] In addition, the presence of antibodies against soluble liver antigen (SLA) and liver and pancreas antigen (LP) as well as to Ro (SSA) may be a risk factor for adverse pregnancy outcomes in women with AIH.[62]

It is reported that up to 20% of women with AIH flare during pregnancy. Flares are often the result of either discontinuing therapy or the dynamic immune state of the pregnant women. Flares are more common, reported to be as high as 52% of women, in the postpartum period when the maternal immune state is reconstituted.[62–64] Some experts advocate preemptively increasing immunosuppressive therapy around 2 weeks before anticipated delivery and maintained through the postpartum period given the high rate of flares after delivery.[64,65] Women should be closely monitored for increased liver tests during the initial postpartum months.

There are no large systematic reviews on the treatment of AIH during pregnancy. The AASLD recommends prednisone monotherapy for pregnant individuals, but it is important to keep in mind that adequate control of the underlying AIH outweighs the minimal risks associated with prednisone or azathioprine use during pregnancy.[62,63,66] Therefore other societies, such as the ACG, recommend continuation of prior treatment with corticosteroids and/or azathioprine during pregnancy. Mycophenolate should be avoided in pregnancy, because it is associated with congenital malformations.[67]

Primary Biliary Cholangitis

There are very limited data on the outcomes and management of primary biliary cholangitis (PBC) during pregnancy.[68–71] Similar to the other chronic diseases, such as AIH and Wilson disease (WD), optimal management of the underlying liver disease before pregnancy is recommended. In general, the onset of PBC is near menopausal age and thus pregnancies are uncommon in this setting. A recent case control study found that pregnant women with PBC overall had favorable maternal outcomes with no higher risk of miscarriage or preterm delivery compared with controls.[71] However, there was a trend toward higher risk of childbirth complications, mainly placenta previa, in that study.

In women with PBC, pregnancy can trigger new-onset pruritus or worsen preexisting pruritus.[71] UDCA can be safely used as treatment during pregnancy and is well tolerated. UDCA should be continued throughout pregnancy to prevent progression of the underlying liver disease.[6]

Wilson Disease

Women with WD commonly have amenorrhea or oligomenorrhea leading to infertility or repeated miscarriages such that these findings may be the initial clinical manifestations of the disease.[72,73] Patients who present with isolated neurologic manifestations at the time of WD diagnosis tend to have significantly more spontaneous abortions than patients with mixed or isolated hepatic symptoms.[74] This finding may be attributed to the propensity of these patients with cerebral copper overload to also have copper deposition in other organs, including the placenta or uterus. Treatment of the underlying disease can restore fertility. Although pregnancy does not seem to alter the course of WD, it is important to optimize the patient's copper status before pregnancy.

There is some concern over the teratogenicity of D-penicillamine, with several reported cases of fetal myelosuppression or embryopathy, including cardiac anomalies.[74] However, treatment discontinuation during pregnancy has a higher risk of maternal hepatic decompensation as well as fetal damage from copper deposition in the placenta and fetal liver.[6,74] Thus, current clinical practice guidelines recommend that chelation treatment of WD should be continued during pregnancy, but dosage reduction is advised for D-penicillamine and trientine, starting in the first trimester, to reduce risk of fetal teratogenicity and throughout pregnancy to promote wound healing at time of delivery.[6,74–76] Zinc therapy seems safe and thus should be continued at regular preconception doses.[5,74] Close and careful monitoring of liver function tests and for neurologic symptoms is recommended during the pregnancy.

Preconception counseling should be provided to all women of childbearing age with WD. Because WD is an inherited disease, genetic counseling and haplotype analysis of the partner should be offered.[5] Contraception agents that contain estrogen should be avoided because estrogens may interfere with biliary copper excretion.[77] In addition, intrauterine devices that contain copper should be avoided. It is also important to discuss the risks and benefits of anticopper therapy along with the risks of uncontrolled WD during pregnancy.[78]

Cirrhosis and Portal Hypertension

Pregnancy in women with underlying cirrhosis is uncommon because disruption of the hypothalamic-pituitary-ovarian axis leads to amenorrhea and reduced fertility. Although not contraindicated, it has been associated with an increase in prematurity, spontaneous abortions, and maternal-fetal mortality.[79–81] Outcomes of pregnancy are related to the degree of liver disease rather than the cause. The preconceptional model for end-stage liver disease (MELD) score can be used to prognosticate cirrhotic women and guide family planning counseling. A MELD greater than or equal to 10 has been found to have 83% sensitivity and specificity for predicting liver decompensation during pregnancy.[82] In contrast, there were no liver-related complications in women with a preconception MELD less than or equal to 6 in that study.

Variceal bleeding is the most frequent and serious complication of portal hypertension during pregnancy, with an increased risk during labor and delivery and the second trimester from the increase in intravascular volume, compression of the inferior vena cava from the gravid uterus, and repeated Valsalva maneuvers during labor.[83] Up to 30% of cirrhotic pregnant women bleed from esophageal varices during pregnancy, and the risk of variceal bleeding increases up to 50% to 78% if there are preexisting varices.[84,85] Patients with noncirrhotic portal hypertension often have better outcomes than cirrhotics with portal hypertension because synthetic function is usually preserved and the reproductive system is often not affected.[1,84]

The management of acute variceal bleeding during pregnancy is similar to that of nonpregnant patients, with a focus on resuscitation, antibiotic prophylaxis, octreotide, and safe and timely endoscopic therapy with band ligation. Limited reports on salvage therapies such as placement of portosystemic shunts and liver transplant have been described when endoscopic options have failed, but are not routinely recommended.

Screening for esophageal varices is strongly recommended and should be scheduled in the second trimester after organogenesis is complete and before the greatest risk of bleeding at delivery.[6] Pregnant women who are found to have large esophageal varices should be treated with β-blockers and/or band ligation, similar to nonpregnant patients. There are limited data on the safety and efficacy of band ligation and β-blockers in this special population. Propranolol and nadolol are both pregnancy category C drugs, but nadolol has a long half-life and thus is not preferred. When β-blockers are used in pregnancy, close fetal monitoring is needed to avoid fetal bradycardia and intrauterine growth retardation.

There are no clear recommendations regarding preferred mode of delivery in patients with portal hypertension because the data are very limited. In the past, vaginal delivery with a short second stage of labor has been advocated along with consideration of forceps or vacuum extraction if needed to avoid excessive straining.[86] Cesarean sections should be performed based on obstetric indications but may also be required for fetal distress or prematurity. However, it carries an increased risk of complications, including bleeding, poor wound healing, and infection, and risk of liver decompensation.

Liver Transplant

Since the first pregnancy in a liver transplant recipient in 1978, pregnancy outcomes have trended toward favorable and survival has reached a reported 20-year survival of 53% in a recent longitudinal study.[87,88] In addition, preconception renal function has been found to predict pregnancy outcomes.[89–91] The deregulation in the hypothalamic-pituitary-ovarian axis associated with end-stage liver disease resolves following transplant. Most women resume regular menstrual cycles within 1 year posttransplant, and some even within the first few months. Thus, preconception family counseling including education about contraception use is crucial before and after liver transplant. The key in posttransplant pregnancy planning is timing, because most experts advocate waiting at least 1 year and some up to 2 years after liver transplant before planning a pregnancy. Delaying pregnancy helps to ensure stable graft function with lower doses of immunosuppression, lower risk of acute cellular rejection, and lower risk of opportunistic infections.[6,92]

The Transplant Pregnancy Registry International (formerly the National Transplantation Pregnancy Registry) has been used to study pregnancy outcomes in all solid organ transplant recipients. The most frequent maternal complication in the post–liver transplant population is hypertension during pregnancy, caused in part by the side effects of immunosuppressive agents. Use of immunosuppressive agents is associated with an increased risk of miscarriage, prematurity, intrauterine growth retardation, and low birth weight.[93] Higher rates of delivery by cesarean section and preterm births compared with the general population have been reported. Pregnancy itself has not been shown to impair graft function or accelerate rejection in patients with stable graft function before pregnancy and receiving appropriate immunosuppressive therapy.[89] Overall the current evidence suggests that pregnancy in liver transplant recipients is safe, common, and can achieve favorable outcomes.

There is no consensus on the optimal maintenance immunosuppression regimen for transplant recipients during pregnancy. It is well established that mycophenolate derivatives are contraindicated during pregnancy owing to the risk of congenital malformations, developmental anomalies, and embryo-fetal toxicity. For women seeking pregnancy on these agents, a strategy of temporary replacement with another agent is strongly advised. Calcineurin inhibitors (cyclosporine and tacrolimus), prednisone, and azathioprine are generally considered safe. The reports of a higher incidence of low birth weight and prematurity in women using calcineurin inhibitors seem to relate to the underlying comorbidities rather than specifically calcineurin inhibitor–related side effects. Compared with tacrolimus and cyclosporine, there are not enough data on the use of everolimus and sirolimus during pregnancy after liver transplant.

Although safety data are overall minimal, breastfeeding is not discouraged in women who are interested, especially given the mounting recognition of the benefits of breastfeeding for both mother and infant. Cyclosporine and tacrolimus are both measurable in breast milk, although in small quantities that are unlikely to cause harm to nursing infants.[93,94] Azathioprine is also considered safe in breastfeeding, with safety data derived from the inflammatory bowel disease population. Breastfeeding while using mycophenolate, everolimus, or sirolimus is not recommended because safety data are lacking.[94]

Acute Hepatitis (Hepatitis A Virus, Hepatitis E Virus, Herpes Simplex Virus)

When a pregnant woman presents with an acute hepatitis, testing for common causes of acute liver injury, including viral hepatitis, hepatitis A virus (HAV), hepatitis E virus (HEV), and herpes simplex virus (HSV), is strongly recommended.[6]

Hepatitis A virus
Pregnancy does not seem to change the course of acute HAV infection. Although acute HAV infection is usually self-limited, it is associated with premature rupture of membranes when presenting in the second half of pregnancy.[95] The presence of anti-HAV immunoglobulin M (IgM) is diagnostic. The US Centers for Disease Control and Prevention recommend HAV immunoglobulin treatment of the neonate if the maternal HAV infection occurs within 2 weeks of delivery. Treatment is otherwise supportive along with passive immunoprophylaxis to the newborn.

Hepatitis E virus
HEV is a single-stranded RNA virus that causes large-scale epidemics of acute viral hepatitis, notably in developing parts of the world such as southeast Asia. Although the disease is usually self-limiting in men and nonpregnant women, it can potentially be more severe and fatal in pregnant women. HEV outbreaks are characteristically associated with a high disease attack rate among pregnant women. Affected pregnant women are more likely to develop fulminant hepatic failure or have a fatal outcome compared with nonpregnant patients.[96] Researchers speculate that diminished cellular immunity and high levels of steroid hormones that influence viral replication during pregnancy may account for the severity of disease.[97,98] However, once fulminant hepatitis develops, the mortality does not differ compared with other causes of severe liver injury.

HEV during pregnancy is associated with prematurity, low birth weight, and an increased risk of perinatal mortality. Pregnant women presenting with an acute hepatitis should be tested for HEV with HEV-IgM and, if present, monitored closely for progression to acute liver failure and potential need for liver transplant evaluation. Treatment is otherwise supportive. There is ongoing research to develop an HEV-directed vaccine.

Herpes simplex virus
HSV infection is rare but can potentially lead to fulminant hepatitis and be fatal. Although only seen in 2% of pregnant women, there is a 40% risk of fulminant liver failure. It usually occurs in the third trimester. The pathognomonic mucocutaneous lesions are only present in less than 50% of cases.[99] Patients can present with nonspecific symptoms of fever and upper respiratory symptoms. Anicteric, or normal or mildly increased bilirubin level, with severely increased transaminase levels should raise suspicion for HSV infection.

Once the diagnosis is suspected, starting acyclovir therapy without delay is recommended because the diagnosis can be difficult to make and acyclovir is well tolerated in pregnancy.[100–102] The HSV-IgM serologic testing has limited specificity and sensitivity and thus HSV polymerase chain reaction should be performed for serologic confirmation.[103] For women with prior HSV infection, the American College of Obstetricians and Gynecologists recommends acyclovir prophylaxis starting at 36 weeks of pregnancy to prevent HSV recurrence and vertical transmission.[103]

REFERENCES

1. Westbrook RH, Dusheiko G, Williamson C. Pregnancy and liver disease. J Hepatol 2016;64:933–45.
2. Joshi D, James A, Quaglia A, et al. Liver disease in pregnancy. Lancet 2010; 375:594–605.
3. Robson SC, Mutch E, Boys RJ, et al. Apparent liver blood flow during pregnancy: a serial study using indocyanine green clearance. Br J Obstet Gynaecol 1990;97:720–3.
4. Henry F, Quatresooz P, Valverde-Lopez JC, et al. Blood vessel changes during pregnancy: a review. Am J Clin Dermatol 2006;7:65–9.
5. Italian Association for the Study of the Liver (AISF). AISF position paper on liver disease and pregnancy. Dig Liver Dis 2016;48:120–37.
6. Tran TT, Ahn J, Reau NS. American College of Gastroenterology (ACG) clinical guideline: liver disease and pregnancy. Am J Gastroenterol 2016;111:176–94.
7. Knox TA, Olans LB. Liver disease in pregnancy. N Engl J Med 1996;335:569–76.
8. Goodwin TM. Hyperemesis gravidarum. Obstet Gynecol Clin North Am 2008;35: 401–17.
9. Tamay AG, Kuscu NK. Hyperemesis gravidarum: current aspect. J Obstet Gynaecol 2011;31:708–12.
10. Pataia V, Dixon PH, Williamson C. Pregnancy and bile acid disorders. Am J Physiol 2017;313:G1–6.
11. Lee RH, Goodwin TM, Greenspoon J, et al. The prevalence of intrahepatic cholestasis of pregnancy in a primarily Latina Los Angeles population. J Perinatol 2006;26:527–32.
12. Lammert F, Marschall HU, Glantz A, et al. Intrahepatic cholestasis of pregnancy: molecular pathogenesis, diagnosis and management. J Hepatol 2000;33: 1012–21.
13. Geenes V, Williamson C. Intrahepatic cholestasis of pregnancy. World J Gastroenterol 2009;15:2049-2066.
14. Walker I, Chappell LC, Williamson C. Abnormal liver function tests in pregnancy. BMJ 2013;347:6055.
15. Williamson C, Hems LM, Goulis DG, et al. Clinical outcome in a series of cases of obstetric cholestasis identified via a patient support group. Br J Obstet Gynaecol 2004;111:676.
16. Glantz A, Marschall HU, Mattsson LA. Intrahepatic cholestasis of pregnancy: relationships between bile acid levels and fetal complication rates. Hepatology 2004;40:467–74.
17. Geenes V, Chappell LC, Seed PT, et al. Association of severe intrahepatic cholestasis of pregnancy with adverse pregnancy outcomes: a prospective population-based case-control study. Hepatology 2014;59:1482–91.
18. Bacq Y, Sentilhes L, Reyes HB, et al. Efficacy of ursodeoxycholic acid in treating intrahepatic cholestasis of pregnancy: a meta-analysis. Gastroenterology 2012; 143:1492–501.

19. Chappell LC, Gurung V, Seed PT, et al. Ursodeoxycholic acid versus placebo, and early term delivery versus expectant management, in women with intrahepatic cholestasis of pregnancy: semifactorial randomised clinical trial. BMJ 2012;344:e3799.

20. Glantz A, Marschall HU, Lammert F, et al. Intrahepatic cholestasis of pregnancy: a randomized controlled trial comparing dexamethasone and ursodeoxycholic acid. Hepatology 2005;42:1399–405.

21. Geenes V, Chambers J, Khurana R, et al. Rifampicin in the treatment of severe intrahepatic cholestasis of pregnancy. Eur J Obstet Gynecol Reprod Biol 2015; 189:59–63.

22. Wikstrom Shemer EA, Stephansson O, Thuresson M, et al. Intrahepatic cholestasis of pregnancy and cancer, immune-mediated and cardiovascular diseases: a population-based cohort study. J Hepatol 2015;63:456–61.

23. Marschall HU, Wikstrom Shemer E, Ludvigsson JF, et al. Intrahepatic cholestasis of pregnancy and associated hepatobiliary disease: a population-based cohort study. Hepatology 2013;58:1385–91.

24. Sibai B, Dekker G, Kupferminc M. Pre-eclampsia. Lancet 2005;365:785–99.

25. American College of Obstetricians and Gynecologists, Task Force on Hypertension in Pregnancy. Hypertension in pregnancy. Report of the American College of Obstetricians and Gynecologists' Task Force on Hypertension in Pregnancy. Obstet Gynecol 2013;122:1122.

26. Weinstein L. Syndrome of hemolysis, elevated liver enzymes, and low platelet count: a severe consequence of hypertension in pregnancy. Am J Obstet Gynecol 2005;193:859.

27. Martin JN Jr, Rose CH, Briery CM. Understanding and managing HELLP syndrome: the integral role of aggressive glucocorticoids for mother and child. Am J Obstet Gynecol 2006;195:914–34.

28. Sibai BM. Diagnosis, controversies, and management of the syndrome of hemolysis, elevated liver enzymes, and low platelet count. Am J Obstet Gynecol 2004;103:981–91.

29. Fitzpatrick KE, Hinshaw K, Kurinczuk JJ, et al. Risk factors, management, and outcomes of hemolysis, elevated liver enzymes, and low platelets syndrome and elevated liver enzymes, low platelets syndrome. Obstet Gynecol 2014; 123:618–27.

30. Mol BWJ, Roberts CT, Thangaratinam S, et al. Pre-eclampsia. Lancet 2016;387: 999–1011.

31. Dani R, Mendes GS, Medeiros Jde L, et al. Study of the liver changes occurring in preeclampsia and their possible pathogenetic connection with acute fatty liver of pregnancy. Am J Gastroenterol 1996;91:292–4.

32. Vigil-De Gracia P, Ortega-Paz L. Pre-eclampsia/eclampsia and hepatic rupture. Int J Gynaecol Obstet 2012;118:186–9.

33. Agatisa PK, Ness RB, Roberts JM, et al. Impairment of endothelial function in women with a history of preeclampsia: an indicator of cardiovascular risk. Am J Physiol Heart Circ Physiol 2004;286:H1389–93.

34. Brownfoot FC, Gagliardi DI, Bain E, et al. Different corticosteroids and regimens for accelerating fetal lung maturation for women at risk of preterm birth. Cochrane Database Syst Rev 2013;(8):CD006764.

35. LeFevre ML, Siu AL, Peters JJ, et al. Low-Dose aspirin use for the prevention of morbidity and mortality from preeclampsia: US Preventive Services Task Force Recommendation Statement. Ann Intern Med 2014;161:819–26.

36. Henderson JT, Whitlock EP, O'Connor E, et al. Low-dose aspirin for prevention of morbidity and mortality from preeclampsia: a systematic review for the U.S. Preventive Services Task Force. Ann Intern Med 2014;160:695–703.

37. Fesenmeier MF, Coppage KH, Lambers DS, et al. Acute fatty liver of pregnancy in 3 tertiary care centers. Am J Obstet Gynecol 2005;192:1416–9.

38. Castro MA, Fassett MJ, Reynolds TB, et al. Reversible peripartum liver failure: a new perspective on the diagnosis, treatment, and cause of acute fatty liver of pregnancy, based on 28 consecutive cases. Am J Obstet Gynecol 1999;181: 389.

39. Knight M, Nelson-Piercy C, Kurinczuk JJ, et al. A prospective national study of acute fatty liver of pregnancy in the UK. Gut 2008;57:951.

40. Nelson DB, Yost NP, Cunningham FG. Acute fatty liver of pregnancy: clinical outcomes and expected duration of recovery. Am J Obstet Gynecol 2013;209: 456.e1-e7.

41. Ibdah JA, Bennett MJ, Rinaldo P, et al. A fetal fatty-acid oxidation disorder as a cause of liver disease in pregnant women. N Engl J Med 1999;340:1723.

42. Den Boer ME, Wanders RJ, Morris AA, et al. Long-chain 3-hydroxyacyl-CoA dehydrogenase deficiency: clinical presentation and follow-up of 50 patients. Pediatrics 2002;109:99.

43. Liu J, Ghaziani TT, Wolf JL. Acute fatty liver disease of pregnancy: updates in pathogenesis, diagnosis, and management. Am J Gastroenterol 2017;112:838.

44. Goel A, Ramakrishna B, Zachariah U, et al. How accurate are the Swansea criteria to diagnose acute fatty liver of pregnancy in predicting hepatic microvesicular steatosis? Gut 2011;60:138–9.

45. Terrault NA, Bzowej NH, Chang KM, et al, American Association for the Study of Liver Diseases. AASLD guidelines for treatment of chronic hepatitis B. Hepatology 2016;63:261–83.

46. Van Zonnevled M, van Nunen AB, Niesters HG, et al. Lamivudine treatment during pregnancy to prevent perinatal transmission of hepatitis B virus infection. J Viral Hepat 2003;10:294–7.

47. Weinbaum CM, Williams I, Mast EE, et al. Recommendations for identification and public health management of persons with chronic hepatitis B virus infection. MMWR Recomm Rep 2008;57:1–20.

48. Brown RS Jr, McMahon BJ, Lok AS, et al. Antiviral therapy in chronic hepatitis B virus infection during pregnancy. A systematic review and meta-analysis. Hepatology 2016;63:319–33.

49. Brown RS Jr, Verna EC, Pereira MR, et al. Hepatitis B virus and human immunodeficiency virus drugs in pregnancy: findings from the antiretroviral pregnancy registry. Hepatology 2012;57:953–9.

50. Samadi Kochaksaraei G, Castillo E, Osman M, et al. Clinical course of 161 untreated and tenofovir-treated chronic hepatitis B pregnant patients in a low hepatitis B virus endemic region. J Viral Hepat 2016;23:15–22.

51. Nguyen V, Tan PK, Greenup AJ, et al. Antiviral therapy for prevention of perinatal HBV transmission: extending therapy beyond birth does not protect against post-partum flare. Aliment Pharmacol Ther 2014;39:1225–34.

52. Patrick SW, Bauer AM, Warren MD, et al. Hepatitis C virus infection among women giving birth – Tennessee and United States, 2009-2014. MMWR Morb Mortal Wkly Rep 2017;66:470–3.

53. Joint Panel from the American Association for the Study of Liver Diseases and the Infectious Diseases Society of America. Recommendations for testing,

managing, and treating hepatitis C. Available at: http://www.hcvguidelines.org/. Accessed August 18, 2018.

54. Society for Maternal-Fetal Medicine (SMFM). Electronic address: pubs@smfm.org, Hughes BL, Page CM, Kuller JA. Hepatitis C in pregnancy: screening, treatment, and management. Am J Obstet Gynecol 2017;43:B2–12.

55. Wijarnpreecha K, Thongprayoon C, Sanguankeo A, et al. Hepatitis C infection and intrahepatic cholestasis of pregnancy: a systematic review and meta-analysis. Clin Res Hepatol Gatroenterol 2017;41:39–45.

56. Gervais A, Bacq Y, Bernuau J, et al. Decrease in serum ALT and increase in serum HCV RNA during pregnancy in women with chronic hepatitis C. J Hepatol 2000;32:293–9.

57. Paternoster DM, Santarossa C, Grella P, et al. Viral load in HCV RNA-positive pregnant women. Am J Gastroenterol 2001;96:751–4.

58. Dunkelberg JC, Berkley EMF, Thiel KW, et al. Hepatitis B and C in pregnancy: a review and recommendations for care. J Perinatol 2014;34:882–91.

59. Benova L, Mohamoud YA, Calvert C, et al. Vertical transmission of hepatitis C virus: systematic review and meta-analysis. Clin Infect Dis 2014;59:765–73.

60. Checa-Cabot CA, Stoszek SK, Quarleri J, et al. Mother-to-child transmission of hepatitis C virus among HIV/HCV-coinfected women. J Pediatr Infect Dis Soc 2013;2:126–35.

61. Westbrook RH, Yeoman AD, Kriese S, et al. Outcomes of pregnancy in women with autoimmune hepatitis. J Autoimmun 2012;38:J239–44.

62. Schramm C, Herkel J, Beuers U, et al. Pregnancy in autoimmune hepatitis: outcome and risk factors. Am J Gastroenterol 2006;101:556–60.

63. Terrabuio DR, Abrantes-Lemos CP, Carrilho FJ, et al. Follow-up of pregnant women with autoimmune hepatitis: the disease behavior along with maternal and fetal outcomes. J Clin Gastroenterol 2009;43:350–6.

64. Buchel E, Van Steenbergen W, Nevens F, et al. Improvement of autoimmune hepatitis during pregnancy followed by flare-up after delivery. Am J Gastroenterol 2002;97:3160–5.

65. Manns MP, Czaja AJ, Gorham JD. Diagnosis and management of autoimmune hepatitis. AASLD practice guidelines. Hepatology 2010;51:1–31.

66. Heneghan MA, Norris SM, O'Grady JG, et al. Management and outcome of pregnancy in autoimmune hepatitis. Gut 2011;48:97–102.

67. Lamers MM, van Oijen MG, Pronk M, et al. Treatment options for autoimmune hepatitis: a systematic review of randomized controlled trials. J Hepatol 2010; 53:191–8.

68. Poupon R, Chretien Y, Chazouilleres O, et al. Pregnancy in women with ursodeoxycholic acid-treated primary biliary cirrhosis. J Hepatol 2005;42:418–9.

69. Trivedi PJ, Kumagi T, Al-Harthy N, et al. Good maternal and fetal outcomes for pregnant women with primary biliary cirrhosis. Clin Gastroenterol Hepatol 2014; 12:1179–85.

70. Goh SK, Gull SE, Alexander GJ. Pregnancy in primary biliary cirrhosis complicated by portal hypertension: report of a case and review of the literature. BJOG 2001;108:760–2.

71. Floreani A, Infantolino C, Franceschet I, et al. Pregnancy and primary biliary cirrhosis: a case-control study. Clin Rev Allergy Immunol 2015;48:236–42.

72. Kaushansky A, Frydman M, Kaufman H, et al. Endocrine studies of the ovulatory disturbances in Wilson's disease (hepatolenticular degeneration). Fertil Steril 1987;47:270–3.

73. Klee JK. Undiagnosed Wilson's disease as cause of unexplained miscarriage. Lancet 1979;2:423.
74. Pfeiffenberger J, Beinhardt S, Gotthardt DN, et al. Pregnancy in Wilson's disease: management and outcome. Hepatology 2018;67:1261–9.
75. European Association for the Study of the Liver. EASL clinical practice guidelines: Wilson's disease. J Hepatol 2012;56:671–85.
76. Roberts EA, Schilsky ML. Diagnosis and treatment of Wilson disease: an update. Hepatology 2008;47:2089–111.
77. Garmizo G, Frauens BJ. Corneal copper deposition secondary to oral contraceptives. Optom Vis Sci 2008;85:E802–7.
78. Kaimov-Kochman R, Ackerman Z, Anteby EY. The contraceptive choice for a Wilson's disease patient with chronic liver disease. Contraception 1997;56: 241–4.
79. Pajor A, Lehoczky D. Pregnancy in liver cirrhosis. Assessment of maternal and fetal risks in eleven patients and review of the management. Gynecol Obstet Invest 1994;38:45–50.
80. Shaheen AA, Myers RP. The outcomes of pregnancy in patients with cirrhosis: a population-based study. Liver Int 2010;30:275–83.
81. Rasheed SM, Abdel Monem AM, Abd Ellah AH, et al. Prognosis and determinants of pregnancy outcome among patients with post-hepatitis liver cirrhosis. Int J Gynaecol Obstet 2013;121:247–51.
82. Westbrook RH, Yeoman AD, O'Grady JG, et al. Model for end-stage liver disease score predicts outcome in cirrhotic patients during pregnancy. Clin Gastroenterol Hepatol 2011;9:694–9.
83. Sandhu BS, Sanyal AJ. Pregnancy and liver disease. Gastroenterol Clin North Am 2003;32:407–36.
84. Pajor A, Lehoczky D. Pregnancy and extrahepatic portal hypertension. Review and report on the management. Gynecol Obstet Invest 1990;30:193–7.
85. Britton RC. Pregnancy and esophageal varices. Am J Surg 1982;143:421–5.
86. Heriot JA, Steven CM, Sattin RS. Elective forceps delivery and extradural anaesthesia in a primigravida with portal hypertension and oesophageal varices. Br J Anaesth 1996;76:325–7.
87. Walcott WO, Derick DE, Jolley JJ, et al. Successful pregnancy in a liver transplant patient. Am J Obstet Gynecol 1978;132:340–1.
88. Schoening WN, Buescher N, Rademacker S, et al. Twenty-year longitudinal follow-up after orthotopic liver transplantation: a single-center experience of 313 consecutive cases. Am J Transplant 2013;13:2384–94.
89. Lim TU, Gonsalkorala E, Cannon MD, et al. Successful pregnancy outcomes following liver transplantation is predicted by renal function. Liver Transpl 2018;24:606–15.
90. Bramham K, Nelson-Piercy C, Gao H, et al. Pregnancy in renal transplant recipients: a UK national cohort study. Clin J Am Soc Nephrol 2013;8:290–8.
91. Sibanda N, Briggs JD, Davison JM, et al. Pregnancy after organ transplantation: a report from the UK transplant registry. Transplantation 2007;83:1301–7.
92. Westbrook RH, Yeoman AD, Agarwal K, et al. Outcomes of pregnancy following liver transplantation: the King's College Hospital experience. Liver Transpl 2015; 21:1153–9.
93. Coscia LA, Constantinescu S, Mortiz MJ, et al. Report from the national transplantation pregnancy registry (NTPR): outcomes of pregnancy after transplantation. Clin Transpl 2010;7:65–85.

94. Sarkar M, Bramham K, Moritz MJ, et al. Reproductive health in women following abdominal organ transplant. Am J Transplant 2018;18:1068–76.

95. Elinav E, Ben-Dov IZ, Sharpia Y, et al. Acute hepatitis A infection in pregnancy is associated with high rates of gestational complications and preterm labor. Gastroenterology 2006;130:1129–34.

96. Bhatia V, Singhal A, Panda SK, et al. A 20-year single-center experience with acute liver failure during pregnancy: is the prognosis really worse? Hepatology 2008;48:1577–85.

97. Jilani N, Das BC, Husain SA, et al. Hepatitis E virus infection and fulminant hepatic failure during pregnancy. J Gastroenterol Hepatol 2007;22:676–82.

98. Navaneethan U, Al Mohajer M, Shasta M. Hepatitis E and pregnancy- understanding the pathogenesis. Liver Int 2008;28:1190–9.

99. Brown ZA, Selke S, Zeh J, et al. The acquisition of herpes simplex virus during pregnancy. N Engl J Med 1997;337:509–15.

100. Stone KM, Reiff-Eldridge R, White AD, et al. Pregnancy outcomes following systemic prenatal acyclovir exposure: conclusions from the international acyclovir pregnancy registry, 1984-1999. Birth Defects Res A Clin Mol Teratol 2004;70:201–7.

101. Navaneethan U, Lancaster E, Venaktesh PG, et al. Herpes simplex virus hepatitis – it's high time we consider empiric treatment. J Gastrointestin Liver Dis 2011;20:93–6.

102. Andrews EB, Yankaskas BC, Cordero JF, et al. Acyclovir in Pregnancy Registry: six years' experience. The Acyclovir in Pregnancy Registry Advisory Committee. Obstet Gynecol 1992;79:7–13.

103. ACOG Committee on Practice Bulletins. ACOG Practice Bulletin. Clinical management guidelines for obstetrician-gynecologists. No. 82 June 2007. Management of herpes in pregnancy. Obstet Gynecol 2007;109:1489–98.

Obstructive Sleep Apnea and the Liver

Malav P. Parikh, MD[a], Niyati M. Gupta, MD[a], Arthur J. McCullough, MD[a,b],*

KEYWORDS

- Nonalcoholic fatty liver disease • Hepatic steatosis • Obstructive sleep apnea
- Chronic intermittent hypoxia and insulin resistance

KEY POINTS

- Chronic intermittent hypoxia (CIH) is the most important factor linking obstructive sleep apnea (OSA) and nonalcoholic fatty liver disease (NAFLD).
- CIH results in a state of systemic inflammation, increased oxidative stress, insulin resistance, and dyslipidemia, predisposing to various manifestations on NAFLD.
- Even though the 2-hit theory has been a popular hypothesis to explain the pathogenesis of NAFLD, current evidence points toward a multiple-hit hypothesis involving complex interplay of environmental and dietary factors, role of insulin resistance, adipose tissue dysfunction, and altered gut microbiota in genetically predisposed subjects.
- The role of continuous positive airway pressure (CPAP) in the management of NAFLD is yet to be established firmly.
- In general, a multifaceted approach to NAFLD with emphasis on diet, life style modification, and weight loss is required, along with sufficiently longer duration of CPAP therapy and appropriate compliance in those with NAFLD and moderate to severe OSA.

INTRODUCTION

Nonalcoholic fatty liver disease (NAFLD) represents a spectrum of liver disorders, including the initial stage of simple fat accumulation (hepatic steatosis); followed by inflammatory changes leading to nonalcoholic steatohepatitis (NASH); and, finally, fibrosis and scaring resulting in liver cirrhosis and its consequences.[1]

The current prevalence of NAFLD is estimated to be 20% to 30%,[2,3] and it has become the second most common indication for liver transplantation in the United States, after chronic hepatitis C.[4] It is projected that over the next 15 years, NASH will become the most common disease cause for liver transplantation.[5] This

Disclosure Statement: The authors have nothing to disclose.
Funded in part by NIH grant U01 DK061732.
[a] Department of Gastroenterology and Hepatology, Digestive Disease and Surgery Institute, Cleveland Clinic Foundation, 9500 Euclid Ave, M2 Annex, Cleveland, OH 44114, USA;
[b] Department of Inflammation and Immunity, Cleveland Clinic Lerner College of Medicine, Case Western University, Cleveland, OH 44195, USA
* Corresponding author.
E-mail address: mcculla@ccf.org

Clin Liver Dis 23 (2019) 363–382
https://doi.org/10.1016/j.cld.2019.01.001
1089-3261/19/© 2019 Elsevier Inc. All rights reserved.

liver.theclinics.com

exponential increase in the incidence and progression of NASH is attributed to the worldwide epidemic of obesity,[6] which has also resulted in an increase in the prevalence of other obesity-related disorders, including metabolic syndrome, type 2 diabetes mellitus (DM), cardiovascular disease, and obstructive sleep apnea (OSA).[7]

OSA is caused by complete or partial obstruction of the upper airway. This results in repetitive episodes of shallow or paused breathing during sleep and causes a reduction in blood oxygen saturation. This nocturnal hypoxia, or chronic intermittent hypoxia (CIH), is the most important factor linking OSA and NAFLD.[8–10] Recent studies have conclusively shown the role of OSA in the development and progression of NAFLD in terms of liver enzyme elevation and histologic alterations (steatosis, lobular inflammation, ballooning degeneration, and fibrosis).[11–19] This article discusses the pathologic mechanisms associating OSA with NAFLD and the impact of OSA treatment on NAFLD outcomes.

OBSTRUCTIVE SLEEP APNEA

OSA is a common clinical condition in which the throat narrows or collapses repeatedly during sleep, resulting in episodes of intermittent oxygen desaturations and nocturnal awakenings.[20,21] It is estimated to be present in 4% to 5% of the general population and is seen twice as commonly in men as in women. Advancing age, male gender, obesity, neck thickness, craniofacial changes, and upper airway soft tissue abnormalities are important risk factors for OSA.[20–22]

The direct consequences of airway collapse are snoring; increased respiratory efforts; hypercapnia; and, most importantly, CIH. This hypoxemia is sensed by carotid body receptors, leading to sympathetic activation; arousal; clearing of the airway; and, eventually, reoxygenation. The cycle of deoxygenation and reoxygenation is repeated several times every night and results in increased catecholamine release, reactive oxygen species (ROS) generation, oxidative stress, and a state of systemic inflammation. Lack of a restorative night sleep also results in excessive daytime sleepiness; morning headaches; concentration difficulties; anxiety; depression; road-traffic accidents; and, in general, a poor quality of life.[20,21,23] OSA is also associated with hypertension, atherosclerosis, coronary artery disease, stroke, insulin resistance, and NAFLD.[24–27]

Polysomnography is the gold standard test for diagnosing OSA and involves recording of several physiologic parameters, including electroencephalogram, electrooculogram, and electromyogram, along with nasal and oral airflow measurements.[28] An episode of apnea is defined by cessation of airflow for greater than 10 seconds despite ongoing inspiratory effort; whereas an episode of hypopnea is defined by greater than 50% reduction in airflow or moderate airflow reduction (<50%) along with either desaturation or electroencephalographic evidence of awakening. The severity of sleep apnea is characterized by the apnea-hypopnea index (AHI), which is simply calculated by dividing the number of events by number of hours of sleep. Accordingly, OSA can be classified as mild (AHI: 5–15), moderate (15–30), and severe (>30).[29] Continuous positive airway pressure (CPAP) is the first-line treatment for OSA. It results in more restful sleep, reduced daytime symptoms, and improved quality of life.[30] However, the effect of CPAP therapy on other chronic conditions, including metabolic syndrome and NAFLD, is less clear (see later discussion).

PATHOGENESIS OF NONALCOHOLIC STEATOHEPATITIS
Two-Hit Hypothesis

Berson and colleagues[31] conducted a pivotal study, during which rat liver mitochondria and rat hepatocytes were exposed to a hepatotoxic drug 4,4′-diethylaminoethoxyhexestrol. This resulted in hepatic steatosis and inhibition of mitochondrial β-oxidation.

Inhibition of mitochondrial respiration caused reduced adenosine triphosphate (ATP) levels and raised levels of ROS. The increased oxidative stress resulted in lipid peroxidation and subsequent cell death.

Day and James[32] proposed the popular 2-hit hypothesis (**Fig. 1**) of steatohepatitis based on this study.[31] The first hit represents hepatic steatosis, which could be related to factors such as excess caloric intake, obesity, or insulin resistance. A subsequent second hit, in the form of an oxidative stress, increased lipid peroxidation, and activation of inflammatory cascade, causes progression to steatohepatitis and fibrosis.

Multiple-hit hypothesis
Although the 2-hit hypothesis remains extremely popular and is often cited, emerging data show that it is too simplistic to explain the complex interplay of the multiple factors involved in the development of NASH. An alternative a multiple-hit hypothesis has been proposed that attempts to take into account several of the underlying mechanisms that may contribute to the pathogenesis of NASH.[33,34]

Genetic predisposition, environmental factors, and dietary habits lead to development of obesity, metabolic syndrome, and insulin resistance. Insulin resistance is a key factor in the progression of NAFLD because it not only leads to increased peripheral lipolysis with increased flux of free fatty acids (FFAs) but also to hepatic de novo lipogenesis (DNL). It also causes adipose tissue dysfunction with altered secretion of adipokines and increased levels of inflammatory cytokines, interleukin (IL)-6, and tumor necrosis factor (TNF)-α.[35] Alteration of gut microbiome causes increased gut permeability, systemic levels of lipopolysaccharides, and absorption of FFAs.[17]

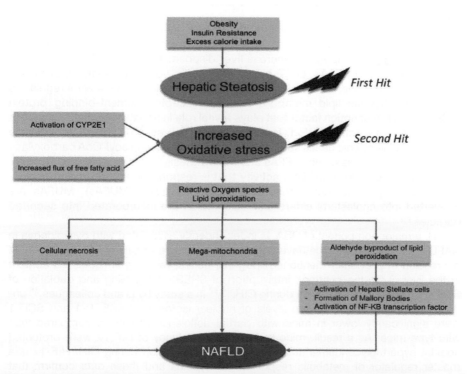

Fig. 1. Two-hit hypothesis. CYP2E1, cytochrome P450 2E1; NF-κB, nuclear factor-κβ.

All of these factors cause an increased flux of FFAs into the liver. This results in excess triglyceride (TG) deposition in the liver (hepatic steatosis) that parallels the generation of lipotoxic metabolites of FFAs. Further, these toxic metabolites cause mitochondrial dysfunction with increased oxidative stress, generation of ROS, and endoplasmic reticulum stress, which manifests in the form of hepatocyte injury and inflammation. Hence, TG accumulation in the hepatocyte is just an innocent bystander or an epiphenomenon in NAFLD pathogenesis, with the toxic metabolites of FFAs being the major mechanism for hepatotoxicity.[33,34]

LINK BETWEEN OBSTRUCTIVE SLEEP APNEA AND NONALCOHOLIC FATTY LIVER DISEASE

Several studies have firmly established the relationship between OSA and NAFLD in adult and pediatric populations (**Table 1**). The severity of sleep apnea and, particularly, its manifestation, CIH, is the most important trigger for increased oxidative stress, generation of ROS, and release of inflammatory cytokines, resulting systemic inflammation that drives the exacerbation of NAFLD and progression to liver fibrosis.[10] CIH causes reduced oxygen tension in the liver, particularly in the hepatocytes surrounding the central vein (zone 3) and results in the expression of hypoxia inducible factors (HIFs), which are the key oxygen sensors that mediate the ability of the cell to respond to a hypoxic environment. HIFs are implicated in the development of dyslipidemia, hepatic steatosis, insulin resistance, and liver fibrosis, and are a key link in the association of OSA and NAFLD.[10,50]

Obstructive Sleep Apnea and Dyslipidemia

Increased de novo lipogenesis

Entry of lipid substrates in the liver occurs through 1 of the following 3 mechanisms: (1) dietary intake of lipids and carbohydrates, (2) de novo lipogenesis, or (3) flux of FFAs from peripheral lipolysis, whereas liver disposes lipids through (1) storage as TGs, (2) oxidation of FAAs, or (3) export of TGs as very-low density lipoproteins (VLDLs) in the peripheral blood (**Fig. 2**).[51] Studies have identified several regulators that control hepatic lipid metabolism. Sterol receptor element-binding protein (SREBP) is a transcription factor that plays a vital role in hepatic DNL.[51,52] It consists of 3 isoforms, of which SREBP-1_c is predominantly expressed in liver. It mediates the expression of lipogenic genes such as fatty acid synthase and acyl-CoA carboxylase and thereby promotes de novo FFAs and TG synthesis.[55] It also increases stearoyl-coenzyme-A desaturase (SCD)-1 activity that is responsible for converting polyunsaturated fatty acids into monounsaturated fatty acids (MUFAs). MUFAs are converted into cholesterol esters and TGs, which are incorporated into secreted particles.[53]

CIH, a major component of OSA, is independently associated with dyslipidemia in NAFLD.[53,54] Studies in mice have shown that exposure to CIH results in enhanced expression of previously mentioned lipogenic genes, resulting in higher TG content in the liver.[55] On the contrary, interruption of SREBP-1 signaling and depletion of SCD-1 prevents hyperlipidemia during CIH.[56,57] In a study by Li and colleagues,[58] under hypoxic conditions, protein levels of nuclear isoforms of SREBP-1 and SCD-1 were significantly lower in mice with partial deficiency of HIF-1α compared with wild-type mice. As a result, mice with partial deficiency of HIF-1α were protected against hypertriglyceridemia and hepatic fat accumulation during CIH. HIF-1α is a master regulator of metabolic responses to hypoxia and these data confirm that CIH increases lipogenesis through the mediation of HIF-1α.

Table 1
Human studies assessing the correlation between obstructive sleep apnea and nonalcoholic fatty liver disease

Reference	Type of Study (Subject Population [n]); Country	NAFLD Assessment	OSA Diagnosis	Important Findings
Tanne et al,[36] 2005	PSG (163); France	LFT or liver biopsy	PSG	Severe OSA is associated with elevation of liver enzymes, insulin resistance, and steatohepatitis.
Kallwitz et al,[37] 2007	Bariatric surgery (85); USA	Liver biopsy	PSG (AHI ≥15/h)	OSA was associated with elevated ALT levels and a trend toward histologic evidence of progressive liver disease (inflammation and fibrosis).
Polotsky et al,[18] 2009	Bariatric surgery (90); USA	LFT or liver biopsy	PSG	Oxygen desaturation >4.6% was associated with 1.5-fold increase in insulin resistance. Significant desaturations may predispose to steatohepatitis.
Daltro et al,[15] 2010	Bariatric surgery (40); Brazil	Liver biopsy	PSG	OSA (AHI ≥15/h) was associated with insulin resistance but not with the severity of NASH.
Aron-Wisnewsky et al,[8] 2012	Bariatric surgery (101); France	Liver biopsy	ODI by nocturnal oximetry	CIH was independently associated with hepatic fibrosis, fibroinflammation, and NAFLD activity score.
Türkay et al,[27] 2012	PSG (71); Turkey	LFT, ultrasound	PSG	AHI, ODI, lowest desaturation values, and percentage of sleep duration with SpO2 <90% were independent predictors of NAFLD.
Corey et al,[38] 2013	Bariatric surgery (159); USA	Liver biopsy	Electronic medical record	Absence of OSA was associated with normal liver histology in subjects undergoing bariatric surgery.
Mir et al,[39] 2013	Population-based study, NHANES database. (NAFLD cases = 1572, controls = 8969); USA	LFT	Sleep Disorders Questionnaire	NAFLD was associated with sleep apnea (OR = 1.39, 0.98–1.97)

(continued on next page)

Table 1
(continued)

Reference	Type of Study (Subject Population [n]); Country	NAFLD Assessment	OSA Diagnosis	Important Findings
Minville et al,[40] 2014	PSG (226); France	SteatoTest, Nash Test, and FibroTest	PSG	On multivariate analysis, nocturnal cumulative time spent at <90% of oxygen saturation was associated with hepatic steatosis but not with NASH.
Sundaram et al,[41] 2014	Obese children aged 10–18 y (25); USA	Liver biopsy or LFT	PSG	Severity of hypoxemia and OSA were associated with transaminitis and advanced liver histology.
Nobili et al,[17] 2014	Children with NAFLD undergoing PSG (65); Italy	LFT or liver biopsy	PSG	Severity of OSA was independently associated with presence of NASH, significant fibrosis, and NAFLD activity score.
Lin et al,[42] 2015	NAFLD subjects undergoing sleep apnea assessment (85); China	Ultrasound	PSG	ODI and average O_2 saturation were independently associated with elevated ALT and AST, respectively.
Agrawal et al,[43] 2015	Subjects from liver clinic with NAFLD and chest clinic with OSA (123); India	Ultrasound, Fibroscan	PSG	OSA severity was an independent predictor of significant hepatic fibrosis in NAFLD subjects.
Corey et al,[14] 2015	Bariatric surgery (213); USA	Liver biopsy	PSG	OSA was independently associated with transaminitis, NASH, and advanced liver histology.
Alkhouri et al,[44] 2015	Obese children evaluated for OSA (58); USA	Circulating markers of hepatic apoptosis or inflammation	PSG	Circulating markers of apoptosis and macrophage activation were significantly increased in obese children with OSA. Treatment reduced markers of macrophage activation.
Petta et al,[45] 2015	NAFLD subjects with elevated ALT, undergoing OSA assessment (126); Italy	LFT, liver biopsy	Cardiorespiratory polygraph	Prevalence of OSA was higher in subjects with F2-F4 fibrosis. Significant fibrosis was associated with nocturnal oxygen saturation (SaO_2) <95%.

Study	Study population	Liver assessment	OSA assessment	Findings
Cakmak et al,[46] 2015	NAFLD subject undergoing OSA assessment (137); Turkey	Ultrasound	PSG	AHI and ODI were significantly higher in subjects with moderate and severe NAFLD. A strong association was noted between reduction in lowest O_2 saturation and increase in NAFLD severity.
Benotti et al,[13] 2016	Bariatric surgery (362); USA	Liver biopsy	PSG	Severity of OSA was associated with NAFLD liver histology.
Qi et al,[47] 2016	Nonobese subjects undergoing PSG and abdominal ultrasound (175); China	Ultrasound	PSG	In nonobese subjects, lowest oxygen saturation was independently associated with NAFLD.
Trzepizur et al,[19] 2016	Multisite cross-sectional study (1285); France	Hepatic steatosis index, LFT, FibroMeter	PSG or home sleep test	Risk of hepatic steatosis increased with severity of OSA and sleep-related hypoxemia.
Asfari et al,[48] 2017	Cross-sectional study using NIS database (OSA subjects = 1490150, non-OSA = 29,222 374); USA	ICD-9-CM	ICD-9-CM	OSA subjects were 3 times more likely to have NASH compared with subjects without OSA.
Ding et al,[49] 2018	Subjects with suspected apnea undergoing OSA and NAFLD assessment (415); China	LFT and ultrasound	PSG	Percentage of total sleep time spent with oxygen saturation of <90%, lowest oxygen saturation, and insulin resistance were associated with NAFLD.

Abbreviations: ICD-9-CM, international classification of diseases, ninth revision, clinical modification; LFT, liver function test; NHANES, National Health And Nutrition Examination Survey; NIS, national inpatient sample; ODI, oxygen desaturation index; PSG, polysomnography.

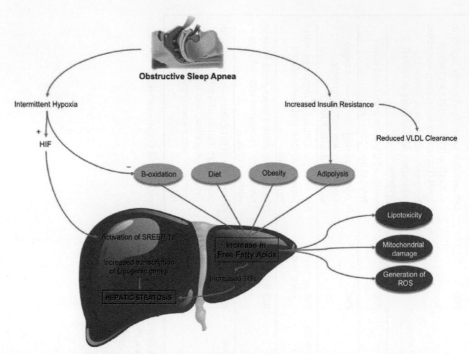

Fig. 2. Increased de novo lipogenesis. SREBP, sterol receptor element-binding protein.

Enhanced peripheral lipolysis and reduced lipoprotein clearance

CIH raises sympathetic activity and induces a state of insulin resistance. This promotes lipolysis in the adipose tissue and increased flux of FFAs in the liver. Under normoxia conditions, FFAs are metabolized by oxygen-dependent mitochondrial combustion through β-oxidation. Hence hypoxia creates a condition of excess FFAs and its reduced utilization through mitochondrial β-oxidation. More FFAs become available for TG and cholesterol synthesis, which eventually results in fatty liver, liver injury through oxidative stress, and NASH. CIH has also been shown to selectively inactivate the adipose tissue lipoprotein lipase and reduce the clearance of VLDL from circulation.[59] In summary, CIH can cause dyslipidemia by upregulating DNL and lipoprotein secretion, and reducing lipoprotein clearance, along with enhanced peripheral lipolysis and influx of FFAs in the liver.

Obstructive Sleep Apnea and Insulin Resistance

OSA is associated with CIH and sleep fragmentation, and an increasing pool of evidence now points toward an association between OSA, insulin resistance, and predisposition to type 2 DM (**Fig. 3**). In a study by Stamatakis and Punjabi,[60] sleep was experimentally fragmented across all stages using auditory and mechanical stimuli in healthy normal volunteers. After 2 nights of sleep fragmentation, they were noted to have reduced insulin sensitivity and glucose effectiveness with an elevated morning cortisol level and increased sympathetic tone. Increase in cortisol levels[61] and raised sympathetic tone[62,63] are well known to promote insulin resistance by reduction of insulin secretion from the pancreas, inhibition of insulin-mediated glucose uptake, and increased hepatic gluconeogenesis. In another study, selective suppression of slow-wave sleep in young healthy adults showed similar results. Sensitivity to insulin was

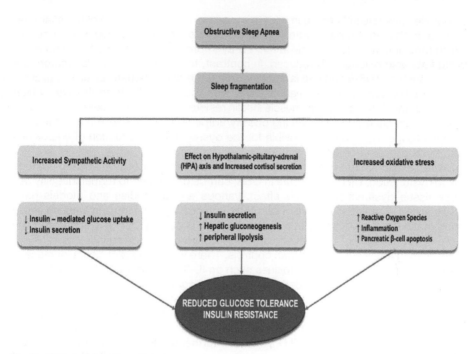

Fig. 3. OSA and insulin resistance.

markedly reduced without adequate compensatory increase in insulin release, leading to reduced glucose tolerance and increased DM risk.[64] In a study by Ip and colleagues,[65] 270 consecutive subjects referred for suspected sleep apnea and no underlying type 2 DM were included and tested for insulin resistance. OSA was associated with insulin resistance as measured by homeostatic model assessment of insulin resistance, independent of body mass index, and progressive increase in insulin resistance was noted per each additional apnea or hypopnea per sleep hour. Mouse models of OSA have further implicated the role of ROS,[66] pancreatic beta cell apoptosis,[67] and inflammation[68] in the development of insulin resistance and predisposition to type 2 DM.[60] Hence, several human and animal studies establish a robust association between OSA and insulin resistance.

Insulin resistance is known to play a crucial role in the pathogenesis of NAFLD. Studies have shown increased adipose tissue and hepatic insulin resistance, and reduced whole-body sensitivity to insulin in NAFLD patients. These are manifested by increased peripheral lipolysis, impaired inhibition of hepatic gluconeogenesis, and reduced glucose disposal, respectively. Further, inability of the insulin to suppress peripheral lipolysis results in increased flux of FFAs to liver and contributes to hepatic DNL. Insulin resistance leads to a state of hyperinsulinemia, which stimulates lipogenic genes via SREBP-1c and further contributes to hepatic steatosis. Overall, hepatic DNL, increased flux of FFAs, and impaired mitochondrial oxidation of FFAs creates a perfect milieu for development and progression of NAFLD.

Obstructive Sleep Apnea and Adipose Tissue Dysfunction

Traditionally considered an inert tissue for pure energy storage, it now clear that adipose tissue is a major endocrine and a signaling organ. During obesity, hypertrophied adipocytes mediate inflammation and harbor an increased proportion of proinflammatory macrophages compared with the antiinflammatory type. Secretion of adiponectin, which mediates a protective role in NAFLD by improving insulin sensitivity and regulating fatty acid oxidation, is reduced. In contrast, the release of proinflammatory cytokines such as TNF-α and IL-6 is increased, which reduces hepatic insulin sensitivity. Peripheral lipolysis is also increased, along with the flux of FFAs to the liver, which further potentiates hepatic and muscle insulin resistance.[69–71] It has been conclusively proven in animal models that during obesity adipose tissue is hypoxic and the local adipose tissue hypoxia is responsible for the dysregulated production of adipokines and metabolic syndrome.[69]

Because inflammation and hypoxia play crucial roles in obesity-mediated adipose tissue dysfunction, CIH, as it occurs in OSA, can be postulated to further intensify adipose tissue dysfunction. To this effect, various animal studies and models have conclusively established the role of intermittent hypoxia (IH) in inducing adipose tissue inflammation and dysfunction, even in the absence of obesity.[70,72] In a recent study by Taylor and colleagues,[73] human adipocytes exposed to IH showed increase in NF-κβ DNA-binding activity compared with controls. There was also a significant increase in the secretion of inflammatory cytokines such as IL-8, IL-6, and TNF-α with IH in adipocytes. Hence, it was concluded that human adipocytes are sensitive to IH, which enhances the expression of inflammatory genes and the release of inflammatory cytokines. Overall, these data provide evidence that IH can mediate adipose tissue dysfunction and the release of proinflammatory adipokines, which are known to be involved in pathogenesis of NAFLD. However, further studies are required in humans to understand the exact underlying mechanisms of IH, especially the impact of obesity.

Obstructive Sleep Apnea and Mitochondrial Dysfunction

Mitochondria are responsible for the production of 95% the cellular energy source, ATP. Under aerobic conditions, mitochondria produce ATP via 3 main biochemical pathways: the tricarboxylic acid cycle or Krebs cycle, oxidative phosphorylation, and fatty acid β-oxidation.[74] In OSA, hypoxia, along with an increased oxidative stress and flux of FAAs, overwhelm these normal mechanisms and result in structural and functional alteration of the mitochondria. Structural alteration is characterized by depletion of mitochondrial DNA[75] and upregulated transcriptional and replication machinery of mitochondrial biogenesis.[76] Increased levels of TNF-α, ROS, and lipid peroxidation products alter the mitochondrial respiratory chain, block the flow of electrons in the respiratory chain, and increase the mitochondrial ROS formation. The resultant oxidative stress further activates inflammatory pathways, contributing to hepatocytes inflammation and the diverse hepatic lesions of NASH.[77]

Obstructive Sleep Apnea and Liver Fibrosis

Stellate cells and portal fibroblasts are important sources of fibrillar collagen and lysyl oxidase (LOX) enzymes in the normal liver and after early hepatic injury (**Fig. 4**).[78] Hypoxia is a potent stimulator of LOX activity, which in turn plays an important role in the covalent cross-linking of collagen and elastin, increasing liver stiffness.[79] This increased stiffness causes increased mechanical tension that is crucial for the differentiation of hepatic stellate cell and portal fibroblasts into myofibroblasts, which are responsible for deposition of extracellular collagen and, eventually, the development of fibrosis.[78] Mesarwi and colleagues[80] have recently demonstrated that serum LOX is elevated in patients with NAFLD-associated hepatic fibrosis, relative to those without fibrosis. These same investigators also proposed the potential role of serum

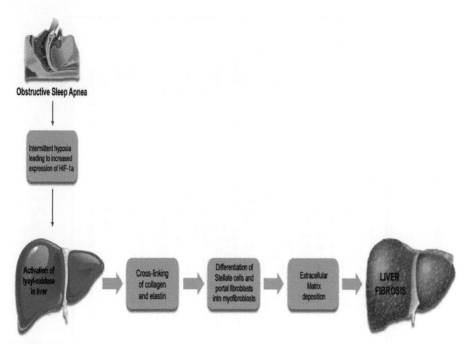

Fig. 4. OSA and liver fibrosis.

LOX as a biomarker of liver fibrosis in patients with severe obesity and OSA. HIF-1α has also been independently implicated in the development of liver fibrosis in a mouse model of NAFLD.[81] Hence, it can be concluded that hypoxia induces HIF-1α, which in turn induces the expression of LOX enzyme and the subsequent development of fibrosis.

Continuous positive airway pressure treatment and impact on nonalcoholic fatty liver disease
CPAP was originally described in 1983 by Sullivan and colleagues[82] and is considered the gold standard therapy for moderate to severe OSA. CPAP therapy acts as a pneumatic support, causing the pharyngeal intraluminal pressure to exceed the surrounding pressure. It also stabilizes the upper airway by increasing the end-expiratory lung volume, thereby preventing the hypoxic events related to the upper airway collapse.[83] Studies have conclusively established the benefits CPAP therapy in decreasing the hypoxic events and daytime sleepiness, lowering the risk of motor-vehicle accidents, and improving hypertension and a better quality of life in general.[84] However, studies have yielded conflicting results about the efficacy of CPAP therapy on metabolic syndrome, including insulin resistance, lipid profile, and body fat composition.[85,86]

Given that CIH plays a vital role in mediation of NAFLD in OSA, treatment with CPAP would be expected to yield unequivocal benefits in NAFLD patients. However, the available studies have yielded mixed results and are listed in **Table 2** and **Table 3**.[80,87–102] In these studies, the impact of CPAP therapy on NAFLD was assessed by means of improvements in liver enzymes, hepatic adiposity, or fibrosis. Importantly, the observational studies that demonstrated the benefits of CPAP (see **Table 2**) were of longer duration than the randomized controlled trials that did not show CPAP to be beneficial (see **Table 3**). Progression of liver fibrosis from 1 stage

Table 2
Studies showing beneficial impact of continuous positive airway pressure in subjects with obstructive sleep apnea and nonalcoholic fatty liver disease

Reference	Study Design	Study Population; Country	Duration of CPAP Therapy	Findings
Impact on liver enzymes				
Chin et al,[87] 2003	Prospective cohort study	40 men; Japan	6 mo	CPAP therapy had beneficial effects on serum aminotransferase abnormalities in obese OSA subjects.
Shpirer et al,[88] 2010	Prospective cohort study	11 subjects; Israel	3 y	Significant reduction in liver enzyme levels and improvement in the mean liver attenuation index in CPAP subjects (n = 6) compared with control group (n = 5).
Hobzova et al,[89] 2015	Prospective cohort study	179 subjects; Czech Republic	13 mo	Significant positive effect on liver enzymes in subjects with moderate to severe OSA.
Kim et al,[90] 2018[a]	Retrospective cohort study	351 subjects; California	6 mo	CPAP treatment was associated with significant biochemical improvement in liver enzymes.
Chen et al,[101] 2018	Prospective cohort study	160 subjects; China	3 mo	CPAP therapy was significantly associated with improvement of ALT and AST levels.
Sundaram et al,[100] 2018	Prospective cohort study	9 subjects; USA	3 mo	CPAP treatment reduces alanine aminotransferase, metabolic syndrome markers, and F (2)-isoprostanes.
Chen et al,[93] 2018	Meta-analysis	5 studies	—	CPAP was associated with a statistically significant decrease in the liver enzyme levels in OSA subjects.
Impact on liver steatosis				
Yoshiro et al,[94] 2014	Retrospective cohort study	61 male subjects; Japan	31 mo	In male OSA subjects with abdominal obesity, significant decrease in liver fat content was observed after long-term CPAP therapy, only when fatty liver was present at baseline.
Buttacavoli et al,[95] 2016	Observational study	15 subjects (3 at 6 mo and 15 at 12 mo follow-up)	6 and/or 12 mo	Long-term CPAP treatment may improve liver steatosis.

Impact on fibrosis

Mesarwi et al,[80] 2015	Prospective cohort study	35 subjects; Brazil	3 mo	A reduction in serum LOX (an enzyme that cross-links collagen and can serve as a biomarker of hepatic fibrosis) was seen in OSA subjects on CPAP.
Hang et al,[99] 2017	Retrospective cohort study	Propensity-matched 5214 subjects; Taiwan	2–10 y	CPAP plays an important role in the delay of the progression of liver disease in OSA subjects and decreases the incidence of liver disease among these groups of subjects.
Kim et al,[90] 2018[a]	Retrospective cohort study	351 subjects; California	6 mo	CPAP treatment was associated with reduction in NAFLD-related fibrosis.

[a] Represents same study with findings in 2 different headings.

Table 3
Studies showing no significant impact of continuous positive airway pressure in subjects with obstructive sleep apnea and nonalcoholic fatty liver disease

Reference	Study Design	Study Population; Country	Duration of CPAP	Findings
Impact on liver enzymes				
Kohler et al,[91] 2009	Randomized controlled trial	94 subjects; United Kingdom	1 mo	CPAP therapy did not improve biochemical markers of potential NAFLD in OSA subjects.
Sivam et al,[92] 2012[a]	Randomized controlled trial	27 subjects; Australia	2 mo	No significant differences were observed in liver enzymes except ALP.
Impact on liver steatosis				
Sivam et al,[92] 2012[a]	Randomized controlled trial	27 subjects; Australia	2 mo	CPAP treatment did not change the adipose tissue distribution in the liver.
Hoyos et al,[96] 2012	Randomized controlled trial	65 men; Australia	12 wk	No significant reduction in liver adiposity was observed with CPAP therapy.
Kritikou et al,[97] 2013	Randomized controlled trial	42 subjects; USA	2 mo	Short-term CPAP treatment did not affect intrahepatic adiposity.
Impact on fibrosis				
Jullian-Desayes et al,[98] 2016	Randomized controlled trial	103 subjects; France	6–12 wk	CPAP therapy did not demonstrate any significant impact on reduction of steatosis, NASH and liver fibrosis.
Labarca et al,[102] 2018	Meta-analysis	5 randomized controlled trials	—	CPAP treatment did not significantly contribute to the improvement in liver histology, liver steatosis, liver fibrosis, and aminotransferase levels.

[a] Represents same study with findings in 2 different headings.

to another takes an average of 7 years in patients with NASH and 14 years in those with NAFLD.[103] Hence it is likely that studies of longer duration will be required to demonstrate the importance of OSA in the pathogenesis of NAFLD and the benefits of CPAP in its treatment. Increasing data indicate that CPAP should be considered as an integral component in the management off NAFLD patients with moderate to severe OSA and that more than 3 months of treatment with appropriate compliance is needed to notice any significant improvements in NAFLD parameters (see **Table 2**). As mentioned earlier, development of NAFLD requires multiple-hits and aberrations in multiple metabolic pathways. Hence, its effective management also needs a multimodal approach with paramount emphasis on diet and lifestyle modification, and weight loss, with CPAP being an essential element in those with NAFLD and moderate to severe OSA.[104]

SUMMARY

CIH is an important risk factor in the pathogenesis of NAFLD in patients with moderate to severe OSA. Reduced oxygen tension induces HIFs, which are implicated in the development of dyslipidemia, hepatic steatosis, insulin resistance, and liver fibrosis, and are a key link in the association of OSA and NAFLD. Given that several metabolic pathways are involved in its pathogenesis, a multipronged approach to NAFLD management is required, with emphasis on weight loss and lifestyle modification. The role of CPAP in the management of NAFLD is yet to be established firmly; however, adequate duration of CPAP therapy with appropriate compliance are important to notice any significant improvements in NAFLD parameters.

REFERENCES

1. Ratziu V, Bellentani S, Cortez-Pinto H, et al. A position statement on NAFLD/NASH based on the EASL 2009 special conference. J Hepatol 2010;53:372–84.
2. Angulo P. Nonalcoholic fatty liver disease. N Engl J Med 2002;346:1221–31.
3. Younossi ZM, Koenig AB, Abdelatif D, et al. Global epidemiology of nonalcoholic fatty liver disease-Meta-analytic assessment of prevalence, incidence, and outcomes. Hepatology 2016;64(1):73–84.
4. Anstee QM, Targher G, Day CP. Progression of NAFLD to diabetes mellitus, cardiovascular disease or cirrhosis. Nat Rev Gastroenterol Hepatol 2013;10:330–44.
5. Parikh ND, Marrero WJ, Wang J, et al. Projected increase in obesity and non-alcoholic-steatohepatitis-related liver transplantation waitlist additions in the United States. Hepatology 2017. [Epub ahead of print].
6. Ogden CL, Carroll MD, Flegal KM. Prevalence of obesity in the United States. JAMA 2014;312(2):189–90.
7. Kopelman PG. Obesity as a medical problem. Nature 2000;404(6778):635–43.
8. Aron-Wisnewsky J, Minville C, Tordjman J, et al. Chronic intermittent hypoxia is a major trigger for non-alcoholic fatty liver disease in morbid obese. J Hepatol 2012;56(1):225–33.
9. Dewan NA, Nieto FJ, Somers VK. Intermittent hypoxemia and OSA: implications for comorbidities. Chest 2015;147(1):266–74.
10. Aron-Wisnewsky J, Clement K, Pépin JL. Nonalcoholic fatty liver disease and obstructive sleep apnea. Metabolism 2016;65(8):1124–35.
11. Jin S, Jiang S, Hu A. Association between obstructive sleep apnea and non-alcoholic fatty liver disease: a systematic review and meta-analysis. Sleep Breath 2018;22(3):841–51.

12. Sundaram SS, Halbower A, Pan Z, et al. Nocturnal hypoxia induced oxidative stress promotes progression of pediatric nonalcoholic fatty liver disease. J Hepatol 2016;65(3):560–9.

13. Benotti P, Wood GC, Argyropoulos G, et al. Impact of obstructive sleep apnea on nonalcoholic fatty liver disease in patients with severe obesity. Obesity (Silver Spring) 2016;24:871–7.

14. Corey KE, Misdraji J, Gelrud L, et al. Obstructive sleep apnea is associated with nonalcoholic steatohepatitis and advanced liver histology. Dig Dis Sci 2015; 60(8):2523–8.

15. Daltro C, Cotrim HP, Alves E, et al. Nonalcoholic fatty liver disease associated with obstructive sleep apnea: just a coincidence? Obes Surg 2010;20(11): 1536–43.

16. Nobili V, Alisi A, Cutrera R, et al. Altered gut liver axis and hepatic adiponectin expression in OSAS: novel mediators of liver injury in pediatric non-alcoholic fatty liver. Thorax 2015;70(8):769–81.

17. Nobili V, Cutrera R, Liccardo D, et al. Obstructive sleep apnea syndrome affects liver histology and inflammatory cell activation in pediatric nonalcoholic fatty liver disease, regardless of obesity/insulin resistance. Am J Respir Crit Care Med 2014;189(1):66–76.

18. Polotsky VY, Patil SP, Savransky V, et al. Obstructive sleep apnea, insulin resistance, and steatohepatitis in severe obesity. Am J Respir Crit Care Med 2009; 179(3):228–34.

19. Trzepizur W, Boursier J, Mansour Y, et al. Association between severity of obstructive sleep apnea and blood markers of liver injury. Clin Gastroenterol Hepatol 2016;14(11):1657–61.

20. Mannarino MR, Di Filippo F, Pirro M. Obstructive sleep apnea syndrome. Eur J Intern Med 2012;23(7):586–93.

21. Lévy P, Kohler M, McNicholas WT, et al. Obstructive sleep apnea syndrome. Nat Rev Dis Primers 2015;1:15015.

22. Strollo PJ Jr, Rogers RM. Obstructive sleep apnea. N Engl J Med 1996;334: 99–104.

23. Azagra-Calero E, Espinar-Escalona E, Barrera-Mora JM, et al. Obstructive sleep apnea syndrome (OSAS). Review of the literature. Med Oral Patol Oral Cir Bucal 2012;17(6):e925–9.

24. Jean-Louis G, Zizi F, Clark LT, et al. Obstructive sleep apnea and cardiovascular disease: role of the metabolic syndrome and its components. J Clin Sleep Med 2008;4(3):261–72.

25. Punjabi NM, Shahar E, Redline S, et al. Sleep-disordered breathing, glucose intolerance, and insulin resistance: the Sleep Heart Health Study. Am J Epidemiol 2004;160:521.

26. Togeiro SM, Carneiro G, Ribeiro Filho FF, et al. Consequences of obstructive sleep apnea on metabolic profile: a Population-Based Survey. Obesity (Silver Spring) 2013;21:847.

27. Türkay C, Ozol D, Kasapoğlu B, et al. Influence of obstructive sleep apnea on fatty liver disease: role of chronic intermittent hypoxia. Respir Care 2012;57:244.

28. American Academy of Sleep Medicine. International classification of sleep disorders. 3rd edition. Darien (IL): American Academy of Sleep Medicine; 2014.

29. The Report of an American Academy of Sleep Medicine Task Force. Sleep-related breathing disorders in adults: recommendations for syndrome definition and measurement techniques in clinical research. Sleep 1999;22:667–89.

30. Giles TL, Lasserson TJ, Smith BJ, et al. Continuous positive airways pressure for obstructive sleep apnea in adults. Cochrane Database Syst Rev 2006;(1):CD001106.

31. Berson A, De Beco V, Lettéron P, et al. Steatohepatitis-inducing drugs cause mitochondrial dysfunction and lipid peroxidation in rat hepatocytes. Gastroenterology 1998;114(4):764–74.

32. Day CP, James OF. Steatohepatitis: a tale of two "hits"? Gastroenterology 1998; 114(4):842–5.

33. Buzzetti E, Pinzani M, Tsochatzis EA. The multiple-hit pathogenesis of nonalcoholic fatty liver disease (NAFLD). Metabolism 2016;65(8):1038–48.

34. Neuschwander-Tetri BA. Hepatic lipotoxicity and the pathogenesis of nonalcoholic steatohepatitis: the central role of nontriglyceride fatty acid metabolites. Hepatology 2010;52(2):774–88.

35. Guilherme A, Virbasius JV, Puri V, et al. Adipocyte dysfunctions linking obesity to insulin resistance and type 2 diabetes. Nat Rev Mol Cell Biol 2008;9:367–77.

36. Tanne F, Gagnadoux F, Chazouilleres O, et al. Chronic liver injury during obstructive sleep apnea. Hepatology 2005;41:1290–6.

37. Kallwitz ER, Herdegen J, Madura J, et al. Liver enzymes and histology in obese patients with obstructive sleep apnea. J Clin Gastroenterol 2007;41(10):918–21.

38. Corey KE, Misdraji J, Zheng H, et al. The absence of obstructive sleep apnea may protect against non-alcoholic fatty liver in patients undergoing bariatric surgery. PLoS One 2013;8(5):e62504.

39. Mir HM, Stepanova M, Afendy H, et al. Association of sleep disorders with nonalcoholic fatty liver disease (NAFLD): a population-based study. J Clin Exp Hepatol 2013;3(3):181–5.

40. Minville C, Hilleret MN, Tamisier R, et al. Nonalcoholic fatty liver disease, nocturnal hypoxia, and endothelial function in patients with sleep apnea. Chest 2014;145(3):525–33.

41. Sundaram SS, Sokol RJ, Capocelli KE, et al. Obstructive sleep apnea and hypoxemia are associated with advanced liver histology in pediatric nonalcoholic fatty liver disease. J Pediatr 2014;164(4):699–706.e1.

42. Lin QC, Chen LD, Chen GP, et al. Association between nocturnal hypoxia and liver injury in the setting of nonalcoholic fatty liver disease. Sleep Breath 2015; 19(1):273–80.

43. Agrawal S, Duseja A, Aggarwal A, et al. Obstructive sleep apnea is an important predictor of hepatic fibrosis in patients with nonalcoholic fatty liver disease in a tertiary care center. Hepatol Int 2015;9(2):283–91.

44. Alkhouri N, Kheirandish-Gozal L, Matloob A, et al. Evaluation of circulating markers of hepatic apoptosis and inflammation in obese children with and without obstructive sleep apnea. Sleep Med 2015;16(9):1031–5.

45. Petta S, Marrone O, Torres D, et al. Obstructive sleep apnea is associated with liver damage and atherosclerosis in patients with non-alcoholic fatty liver disease. PLoS One 2015;10(12):e0142210.

46. Cakmak E, Duksal F, Altinkaya E, et al. Association between the severity of nocturnal hypoxia in obstructive sleep apnea and non-alcoholic fatty liver damage. Hepat Mon 2015;15(11):e32655.

47. Qi JC, Huang JC, Lin QC, et al. Relationship between obstructive sleep apnea and nonalcoholic fatty liver disease in nonobese adults. Sleep Breath 2016; 20(2):529–35.

48. Asfari MM, Niyazi F, Lopez R, et al. The association of nonalcoholic steatohepatitis and obstructive sleep apnea. Eur J Gastroenterol Hepatol 2017;29(12): 1380–4.

49. Ding H, Huang JF, Xie HS, et al. The association between glycometabolism and nonalcoholic fatty liver disease in patients with obstructive sleep apnea. Sleep Breath 2018. [Epub ahead of print].

50. Shin MK, Drager LF, Yao Q, et al. Metabolic consequences of high-fat diet are attenuated by suppression of HIF-1α. PLoS One 2012;7(10):e46562.

51. Suzuki T, Shinjo S, Arai T, et al. Hypoxia and fatty liver. World J Gastroenterol 2014;20(41):15087–97.

52. Raghow R, Yellaturu C, Deng X, et al. SREBPs: the crossroads of physiological and pathological lipid homeostasis. Trends Endocrinol Metab 2008;19(2):65–73.

53. Drager LF, Jun JC, Polotsky VY. Metabolic consequences of intermittent hypoxia: relevance to obstructive sleep apnea. Best Pract Res Clin Endocrinol Metab 2010;24(5):843–51.

54. Adedayo AM, Olafiranye O, Smith D, et al. Obstructive sleep apnea and dyslipidemia: evidence and underlying mechanism. Sleep Breath 2012;18(1):13–8.

55. Li J, Thorne LN, Punjabi NM, et al. Intermittent hypoxia induces hyperlipidemia in lean mice. Circ Res 2005;97(7):698–706.

56. Li J, Nanayakkara A, Jun J, et al. Effect of deficiency in SREBP cleavage activating protein on lipid metabolism during intermittent hypoxia. Physiol Genomics 2007;31(2):273–80.

57. Savransky V, Jun J, Li J, et al. Dyslipidemia and atherosclerosis induced by chronic intermittent hypoxia are attenuated by deficiency of stearoyl coenzyme A desaturase. Circ Res 2008;103(10):1173–80.

58. Li J, Bosch-Marce M, Nanayakkara A, et al. Altered metabolic responses to intermittent hypoxia in mice with partial deficiency of hypoxia inducible factor-1alpha. Physiol Genomics 2006;25(3):450–7.

59. Drager LF, Li J, Shin M-K, et al. Intermittent hypoxia inhibits clearance of triglyceride-rich lipoproteins and inactivates adipose lipoprotein lipase in a mouse model of sleep apnea. Eur Heart J 2012;33(6):783–90.

60. Stamatakis KA, Punjabi NM. Effects of sleep fragmentation on glucose metabolism in normal subjects. Chest 2010;137(1):95–101.

61. Andrews RC, Walker BR. Glucocorticoids and insulin resistance: old hormones, new targets. Clin Sci (Lond) 1999;96(5):513–23.

62. Deibert DC, DeFronzo RA. Epinephrine-induced insulin resistance in man. J Clin Invest 1980;65(3):717–21.

63. Avogaro A, Toffolo G, Valerio A, et al. Epinephrine exerts opposite effects on peripheral glucose disposal and glucose-stimulated insulin secretion. A stable label intravenous glucose tolerance test minimal model study. Diabetes 1996; 45(10):1373–8.

64. Tasali E, Leproult R, Ehrmann DA, et al. Slow-wave sleep and the risk of type 2 diabetes in humans. Proc Natl Acad Sci U S A 2008;105(3):1044–9.

65. Ip MS, Lam B, Ng MM, et al. Obstructive sleep apnea is independently associated with insulin resistance. Am J Respir Crit Care Med 2002;165(5):670–6.

66. Peng YJ, Yuan G, Ramakrishnan D, et al. Heterozygous HIF-1alpha deficiency impairs carotid body-mediated systemic responses and reactive oxygen species generation in mice exposed to intermittent hypoxia. J Physiol 2006;577(Pt 2):705–16.

67. Xu J, Long YS, Gozal D, et al. Beta-cell death and proliferation after intermittent hypoxia: role of oxidative stress. Free Radic Biol Med 2009;46(6):783–90.

68. Ryan S, Taylor CT, McNicholas WT. Selective activation of inflammatory pathways by intermittent hypoxia in obstructive sleep apnea syndrome. Circulation 2005;112(17):2660–7.
69. Hosogai N, Fukuhara A, Oshima K, et al. Adipose tissue hypoxia in obesity and its impact on adipocytokine dysregulation. Diabetes 2007;56(4):901–11.
70. Ryan S. Adipose tissue inflammation by intermittent hypoxia: mechanistic link between obstructive sleep apnea and metabolic dysfunction. J Physiol 2017; 595(8):2423–30.
71. Trayhurn P, Wang B, Wood IS. Hypoxia and the endocrine and signaling role of white adipose tissue. Arch Physiol Biochem 2008;114(4):267–76.
72. Poulain L, Thomas A, Rieusset J, et al. Visceral white fat remodeling contributes to intermittent hypoxia-induced atherogenesis. Eur Respir J 2014;43(2):513–22.
73. Taylor CT, Kent BD, Crinion SJ, et al. Human adipocytes are highly sensitive to intermittent hypoxia induced NF-kappaB activity and subsequent inflammatory gene expression. Biochem Biophys Res Commun 2014;447(4):660–5.
74. Sharpe AJ, McKenzie M. Mitochondrial fatty acid oxidation disorders associated with short-chain Enoyl-CoA Hydratase (ECHS1) deficiency. Cells 2018;7(6):46.
75. Kim YS, Kwak JW, Lee KE, et al. Can mitochondrial dysfunction be a predictive factor for oxidative stress in patients with obstructive sleep apnea? Antioxid Redox Signal 2014;21(9):1285–8.
76. Lacedonia D, Carpagnano GE, Crisetti E, et al. Mitochondrial DNA alteration in obstructive sleep apnea. Respir Res 2015;16(1):47.
77. Pessayre D, Fromenty B. NASH: a mitochondrial disease. J Hepatol 2005;42: 928–40.
78. Kagan HM. Lysyl oxidase: mechanism, regulation and relationship to liver fibrosis. Pathol Res Pract 1994;190(9–10):910–9.
79. Liu SB, Ikenaga N, Peng ZW, et al. Lysyl oxidase activity contributes to collagen stabilization during liver fibrosis progression and limits spontaneous fibrosis reversal in mice. FASEB J 2016;30(4):1599–609.
80. Mesarwi OA, Shin MK, Drager LF, et al. Lysyl oxidase as a serum biomarker of liver fibrosis in patients with severe obesity and obstructive sleep apnea. Sleep 2015;38(10):1583–91.
81. Mesarwi OA, Shin MK, Bevans-Fonti S, et al. Hepatocyte hypoxia inducible factor-1 mediates the development of liver fibrosis in a mouse model of nonalcoholic fatty liver disease. PLoS One 2016;11(12):e0168572.
82. Sullivan C, Berthon-Jones M, Issa F. Nocturnal nasal-airway pressure for sleep apnea. N Engl J Med 1983;309:112.
83. Jordan AS, McSharry DG, Malhotra A. Adult obstructive sleep apnea. Lancet 2014;383:736.
84. Kryger MH, Malhotra A. Management of obstructive sleep apnea in adults. In: Collop N, editor. UpToDate, Available at: https://www.uptodate.com/contents/management-of-obstructive-sleep-apnea-in-adults. Accessed November 24, 2018
85. Spicuzza L, Caruso D, Di Maria G. Obstructive sleep apnea syndrome and its management. Ther Adv Chronic Dis 2015;6(5):273–85.
86. Liu X, Miao Y, Wu F, et al. Effect of CPAP therapy on liver disease in patients with OSA: a review. Sleep Breath 2018;22(4):963–72.
87. Chin K, Nakamura T, Takahashi K, et al. Effects of obstructive sleep apnea syndrome on serum aminotransferase levels in obese patients. Am J Med 2003; 114(5):370–6.

88. Shpirer I, Copel L, Broide E, et al. Continuous positive airway pressure improves sleep apnea associated fatty liver. Lung 2010;188(4):301–7.
89. Hobzova M, Ludka O, Stepanova R, et al. Continuous positive airway pressure treatment and liver enzymes in sleep apnea patients. Sleep Med 2015;16:215–6.
90. Kim D, Ahmed A, Kushida C. Continuous positive airway pressure therapy on nonalcoholic fatty liver disease in patients with obstructive sleep apnea. J Clin Sleep Med 2018;14(8):1315–22.
91. Kohler M, Pepperell JC, Davies RJ, et al. Continuous positive airway pressure and liver enzymes in obstructive sleep apnea: data from a randomized controlled trial. Respiration 2009;78(2):141–6.
92. Sivam S, Phillips CL, Trenell MI, et al. Effects of 8 weeks of continuous positive airway pressure on abdominal adiposity in obstructive sleep apnea. Eur Respir J 2012;40(4):913–8.
93. Chen LD, Lin L, Zhang LJ, et al. Effect of continuous positive airway pressure on liver enzymes in obstructive sleep apnea: a meta-analysis. Clin Respir J 2018; 12(2):373–81.
94. Yoshiro T, Kimihiko M, Masanori A, et al. Impacts of long- term CPAP therapy on fatty liver in male OSA patients with abdominal obesity. Eur Respir J 2014;44: S4661.
95. Buttacavoli M, Gruttad'Auria CI, Olivo M, et al. Liver steatosis and fibrosis in OSA patients after long-term CPAP treatment: a preliminary ultrasound study. Ultrasound Med Biol 2016;42(1):104–9.
96. Hoyos CM, Killick R, Yee BJ, et al. Cardiometabolic changes after continuous positive airway pressure for obstructive sleep apnea: a randomized sham-controlled study. Thorax 2012;67(12):1081–9.
97. Kritikou I, Basta M, Tappouni R, et al. Sleep apnea and visceral adiposity in middle-aged male and female subjects. Eur Respir J 2013;41(3):601–9.
98. Jullian-Desayes I, Tamisier R, Zarski JP, et al. Impact of effective versus sham continuous positive airway pressure on liver injury in obstructive sleep apnea: data from randomized trials. Respirology 2016;21(2):378–85.
99. Hang LW, Chen CF, Wang CB, et al. The association between continuous positive airway pressure therapy and liver disease development in obstructive sleep apnea/hypopnea syndrome patients: a nationwide population-based cohort study in Taiwan. Sleep Breath 2017;21(2):461–7.
100. Sundaram SS, Halbower AC, Klawitter J, et al. Treating obstructive sleep apnea and chronic intermittent hypoxia improves the severity of nonalcoholic fatty liver disease in children. J Pediatr 2018;198:67–75.e1.
101. Chen LD, Zhang LJ, Lin XJ, et al. Association between continuous positive airway pressure and serum aminotransferases in patients with obstructive sleep apnea. Eur Arch Otorhinolaryngol 2018;275(2):587–94.
102. Labarca G, Cruz R, Jorquera J. Continuous positive airway pressure in patients with obstructive sleep apnea and non-alcoholic steatohepatitis: a systematic review and meta-analysis. J Clin Sleep Med 2018;14(1):133–9.
103. Singh S, Allen AM, Wang Z, et al. Fibrosis progression in nonalcoholic fatty liver vs nonalcoholic steatohepatitis: a systematic review and meta-analysis of paired-biopsy studies. Clin Gastroenterol Hepatol 2014;13(4):643–54.e1-9 [quiz: e39–40].
104. Chirinos JA, Gurubhagavatula I, Teff K, et al. CPAP, weight loss, or both for obstructive sleep apnea. N Engl J Med 2014;370(24):2265–75.

Moving?

Make sure your subscription moves with you!

To notify us of your new address, find your **Clinics Account Number** (located on your mailing label above your name), and contact customer service at:

Email: journalscustomerservice-usa@elsevier.com

800-654-2452 (subscribers in the U.S. & Canada)
314-447-8871 (subscribers outside of the U.S. & Canada)

Fax number: 314-447-8029

**Elsevier Health Sciences Division
Subscription Customer Service
3251 Riverport Lane
Maryland Heights, MO 63043**

*To ensure uninterrupted delivery of your subscription, please notify us at least 4 weeks in advance of move.

Printed and bound by CPI Group (UK) Ltd, Croydon, CR0 4YY

03/10/2024

01040404-0002